MEDICAL
INTELLIGENCE
UNIT

The Carotid Body Chemoreceptors

Constancio González
Universidad de Valladolid
Valladolid, Spain

Springer
New York Berlin Heidelberg London Paris
Tokyo Hong Kong Barcelona Budapest

LANDES BIOSCIENCE
AUSTIN, TEXAS
U.S.A.

Medical Intelligence Unit

The Carotid Body Chemoreceptors

LANDES BIOSCIENCE
Austin, Texas, U.S.A.

Please address all inquiries to the Publishers:
Landes Bioscience, 810 South Church Street, Georgetown, Texas, U.S.A. 78626
Phone: 512/ 863 7762; FAX: 512/ 863 0081

International distributor (except North America):
Springer-Verlag GmbH & Co. KG
Tiergartenstrasse 17, D-69121 Heidelberg, Germany

Springer

International ISBN: 3-540-61948-8

Library of Congress Cataloging-in-Publication Data

The carotid body chemoreceptors / [edited by] Constancio González
p. cm. — (Medical intelligence unit)
Includes bibliographical references and index.
ISBN 1-57059-465-1 (alk. paper)
1. Carotid body. 2. Chemoreceptors. I. González, Constancio.
II. Series.
[DNLM: 1. Carotid Body — physiology. 2. Receptors, Sensory-
-physiology. WL 102.9 C293 1997]
QP368.8.C37 1997
612.4'92 — dc21
DNLM/DLC
for Library of Congress 97-19788
CIP

Publisher's Note

Landes Bioscience Publishers produces books in six Intelligence Unit series: *Medical, Molecular Biology, Neuroscience, Tissue Engineering, Biotechnology* and *Environmental.* The authors of our books are acknowledged leaders in their fields. Topics are unique; almost without exception, no similar books exist on these topics.

Our goal is to publish books in important and rapidly changing areas of bioscience for sophisticated researchers and clinicians. To achieve this goal, we have accelerated our publishing program to conform to the fast pace at which information grows in bioscience. Most of our books are published within 90 to 120 days of receipt of the manuscript. We would like to thank our readers for their continuing interest and welcome any comments or suggestions they may have for future books.

Shyamali Ghosh
Publications Director
Landes Bioscience

Dedication

To my wife Ana Obeso
To our children Elvira, Ana and Constancio

CONTENTS

EDITOR

Constancio González, MD, PhD
Departamento de Bioquímica y
Biología Molecular y Fisiología
IBGM. Facultad de Medicina
Universidad de Valladolid
Valladolid, Spain
Chapters 2, 3, 5

CONTRIBUTORS

Laura Almaraz, MD, PhD
Departamento de Bioquímica y
Biología Molecular y Fisiología
Universidad de Valladolid
Valladolid, Spain
Chapter 8

Theresa Brosenitsch
Department of Neurosciences
Case Western Reserve University
School of Medicine
Cleveland, Ohio, USA
Chapter 9

Bruce Dinger, PhD
Department of Physiology
University of Utah
Salt Lake City, Utah, USA
Chapters 3, 8

David F. Donnelly, PhD
Department of Pediatrics
Yale University School of Medicine
New Haven, Connecticut, USA
Chapter 11

Jeffrey T. Erickson, PhD
Department of Neurosciences
Case Western Reserve Unversity
School of Medicine
Cleveland, Ohio, USA
Chapter 9

Carlos Eyzaguirre, MD
Department of Physiology
University of Utah
Salt Lake City, Utah, USA
Prologue

James C.W. Finley, MD, PhD
Department of Medicine
Case Western Reserve University
School of Medicine
Cleveland, Ohio, USA
Chapter 9

Salvatore J. Fidone, PhD
Department of Physiology
University of Utah
Salt Lake City, Utah, USA
Chapters 3, 8

Robert S. Fitzgerald, PhD
Dept. Environmental
Health Sciences
Division of Environmental
Physiology
The Johns Hopkins University
Baltimore, Maryland, USA
Chapter 10

Benito Herreros, MD, PhD
Departamento de Bioquímica y
Biología Molecular y Fisiología
Universidad de Valladolid
Valladolid, Spain
Chapter 2

David M. Katz, PhD
Department of Neurosciences
Case Western Reserve University
School of Medicine
Cleveland, Ohio, USA
Chapter 9

José Ramón López-López, MD, PhD
Departamento de Bioquímica y
Biología Molecular y Fisiología
Universidad de Valladolid
Valladolid, Spain
Chapter 4

Ana Obeso, MD, PhD
Departamento de Bioquímica y
Biología Molecular y Fisiología
Universidad de Valladolid
Valladolid, Spain
Chapter 2

Rosario Pásaro, PhD
Departamento de Fisiología Animal
Laboratorio de Neurobiología
Sevilla, Spain
Chapter 12

Chris Peers, PhD
Institute for Cardiovascular Research
Leeds University
Leeds, UK
Chapter 4

María Teresa Pérez-García, MD, PhD
Departamento de Bioquímica y
Biología Molecular y Fisiología
Universidad de Valladolid
Valladolid, Spain
Chapter 5

Juan Ribas, MD, PhD
Departamento de Fisiología
Facultad de Medicina
Avda. Sánchez Pizjuan 4
Sevilla, Spain
Chapter 12

Asunción Rocher, PhD
Departamento de Bioquimica y
Biologia Molecular y Fisiologia
IBGM. Facultad de Medicina
Universidad de Valladolid
Valladolid, Spain
Chapter 2

Machiko Shirahata, MD, DMSc
Dept. Environmental
Health Sciences
Division of Environmental
Physiology
The Johns Hopkins University
Baltimore, Maryland, USA
Chapter 10

Alain Verna, MD
Director of the Microscopy Center
Laboratoire de Cytologie
Universite de Bourdeaux II
Talence, France
Chapter 1

Z.-Z. Wang, PhD
Laboratory of Cell Biology
National Institute of Mental Health
Bethesda, Maryland, USA
Chapter 8

Patricio Zapata, MD
Laboratorio de Neurobiologia
Universidad Catolica de Chile
Santiago, Chile
Chapters 6, 7

PREFACE

When Landes Bioscience offered me the opportunity to edit a book on The Carotid Body Chemoreceptors, I had mixed feelings about the wish and the effort. Professors Zapata, Eyzaguirre and Fidone encouraged me to accept the challenge.

In designing the book I have attempted to cover all topics in current carotid body research. I asked the contributors to avoid a mere juxtaposition of data and also encouraged them to express personal opinions on the data to obtain an animated book.

I wanted Prof. Carlos Eyzaguirre to write the introductory chapter, the Prologue, as a small tribute to his contribution to the field. Prof. Eyzaguirre drove the carotid body from the complexity of the intact mammalian organism to a simple superfusing bath, where it was possible to control every experimental variable. He has carried the torch of arterial chemoreception from his pioneer work in the early 1960s until now. The number of disciples around the world, whether in the first or second generation, now outnumbers his nearly 40 years dedication to the field.

The first part of the book is devoted to the cellular aspects of the function of the carotid body chemoreceptors. From a neat description of the carotid body structure (Alain Verna, chapter 1), the book moves to the energy metabolism in the carotid body (Obeso et al, chapter 2). This second chapter is intentiionally iconoclastic—breaking myths on the ill-defined uniqueness of the glomic tissue metabolism, while underlining the particularities of a tissue designed to be active in direct proportion to the degree of the prevailing hypoxia. González, Dinger and Fidone summarize in chapter 3 current concepts on neurotransmission at the sensory synapse of the carotid body with major emphasis on the biochemical aspects of the neurotransmitters. López-López and Peers (chapter 4) describe the electrical properties of chemoreceptor cells and dissect differences between species and developmental stages. Pérez-García and González (chapter 5) frame their discussion on the transduction mechanisms in the carotid body chemoreceptors within the concept of physiological hypoxia, and in light of the known mechanisms in other cells endowed with physiological sensitivity to oxygen tension decrease. Patricio Zapata in chapters 6 and 7 provides an extensively documented account of the output of the carotid body in terms of action potential frequency in the sensory nerve of the organ. Almaraz, Dinger and Fidone (chapter 8) present, for the first time in literature, a coherent view on the mechanisms of the elusive efferent control of the carotid body chemoreceptor function.

The second part of the book is devoted to the systemic effects evoked from the carotid body chemoreceptors. In describing where in the brainstem the central projections of the carotid sinus nerve terminate, Katz et al in chapter 9 set the basis for understanding the full array of systemic responses evoked by stimulating the carotid body. Fitzgerald and Shirahata in chapter 10 describe those responses at every peripheral target of the chemoreflex, and emphasize the interplay of orders originating in the carotid body and in other sensory receptors. Donnelly in chapter 11 tells us what the carotid body does before air-breathing starts, and describes how the organ acquires functional maturity in the postnatal period. Chapter 12, coauthored by Pásaro and Ribas, summarizes what can go wrong with carotid body function, and emphasize the possible significance of this chemoreceptor organ, or its connections, in the genesis of sudden death in neonates.

Every chapter has a final section in which the authors suggest what they consider to be crucial experiments in future developments of the carotid body chemoreception field. We hope that the book provides support to current research and encourages new trends in this specialized area of physiology.

I want to express my gratitude to the contributors for their efforts in making their chapters well organized and up-to-date. I also want to thank them for their kind acceptance of imposed deadlines.

Finally, I want to thank Mª de los Llanos Bravo and Josefina Revuelta for secretarial assistance. Also, thanks to my coworkers, Drs. Almaraz, López-López, Obeso, Pérez-García, Rigual, Rocher and Vicario, who tolerated in good humor the drain on my time during the preparation of the book.

Constancio González
Valladolid, March 1997

PROLOGUE

Some Thoughts About Mechanisms Involved in Carotid Body Chemoreception

Carlos Eyzaguirre

This prologue is not a review and, consequently, does not cover all aspects of carotid body physiology. It is simply an introduction to the excellent chapters that follow, and includes the biases and opinions of this writer regarding carotid body functions.

The carotid body plays an essential role in the control of ventilation during hypoxia, and is the only organ in the body that can do this task. Consequently, it has attracted a great deal of attention throughout the years. Experimentation has evolved from the study of reflexes using a smoked drum to modern and more sophisticated approaches involving biophysics, biochemistry and molecular biology (for general references see González et al[1]).

In spite of many efforts by competent investigators, we are still far from resolving a crucial question—how the sensory discharges of the carotid nerve originate. There is general agreement that different "natural" stimuli (hypoxia, hypercapnia and acidity) increase the sensory nerve discharges that ultimately elicit reflexes in the central nervous system (CNS). However, we do not know how the nerve discharges come about. Many hypotheses or theories have been put forward in trying to resolve this question. A few hypotheses come to mind such as the metabolic, the acidic and transmitter hypotheses, all of which have been intellectual efforts to explain the inexplicable. Why has this been so difficult?

First, the morphology of the carotid body is complex. We have a miniscule organ (about 1 mm^3) formed by lobules (glomera) containing the glomus (type I, chief or chemoreceptor) cells, innervated by branches of the carotid nerve (itself a branch of the glossopharyngeal nerve). The contacts between the nerve terminals and glomus cells form sensory synapses that are not uniformly polarized. Morphologically, some junctions are polarized from glomus cell to nerve ending, from nerve endings to glomus cell and others are bidirectional. Sometimes, differences in synaptic polarity occur within a few Ångstroms in one junction. In addition, glomus cells are not independent units since there are gap junctions between them that allow intercellular passage of substances and currents. The glomus cells and the synaptic junctions are enveloped by processes of glial-like sustentacular (type II) cells.[2,3] Furthermore, carotid nerve fibers branch to innervate more than one glomus cell and type I cells receive more than one nerve fiber.[4-6] Recently, gap junctions have been found between type I and type II cells and between glomus cells and nerve terminals.[7] Clearly, this morphological complexity precludes a simple and unified explanation of the mechanisms involved in the generation of the sensory impulses.

Another complication is the nature of glomus cells. As elegantly demonstrated by Douarin and colleagues,[8] these cells originate from the neural crest (like sympathetic neurons and chromaffin cells of the adrenal medulla) and migrate toward the peripheral blood vessels. This has been shown in birds, but a similar situation seems to occur in mammals.[9] Once in place, the glomus cells retain some neuronal properties but also lose and develop others. For instance, type I cells appear to have plenty of voltage-gated K^+ channels. However, Na^+ and Ca^{2+} channels, described in rabbit glomus cells, are rare or nonexistent in rat or mouse cells.[10-15] Nevertheless, the main function of these cells is secretory. They contain many chemicals (catecholamines—especially dopamine—acetylcholine and neuropeptides) released during stimulation toward the sensory terminals (see refs. 1,16-18). Therefore, these "wannabe" neurons act like glands without a duct!

The pharmacology of synaptic transmission between glomus cells and carotid nerve terminals has been a major headache for researchers in this field. Proponents of a cholinergic origin of the discharges (including this writer) have had problems supporting this view. If ACh, released from the cells, is the transmitter one would expect cholinergic blockers to block the increased discharge occurring during stimulation; however, this does not happen. At best one obtains a reduced discharge increase. Proponents of a catecholaminergic (dopaminergic) origin of the afferent discharge also have had problems. One is that exogenously applied dopamine (DA) blocks the sensory discharge in cat carotid bodies while it increases the discharge in rabbit chemoreceptors.[19] The other is that DA blockers do not wipe out these effects. Finally, preparations bathed in zero $[Ca^{2+}]_o$ (that should eliminate transmitter release) show a reduced discharge, but it is still there.[1,16-18] Consequently, a "transmitter hypothesis," while being attractive, does not fully explain the origin of the afferent discharge. Perhaps the released chemicals act as modulators (not transmitters), as suggested by Zapata.[18] This idea gains strength from the recent finding of gap junctions between type I cells and nerve terminals in the rat.[7] When such research is expanded to cover other species, and we know the extent and nature of such junctions, we may have an explanation of the "transmitter puzzle." Indeed, if there is intercellular communication (chemical and current spread) between glomus cells and nerve terminals, it should not be surprising that synaptic blockers are rather ineffective. For instance, if calcium and/or other ions move from the cells to the nerve terminal, they could cause nerve depolarization, affecting the onset of the sensory discharge.[20,21]

With the arrival of voltage-clamping with a single electrode (whole-cell, perforated patch, and cell-attached configurations), a great deal of work has been done on cultured glomus cells. This effort has resulted in considerable advances in our knowledge of glomus cell behavior. Practically all investigators have voltage-clamped the cells at a very negative potential (about -70 mV) and have used increasingly positive pulses to measure the resulting currents. These experiments have revealed the presence of significant outward currents, mainly through K^+ channels.[10] Only one study has explored the presence of Cl^- currents,[22] although chloride ions are important in the normal resting potential of glomus cells.[23] What differentiates glomus cells from neurons is that inward currents (Na^+ and Ca^{2+}) have not been recorded equally well in glomus cells of different species. For instance, rabbit cells have many Na^+ and Ca^{2+} channels, something that does not occur in rat or mouse cells[11,24] (also, Jiang and Eyzaguirre, unpublished). Published data from cat glomus cells is very scant. In addition, the age of the animal used as a provider of glomus cells seems to have an influence in the presence or absence of inward current channels. It appears that these channels occur more frequently in glomus cells harvested from embryos or newborn animals as compared with cells obtained from adults (see chapter 4).

These results have important implications since they show that type I cells of different species do not behave identically and that age changes glomus cell behavior. The older the animal, the less neuron-like these cells become . Thus, one may ask if species differences in glomus cell behavior are related to normal differences in development. If this is the case, one could speculate that rats and mice develop much faster than rabbits, and perhaps cats. Stretching this reasoning, one may hypothesize that glomus cells from human or nonhuman primate infants (that develop much slower than lower mammals) would show quite an array of outward and inward current channels, a property lost in adults. At present, we know nothing about the behavior of human or primate type I cells.

An interesting phenomenon observed by many investigators is that hypoxia depresses, but does not block, the outward and voltage-gated K^+ currents and a great deal of significance has been attached to this fact (see ref. 1 and references therein). It has been suggested that inhibition of K^+ currents depolarizes the glomus cells, leading to calcium influx (also through voltage-gated channels) and consequent release of transmitters toward the nerve terminals. This assumption requires five premises: (1) that glomus cells depolarize during stimulation; (2) that the voltage-gated calcium current will increase; (3) that all glomus cells have identical behavior; (4) that the enveloping sustentacular cells do not play a significant role in these phenomena; and (5) that blockers of K^+ channels should increase the sensory discharge as hypoxia does. However, several observations do not favor the idea that depression of the outward K^+ current is the only mechanism responsible for the increased discharge during stimulation:

1) Different stimuli (hypoxia, hypercapnia, acidity) depolarize about one-half of the cells while the others undergo hyperpolarization. This effect is conditioned by the presence of sustentacular cells when the glomus cells are clustered and their absence when type I cells are isolated.[25]

2) Earlier observations showed that the voltage-gated inward Ca^{2+} current was not affected by hypoxia.[12,14] However, more recent ones have shown that this current is depressed by hypoxia.[13] This occurs even when there is a marked increase in intracellular calcium during hypoxia and other stimuli. It has been suggested that $[Ca^{2+}]_i$ increase is mostly due to calcium inflow.[1] This is probably the case, although it cannot happen through unaffected or depressed voltage-gated calcium channels. Intracellular calcium must increase either by influx through other channels (see later) or it may come from intracellular stores.[62] Thus, it is necessary to explore further this point, which is crucial, to reconcile apparently contradictory observations.

3) Glomus cells do not behave identically in their electric responses. This suggests a nonuniform population,[26] bringing back old morphological observations suggesting the same.[2] It also supports the findings with microelectrodes (see later).

4) The sustentacular cells do not seem to be just enveloping bags. They are glial-like[27] and may possess many properties of glia in the CNS where they influence neuronal behavior.[28]

5) Recent evidence has shown that application of TEA (a classic cholinergic-ganglionic- and potassium channel blocker) depresses the outward K^+ current without influencing the sensory discharge, simultaneously recorded.[29] This is not strange since this agent and other cholinergic blockers have been used in the past to test (and reject) the cholinergic hypothesis of chemoreception. In fact, TEA eliminates the nerve responses to applied ACh but does not substantially modify the effects of "natural" carotid body stimuli on the carotid nerve discharge or reflexes induced by it.[30,31]

Practically all work with voltage-clamping has employed voltage-gating. One should reflect, however, if this should be the only approach. Electrophysiologically, the carotid body reacts slowly to different stimuli when compared with nerve or muscle. Therefore, it may be profitable to steadily voltage-clamp at different levels, apply the stimuli and observe the currents developed. We know from several studies that hypoxia mostly induces increases in $[Ca^{2+}]_i$[1], $[Na^+]_i$ and $[Cl^-]_i$ and a decrease in $[K^+]_i$ (see refs. 32,33; also, Zhang, Jiang and Eyzaguirre, unpublished). It is likely that intracellular ionic changes are produced mainly by ion fluxes in and out of the cells. These fluxes should be accompanied by correspondingly increased ionic currents. Due to the reservations expressed about voltage-gated channels, one should look at other pathways such as ligand-gated and passive channels, responsible for the membrane potential.[63] For instance, the available evidence shows that hypoxia depresses the potassium and calcium voltage-gated channels although it probably increases the fluxes of these ions, which must use a pathway that is not voltage-dependent.

A well known and very important area has not been explored in glomus cell research. It is the presence of metabolically dependent ion pumps (electrogenic or neutral), responsible for maintaining the resting potential of cells.[34,35] It is conceivable that oxygen deprivation alters the functioning of pumps, allowing ions to flow according to their concentration gradients. This is precisely what happens. For instance, severe hypoxia decreases $[K^+]_i$ from about 30-50 mM ($[K^+]_o$ 3-4 mM) to 20-30 mM, suggesting that this ion flowed out of the cells.[33] The same stimulus significantly increased $[Cl^-]_i$ from about 30 mM ($[Cl^-]_o$ about 106 mM) to more than 40 mM, suggesting Cl^- inflow.[32] Similarly, it has been widely reported that hypoxia and other stimuli (acidity) markedly increase intracellular calcium.[1] More recently, we have found that hypoxia increases (about 2x) $[Na]_i$ from a resting level of <20 mM ($[Na]_o$ 121 mM) (Zhang, Jiang and Eyzaguirre, unpublished). These experiments suggest that stimuli (especially hypoxia) contribute to a breakdown of forces maintaining normal ionic balances across the cell membrane. All these experiments were conducted without voltage-activation of membrane channels.

An important element in the carotid body receptor complex is the highly neglected sustentacular (type II) cells. As indicated before, these cells send processes that surround most glomus cells and the synaptic contacts with carotid nerve terminals. Sustentacular cells have been identified as belonging to the glia family.[27] As such, they should have an array of metabolically active pumps and exchange mechanisms that are bound to influence the electrical behavior and ionic exchanges in the glomus cells.[28] We know that, electrically, they behave like glia having very negative resting potential, very small capacitance and do not generate action potentials.[36] Recently, it has been found that there are gap-like connections between sustentacular and glomus cells.[7] This finding has important connotations. First, gap connections between neurons and glia have not been found in the CNS of mammals[37] and their presence in the carotid body is unusual. Second, the normal exchange of substances and information across the space between glial and neuronal cells should be much more effective when gap junctions also occur between them.

We know almost nothing about the influences of sustentacular cells on glomus cell functions. However, some clues are available. Clustered glomus cells in culture (retaining their sustentacular envelope) behave differently from isolated cells that do not.[36] For instance, the resting potential (E_M) of clustered rat glomus cells was not influenced by extracellular potassium whereas the E_M of isolated cells was clearly related to $[K^+]_o$.[33,38] Oxygen deprivation depolarized about 80% of clustered cells but did not change significantly their pH_i.[39-42] On the other hand, isolated cells were mostly hyperpolarized by hypoxia and their pH_i decreased.[25,39] Clustered and isolated glomus cells have, however, some similar properties. During hypoxia, changes in $[K^+]_i$ and $[Na^+]_i$ are similar in clusters and in isolation[33] (also, Zhang, Jiang and Eyzaguirre, unpublished). Still, it remains to be established if differences in behavior between clustered and isolated glomus cells are entirely due to the presence or absence of the sustentacular envelope.

Concerning the previous paragraph it should be pointed out that other authors working with whole-cell clamping have reported only glomus cell depolarization with hypoxia.[43] Also, Weiss and Donnelly[44] have shown that depolarization is crucial to chemical release from these cells. It is not known whether differences with microelectrode recordings have occurred because of different techniques, animal species and age, or other factors. It is easier to explain the fact that other authors, working with the whole carotid body or clustered glomus cells, have reported no effects of hypoxia on pH_i.[45,46] These investigators used pH-sensitive dyes applied to the whole preparation or cultured cell clusters. When we recorded pH_i from individual cells in clusters we found that about one-half of the cells became more acidic whereas the rest became more alkaline.[39] Thus, recording pH_i from all the cells (dye experiments) should result in an average response: pH shifts toward acidity in some cells would be canceled by the alkalinization of the others.

An important aspect of carotid body physiology is the nature of the oxygen sensor in these receptors. In some ways it is like trying to find the philosophers' stone since such finding would turn everything into gold. Two lines of thought have evolved. One suggests that the oxygen-sensitive site be located in the cytoplasm, probably involving a heme-like protein.[47] The other, locates this function in the glomus cell membrane.[1,48] At present, we do not have enough information to favor one or the other proposition. However, the possibility exists that both membrane and cytoplasmic sites are involved, working together to detect oxygen lack. This problem is so crucial in understanding oxygen chemoreception that one would hope that further work is done in this important area.

Glomus cells are dye and electrically coupled.[49-54] Some cells are tightly coupled, although most of them are only loosely coupled. As indicated earlier, we do not know how many cells are coupled and whether this phenomenon occurs in all species since only rat glomus cells have been studied. During activation, most (but not all) cells show partial uncoupling.

It is important to find a physiological meaning to coupling or intercellular communication. In vertebrates, most cells in the body are interconnected except nerves, skeletal muscle and most neurons in the CNS. In the carotid body, one could assume that cells are in communication because of their secretory nature. Secretion of glandular cells runs in parallel with changes in their coupling, whatever the direction of the latter phenomenon. Cells in exocrine glands usually uncouple during secretion although some endocrine cells become more tightly coupled during this process.[55]

One may hypothesize that different degrees of intercellular coupling between "resting" glomus cells serves to maintain a certain level of transmitters (modulators) in sufficient supply for release during stimulation. Thus, poorly coupled cells would be releasing certain amount, of chemicals, necessary to maintain a baseline discharge in the carotid nerve. The tightly coupled glomus cells would be saving the chemicals for future use. During stimulation, the more tightly coupled cells "at rest" would uncouple and release their chemical content toward the nerve terminals. Initially poorly coupled cells would become more tightly coupled and stop releasing transmitters that would accumulate in their cytoplasm. This hypothesis suggests that glomus cells function like a push-pull pump. This assumption is not unreasonable since a short and strong stimulus would not deplete the chemical contents in all the cells. If that happened, the organ could not respond to a series of stimuli or to prolonged activation. However, there is no evidence that the proposed mechanism really occurs since the opposite situation (like in endocrine glands) may happen. However, during stimulation most glomus cells become less tightly coupled, suggesting that the proposed mechanism may be the correct one.[21]

The immediate question is, can we test this model? I believe that we can. Several years ago, intracellular recordings from carotid nerve terminals showed many small depolarizing potentials (s.d.p.s) in unstimulated preparations. During stimulation with NaCN or ACh the frequency of these potentials increased to the point of fusion, resulting in a larger total depolarization accompanying the increased sensory discharge. The s.d.p.s. probably resulted from minute leakages of transmitters from the glomus cells, impinging on the nerve terminals. The stimuli probably increased transmitter release, resulting in more frequent occurrences of the s.d.p.s, a larger depolarization and increased discharge.[57] This assumption was based on the similarity of this phenomenon with what occurs in the neuromuscular junction. In such preparation resting transmitter leakage results in the miniature end-plate potentials (m.e.p.s) that fuse during stimulation and lead to the generation of the end-plate potential.[56] However, the amplitude of the s.d.p.s was larger than that of the m.e.p.s. In our case, it was assumed that the nerve ending depolarization was the equivalent of a receptor or generator potential since it was resistant to local anesthetics (such as procaine) and tetrodotoxin (TTX), as occurs in other receptor organs.[5]

These experiments were extremely difficult to do because the nerve terminals (although large enough to be impaled with microelectrodes) were often pushed away by the pipette and impalements were usually unsuccessful. To avoid these problems, we cocultured glomus cells with nodose ganglion neurons to promote synaptic contacts between the neurons and the glomus cells. Cultured neurons are easy to impale and we partially succeeded since several cocultured neurons showed receptor-like potentials with an increased sensory discharge.[58] However, s.d.p.s were not obtained, probably because the neuronal processes were too long and thin to properly allow the electrotonic spread of the very small s.d.p.s. More recently, Alcayaga and Arroyo[59] and Zhong and Nurse[60] have succeeded in recording from cocultures of petrosal ganglio neurons and glomus cells. Alcayaga and Arroyo[59] have succeeded in obtaining results similar to those of Alcayaga and Eyzaguirre[58] whereas Zhong and Nurse[60] have presented recordings that look similar to the s.d.p.s recorded from the whole carotid body.[57] Consequently, cocultures of petrosal neurons and type I cells provide an ideal situation to study the coupling hypothesis presented above. It is a matter of impaling adjacent, and coupled, glomus cells besides the cocultured neuron. Such experiments would inform us of the changes in glomus cell intercellular coupling and of the s.d.p.s during stimulation. The latter would be an indication of chemical release, which can be confirmed (at least for dopamine) with voltammetric methods. Furthermore, this preparation should allow researchersto further test the idea that glomus cell depolarization is a *sine qua non* condition for chemical release. Such phenomenon should be accompanied by increased frequency and total amplitude of the s.d.p.s.

Concerning the methods used for studying the electric properties of glomus cells, this writer has several qualms: (1) Whole-cell voltage clamping profoundly alters the intracellular environment. We know that second messengers such as Ca^{2+} ions and cAMP (see refs. 1,61, and other chapters in this book) are important factors in oxygen chemoreception, together with other second messengers. These agents are dialyzed during whole-cell clamping. It would be much better to routinely use the perforated patch technique that at least respects the cell cytoplasm.[24] Even this technique has problems since the electric responses of the cells will be conditioned by the ions in the recording electrode. Little effort has been made to fill the recording pipettes with solutions that resemble the intracellular ion concentrations. (2) Not enough attention has been paid to establish differences between clustered and isolated glomus cells. As mentioned above, sustentacular cells do change some responses of glomus cells to hypoxia. (3) It is important to consider that freshly harvested and dissociated glomus cells may not behave identically to cells that have been in culture for some time. (4) The age of the animals (embryos, newborns or adults) from which the cultures were obtained should be carefully considered since this factor alone may be responsible for some differences seen in the behavior of glomus cells. (5) Careful attention should be paid to species differences since, as mentioned above, not all glomus cells from different animals behave similarly.

Finally, we must be aware that cultured glomus cells, and for that matter preparations in vitro, do not necessarily behave the same as glomus cells in the animal. Certainly, without in vitro and cultured cell preparations many important features of carotid body physiology could not have been detected. However, it is important to recognize the value of early work with humans and animals in which the natural environment of the carotid body is better preserved. Similarly, the classical morphologists and electron microscopists have given us extremely valuable building blocks upon which we have organized and pursued research at the cellular level.

References

1. González C, Almaraz L, Obeso A, Rigual R. Carotid body chemoreceptors: From natural stimuli to sensory discharges. Physiol Rev 1994; 74:829-898.
2. McDonald DM. Peripheral chemoreceptors: Structure-function relationships of the carotid body. In: Hornbein TF, Lenfant C, eds. Regulation of Breathing. Vol. 17. Lung Biology in Health and Disease. New York: Dekker, 1981:105-320.
3. Verna A. The mammalian carotid body: Morphological data In: González,C, ed. The Carotid Body Chemoreceptors. Austin: Landes Bioscience, 1997:1-29.
4. De Castro F. Nuevas observaciones sobre la inervación de la región carotídea. Los quimio y preso-receptores. Trab Lab Invest Biol Univ Madrid 1940; 32:297-385.
5. Eyzaguirre C, Gallego A. An examination of de Castro's original slides. In: Purves MJ, ed. The Peripheral Arterial Chemoreceptors. London: Cambridge University Press, 1975:1-23.
6. Kondo H. Innervation of the carotid body of the adult rat; A serial ultrathin section analysis. Cell Tiss Res 1976; 173:1-15.
7. Kondo H, Iwasa H. Re-examination of the carotid body ultrastructure with special attention to intercellular membrane appositions. Adv Exp Med Biol 1996; 410:45-50.

8. Le Douarin N. The Neural Crest. London: Cambridge University Press 1982.
9. Kondo H. A light and electron microscopic study on the embryonic development of the rat carotid body. Am J Ant 1975; 144:275-294.
10. López-López JR, Peers C. Electrical properties of carotid body chemoreceptor cells. Effects of antural stimuli In: González C, ed. The Carotid Body Chemoreceptors. Austin: Landes Bioscience, 1997:65-76.
11. Fieber LA, McCleskey EW. L-Type calcium channels in Type I cells of the rat carotid body. J Neurophysiol 1993; 7:1378-1384.
12. López-Barneo J, López-López JR, Ureña J, González C. Chemotransduction in the carotid body: K^+ current modulated by PO_2 in type I chemoreceptor cells. Science 1988; 241:580-582.
13. López-Barneo J. Oxygen-sensing by ion channels and the regulation of cellular functions. TINS 1996; 19:435-440.
14. Hescheler J, Delpiano MA, Acker H, Pietruschka F. Ionic currents on type I cells of the rabbit carotid body measured by voltage-clamp experiments and the effect of hypoxia. Brain Res 1989; 486:79-88.
15. Delpiano MA, Hescheler J. Evidence for a PO_2-sensitive channel in the type-I cell of the rabbit carotid body. FEBS Lett 1989; 249:195-198.
16. Eyzaguirre C, Fitzgerald RS, Lahiri S, Zapata P. Arterial chemoreceptors. In: Shepherd JT, Abbout FM, eds. Peripheral Circulation and Organ Blood Flow: The Cardiovascular System. Handbook of Physiology: Am Physiol Soc 1993:557-621.
17. Fidone SJ, González C. Initiation and control of chemoreceptor activity in the carotid body. In: Fishman AP, ed. Handbook of Physiology, The Respiratory System. Vol. II, sect. 3. Bethesda: Am Physiol Soc 1986:247-312.
18. Eyzaguirre C, Zapata P. Perspectives in carotid body research. J Appl Physiol 1984; 57:931-957.
19. Monti-Bloch L, Eyzaguirre C. A comparative physiological and pharmacological study of cat and rabbit carotid body chemoreceptors. Brain Res 1980; 193:449-470.
20. Eyzaguirre C, Abundara V. Possible role of coupling between glomus cells in carotid body chemoreception. Biol Signals 1995; 4:263-270.
21. Eyzaguirre C, Abundara V. Reflections on the carotid nerve sensory discharge and coupling between glomus cells. Adv Exp Med Biol 1996; 41:159-168.
22. Stea A, Nurse C. Chloride channels in cultured glomus cells of the rat carotid body. Am J Physiol Cell Physiol 1989; 26: C174-C181.
23. Oyama Y, Walker JL, Eyzaguirre C. The intracellular chloride activity of glomus cells in the isolated rabbit carotid body. Brain Res 1986; 368:167-169.
24. Stea A, Nurse C. Whole-cell and perforated patch recordings from O_2-sensitive rat carotid body cells grow in short and long-term cultures. Pfluegers Arch 1991; 418:93-101.

25. Pang L, Eyzaguirre C. Different effects of hypoxia on the membrane potential and input resistance of isolated and clustered carotid body glomus cells. Brain Res 1992; 575:167-173.
26. Donnelly DF. Response to cyanide of two types of glomoid cells in mature rat carotid body. Brain Res 1993; 630:157-168.
27. Kondo H, Iwanaga T, Nakajima T. Immunocytochemical study on the localization of neuron-specific enolase and S-protein in the carotid body of rats. Cell Tiss Res 1982; 227:291-295.
28. Abbott NJ (De). Glial-Neuronal Interaction. Ann NY Acad Sci 1991:(633).
29. Chen PM, Donnelly DF. Relationship between changes of glomus cell current and neural response of rat carotid body. J Neurophysiol 1995; 74:2077-2611.
30. Moe GK, Capo LR, Peralta B. Action of tetraethylammonium on chemoreceptor and stretch receptor mechanisms. Am J Physiol 1948; 153:601-605.
31. Anichkov SV, Belen'kii ML. Pharmacology of the Carotid Body Chemoreceptors. New York: Pergamon Press 1963.
32. Pang C, Eyzaguirre C. Effect of hypoxia on the intracellular chloride activity of cultured glomus cells in the rat carotid body. Biol Res 1993; 26:365-370.
33. Zhang XQ, Pang L, Eyzaguirre C. Effects of hypoxia on the intracellular K^+ of clustered and isolated glomus cells of mice and rats. Brain Res 1995; 676:413-420.
34. Thomas RC. Electrogenic sodium pumps in nerve and muscle cells. Physiol Rev 1972; 52:563-594.
35. Läuger P. Electrogenic Ion Pumps, Sunderland MA: Sinauer, 1991.
36. Duchen MR, Caddy KWT, Kirby GC, Patterson DL, Ponte JL, Biscoe TJ. Biophysical studies of the cellular elements of the rabbit carotid body. Neuroscience 1988; 26:291-311.
37. Murphy TH, Blatter LA, Weir WG, Baraban JM. Rapid communication between neurons and astrocytes in primary cortical cultures. J Neurosci 1993; 13:2672-2679.
38. Oayama Y, Walker JL, Eyzaguirre C. Intracellular potassium activity, potassium equilibrium potential and membrane potential of carotid body glomus cells. Brain Res 1986; 381:405-408.
39. Pang L, Eyzaguirre C. Hypoxia affects differently the intracellular pH of clustered and isolated glomus cells of the rat carotid body. Brain Res 1993; 623:349-355.
40. He SF, Wei JY, Eyzaguirre C. Effects of relative hypoxia and hypercapnia on intracellular pH and membrane potential of cultured carotid body cells. Brian Res 1991; 556:333-338.
41. He SF, Wei JK, Eyzaguirre C. Intracellular pH and some membrane characteristics of cultured carotid body cells. Brain Res 1991; 547:258-286.
42. He SF, Wei JY, Eyzaguirre C. Influence of intracellular pH on the membrane potential of cultured carotid body glomus cells. Brain Res 1993; 601:353-357.

43. Buckler KJ, Vaughan-Jones RD. Effects of hypoxia on membrane potential and intracellular calcium in rat neonatal carotid body type I cells. J Physiol (Lond) 1994; 476:423-428.
44. Weiss N, Donnelly DF. Depolarization is a critical event in hypoxia-induced glomus cell secretion. Adv Exp Med Biol 1996; 410:181-188.
45. Iturriaga R, Rumsey WL, Lahiri S, Spergel D, Wilson DF. Intracellular pH and oxygen chemoreception in the cat carotid body in vitro. J Appl Physiol 1992; 72:2259-2262.
46. Wilding TJ, Cheng B, Ross A. pH regulation in adult rat carotid body glomus cells. J Gen Physiol 1992; 100:593-608.
47. Cross R, Henderon L, Jones TG, Delpiano M, Hentschel J, Acker H. Involvement of an NAD(P)H oxidase as a pO_2 sensor protein in the rat carotid body. Biochem J 1990; 272:743-747.
48. Lahiri S, Buerk DG, Chugh D, Osani S, Mokashi A. Reciprocal photolabile O_2 consumption and chemoreceptor excitation by carbon monoxide in the cat carotid body: Evidence for cytochrome a_3 as the primary O_2 sensor. Brain Res 1995; 684:194-200.
49. Baron M, Eyzaguirre C. Effects of temperature on some membrane characteristics of carotid body cells. Am J Physiol Cell Physiol 1977; 2: C35-C46.
50. Monti-Bloch L, Eyzaguirre C. Effects of different stimuli and transmitters on glomus cell membranes and intracellular communications. In: Eyzaguirre C, Fidone SJ, Fitzgerald RS, Lahiri S, McDonald DM, eds. Arterial Chemoreception. New York: Springer, 1990: 157-167.
51. Monti-Bloch L, Abundara V, Eyzaguirre C. Electrical communication between glomus cells of the rat carotid body. Brain Res 1993; 622:119-131.
52. Abudara V, Eyzaguirre C. Electrical coupling between cultured glomus cells of the rat carotid body: observations with current and voltage clamping. Brain Res 1994; 664:257-265.
53. Abudara V, Eyzaguirre C. Effects of calcium on the electric coupling of carotid body glomus cells. Brain Res 1996; 725:125-131.
54. Abudara V, Eyzaguirre C. Effects of hypoxia on the intercellular channel activity of cultured glomus cells. Adv Exp Med Biol 1996; 410:151-158.
55. Meda P. Gap junctional coupling and secretion in endocrine and exocrine pancreas. In: Sperelakis N, Cole WC, eds. Cell Interactions and Gap Junctions. Vol. 1. Boca Raton: CRC Press1989:59-84.
56. Katz B. Nerve, Muscle and Synapse. MacGraw-Hill: New York, 1966.
57. Hayashida Y, Koyano H, Eyzaguirre C. An intracellular study of chemosensory fibers and endings. J Neurophysiol 1980; 44:1077-1088.
58. Alcayaga J, Eyzaguirre C. Electrophysiological evidence for the reconstitution of chemosensory units in cocultures of carotid body and nodose ganglion neurons. Brain Res 1990; 534:324-328.

59. Alcayaga J, Arroyo J. Responses of cat petrosal ganglion neurons are modified by the presence of carotid body cells in tissue cultures. Adv Exp Med Biol 1996; 410:195-201.
60. Zhong H, Nurse C. Cocultures of rat petrosal neurons and carotid body type I cells. Adv Exp Med Biol 1996; 410:189-193.
61. Obeso A, González C, Dinger B, Fidone S. Metabolic activation of carotid body glomus cells by hypoxia. J Appl Physiol 1989; 67:484-487.
62. Biscoe TJ, Duchen MR. Responses of type I cells dissociated from the rabbit carotid body to hypoxia. J Physiol (Lond) 1990; 428:39-59.
63. Edwards C. The selectivity of ion channels ion nerve and muscle. Neuroscience 1982; 7:1335-1366.

CHAPTER 1

The Mammalian Carotid Body: Morphological Data

Alain Verna

INTRODUCTION

The carotid body (CB) is a very small organ (around 2 mm diameter in man, less than 1 mm diameter in laboratory animals) located at the level of the bifurcation of the common carotid artery (Fig. 1.1). It receives arterial blood from a short artery which may be a branch of the internal carotid artery, external carotid artery or occipital artery, depending on the species considered. Individual variations in the organization of the blood supply are also common.[1] The carotid body artery divides to generate a dense capillary network. This fine network is responsible for the pinky appearance of the carotid body. A venous plexus is often visible at the CB surface and one or several veins join the internal jugular vein or one of its branches. Careful dissection also shows that the CB is innervated by a branch of the glossopharyngeal nerve, Hering's nerve or the carotid sinus nerve, and by one or several nerves coming from the sympathetic superior cervical ganglion. A comparative study of CB anatomy, blood supply and nerve supply can be found in Adams,[2] with historical considerations (discovery, denomination, first interpretations...).

Discussions with nonspecialists, more especially from medical origin, reveal that the CB is frequently confused with the carotid sinus. This is understandable because both organs are located close to each other and receive nerve fibers from the same origin, but their respective roles are very different. To avoid any confusion, let me introduce briefly, the essential aspects:

1) The carotid sinus is a dilation of the internal carotid artery, near its origin, characterized by the presence, in the arterial wall, of "free" nerve endings which sense the arterial blood pressure; these nerve endings are baroreceptors. Baroreceptors are, functionally speaking primary sensory receptors since sensory neurons detect, transduce and transmit the information.

The Carotid Body Chemoreceptors,
edited by Constancio González.

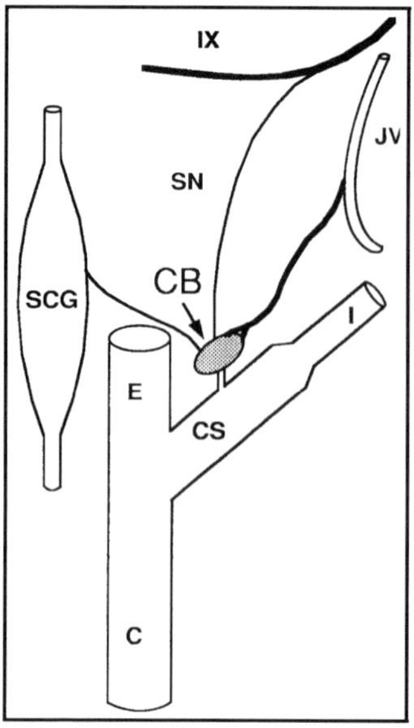

Fig. 1.1. Vasculo-nervous connections of the carotid body. CB: carotid body; C: common carotid artery; CS: carotid sinus; E: external carotid artery; I: internal carotid artery; JV: internal jugular vein; SCG: superior cervical ganglion; SN: sinus nerve; IX: glossopharyngeal nerve.

2) The carotid body is a small mass of tissue, containing specialized cells innervated by sensory nerve fibers and which senses the concentration of chemicals in the arterial blood, more especially blood gases; it is a chemoreceptor. The CB is therefore a secondary receptor since specialized cells detect and transduce stimuli, whereas a second cell (a neuron) transmits the message (see chapter 5).

A histological section through the CB immediately shows the four principal components of the organ: blood vessels, connective tissue, cell clusters, nerve fibers (Fig. 1.2). We will consider these components, as they appear in the light or electron microscope, focusing on the most recent results since many reviews concerning CB morphology have been published.[3-6]

BLOOD VESSELS

The CB has a spongy appearance, in section, due to the abundance of the blood vessels. In the cat, the ratio of the vascular volume to the total volume of the CB is between 15-20%.[7-9] These numerous blood vessels probably explain the organ's enormous blood flow, relative to its size. In the adult cat CB, the blood flow is estimated to be around 2000 ml/min/100 g (see ref. 10; see chapter 2). It is well known that blood flow variations modify the chemoafferent activity. A detailed knowledge of the CB vascular bed is therefore necessary to understand CB physiology.

Arteries

The CB artery and its branches are characterized by elastic laminae and a few layers of smooth muscle cells. In fact, the term "CB artery" is misleading since branches of this artery supply nearby structures such as the carotid sinus, nodose ganglion and superior cervical ganglion. A sphincter-like intimal cushion is present at the origin of the CB artery in the rat and mouse,[1,11] but this does not exist in other species.

The structure of these vessels does not deserve any special comment; the endothelium is not fenestrated. Nerve endings are frequent around CB arteries and arterioles, the highest innervation density being, in the rat, on third- to fifth-order arterioles.[12] In connection with this thin wall, it must be added that there exist both morphological and electrophysiological evidence for the occurrence of some barosensory nerve fibers around glomic arteries.[1,13]

Capillaries

Most of the blood vessels in the CB are capillaries, showing a very convoluted trajectory, and large variations in diameter. They are characterized by a thin endothelium (sometimes fenestrated; Fig. 1.5) and are more or less surrounded by pericyte processes. There are two types of capillaries in the CB according to de Castro and Rubio[14] and McDonald.[12] In the rat, type I capillar-

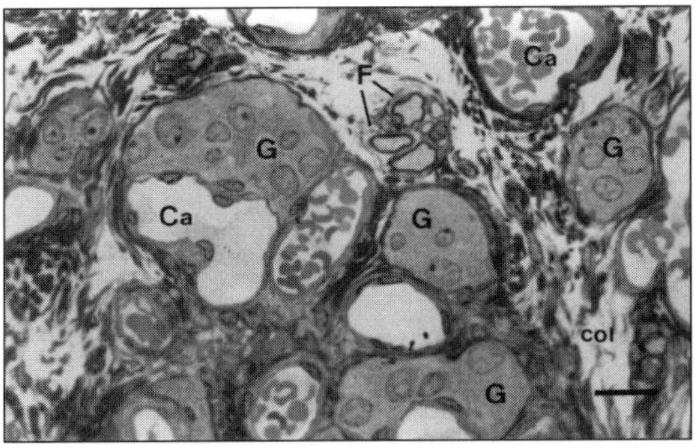

Fig. 1.2. Semi-thin section through the rabbit carotid body. G: glomus cells; F: myelinated nerve fibers; Ca: capillaries; col: collagen. Bar 15 μm.

ies (the most abundant) are closely associated to glomus cells, are tortuous and their diameter varies from 8 to more than 20 μm; they are therefore unusually large. Type II capillaries have a more constant diameter (less than 10 μm), they have straight as well as curved regions and they are not strictly associated with glomus cells.[11,12,15]

Arteriovenous Anastomoses

The existence of arteriovenous anastomoses in the CB has been long debated. The most convincing evidence is a serial section analysis by McDonald and Larue[11] which clearly identify some arterioles directly connected to small venules. Thus, arteriovenous anastomoses really do exist in the CB, at least in the rat.

Venules, Veins and Lymphatics

Venules are very numerous and emerge from the CB to form a dense venous plexus on its surface. They have a thicker endothelium than capillaries and show fewer fenestrations. Their diameter varies from about 10 μm to more than 100 μm. Most venules are interconnected with one another. Veins from the CB join other organs to drain into the internal and external jugular vein.

Although often ignored, lymphatic vessels are also present in the CB. They are characterized by a very thin unfenestrated endothelium. According to McDonald and Larue[11] lymphatics are more numerous at the surface of the rat CB than in deeper regions.

Functional Aspects

The importance and complexity of the vascular compartment is a conspicuous feature of the CB, and suggests an important role in the physiology of this organ. It is well known that chemoafferent activity is modified by variations in blood flow and several studies have suggested that local blood flow (at the level of glomus cells) may be regulated independently of total blood flow through the organ.[16,17] The effects of chronic hypoxia also suggest that CB vasculature and chemoafferent activity are linked: after chronic hypoxia, there is a dramatic increase in capillary diameters[18] and a growth of new blood vessels.[8] However, it must be kept in mind that superfused arterial chemoreceptors perfectly detect hypoxia (and other stimuli) in vitro, showing that vascular integrity is not a necessary condition for the transduction phenomenon. It seems, therefore, that the vascular complexity of the CB is not, in itself, responsible for the transduction mechanism, but may be involved in fine adjustments related to the physiological state of the animal.

CONNECTIVE TISSUE

The connective tissue constitutes a large fraction of the total volume of the CB[19,20] (around 50-60%), but there are significant species differences. Thus, for example, the connective tissue is more abundant in the rabbit CB than in the rat or human CB.

The principal components of the CB connective tissue are fibrocytes and collagen fibers. Fibrocytes do not deserve any special comment. They are characterized by very elongated and ramified cytoplasmic processes. Some of them, located close to glomus cell groups, may be confused with sustentacular cells at the light microscope level but such confusion is impossible with the electron microscope since fibrocytes are devoid of basal lamina, in addition to the absence of contacts with glomus cells and nerve fibers.

Mastocytes may be present within the connective tissue of the human and rat CB. This is important for those interested in the serotonin content of the CB, since mastocytes contain serotonin.

According to Kondo and Yamamoto[21] glomus cell clusters are surrounded by a sheath of flattened perineurial cells which may be identified, immunocytochemically, by the presence of nerve growth factor receptors on their surface. The authors suggested that the CB is a multiunit structure, each unit being made of glomus cells, sustentacular cells and nerve fibers, surrounded, as a whole, by a sheath of perineurial cells.

CELL CLUSTERS

In addition to its extensive vascular supply, the CB is characterized by the occurrence of cell clusters of variable size, closely related to capillaries and dispersed in a stroma made of fibrocytes and collagen fibers (Fig. 1.3). Each cell cluster is made of two types of cells, known for a long time: glomus cells and sustentacular cells (also known as type I or chemoreceptor and type II cells, respectively) (Fig. 1.4). Since many studies were devoted to the structure of these cells, I will develop only what seems important to me and some recent developments.

Sustentacular Cells

Sustentacular cells may be compared to the satellite cells which surround ganglionic neurons in the peripheral nervous system. They surround glomus cells (although not totally; Fig. 1.5) with a thin cytoplasmic layer containing the usual organelles, among which cytoskeletal elements are abundant. It has been shown immunocytochemically that sustentacular cells, like Schwann and glial cells, contain S 100 protein and glial fibrillary acidic protein.[22,22a] Sustentacular cells do not contain secretory granules and are therefore easy to differentiate from glomus cells with the electron microscope since only glomus cells contain dense-cored vesicles. The problem is more difficult at the light microscope level: sustentacular cells may be identified by their location at the periphery of cell clusters and the flattened or curved shape of their nucleus, often more darkly stained than the nucleus of glomus cells. However, Schwann cells and, to a lesser extent, fibrocytes, are also present at the periphery of cell clusters, and also show a flattened and heavily stained nucleus. It is, therefore, sometimes impossible to unambiguously identify a sustentacular cell with the light microscope. Sustentacular cells are, morphologically, less sensitive to hypoxia than glomus cells.[23] The extracellular space

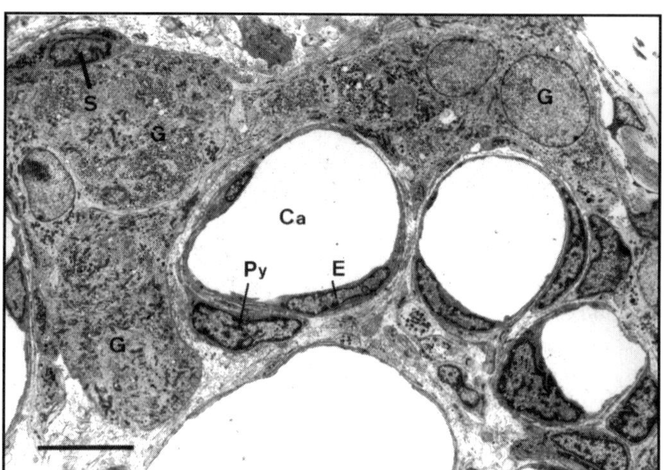

Fig. 1.3. Thin section through the rabbit carotid body showing the relationships between glomus cell clusters and blood vessels. G: glomus cells; S: sustentacular cells; Ca: capillaries; E: endothelial cell; Py: pericyte. Bar: 4 μm.

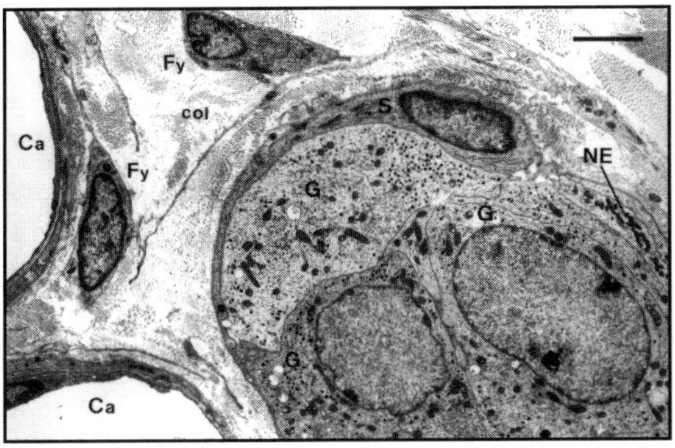

Fig. 1.4. Rabbit carotid body. This electron micrograph shows the principal components of the chemoreceptor tissue: G: glomus cells; S: sustentacular cells; NE: nerve endings; Ca: Capillaries. Fy: fibrocytes; Col: collagen. Bar: 2 μm.

between glomus cells and sustentacular cells does not seem to be closed, by tight junctions for example. Furthermore, tracer studies have shown this space to be easily accessible to large molecules.[24,25]

Glomus Cells

Histologically, glomus cells are characterized by a round and pale nucleus. Their size and shape are difficult to determine since they frequently show cytoplasmic processes intermingled within a given cluster. Their cytoplasmic organelles are well known (Fig. 1.6) and it does not seem necessary to add new comments on the aspects of mitochondria, reticulum, Golgi apparatus and so on. I just would like to mention the existence of a well developed cytoskeleton, which is often ignored. Surprisingly, there are only a few descriptions of gap-junctions[4] in spite of observations showing dye spreading from a glomus cell to a neighboring cell[26] and physiological data suggesting electrical coupling between glomus cells.[27-31] Several explanations are possible: gap junctions were not searched for with sufficient attention (we find only what we are looking for!); alternatively, fixation procedure using aldehydes may uncouple glomus cells (we must not forget we are working on a chemoreceptor!). Quick-freezing followed by freeze-fracture would be the method of choice to solve this problem. A recent paper by Kondo and Iwasa[32] seems very promising: these authors used a freeze-substitution protocol after chemical fixation and cryoprotection with glycerol; they observed numerous structures similar to gap junctions between adjacent glomus cells, between glomus cells and sustentacular cells, and also between glomus cells and nerve endings. Unfortunately the results are not convincing because freezing may induce artifacts looking alike to gap junctions (Verna, unpublished observations). The authors themselves concede very honestly, that freeze-fracture studies and immunocytochemistry for connexins are necessary to confirm their results.

The distinctive feature of glomus cells is the presence of numerous dense-core vesicles in the cytoplasm. During the period 1970-1980, many studies demonstrated that

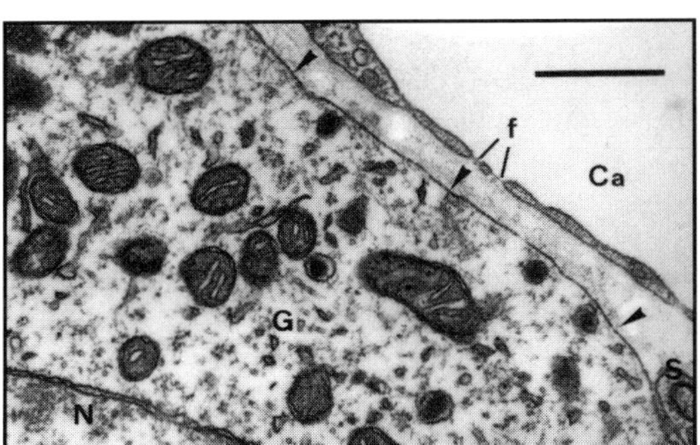

Fig. 1.5. Rabbit carotid body. Glomus cells are not totally covered by sustentacular cells. In this example, a large part of a glomus cell membrane is directly exposed to the extracellular spaces (arrowheads), at a short distance from the fenestrated endothelium of a capillary. G: glomus cell; Ca: capillary F: endothelium fenestrations; N: glomus cell nucleus S: sustentacular cell process. Bar: 0.5 μm.

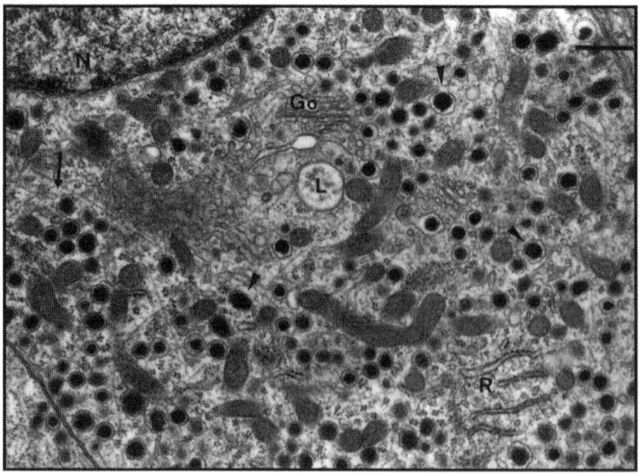

Fig. 1.6. Rabbit carotid body. Electron micrograph showing the organelles of glomus cells. G: Golgi saccules; L: lysosome; N: nucleus; R: rough endoplasmic reticulum; arrow: microtubules; arrowheads: dense-core vesicles. Bar: 0.5 μm.

these vesicles are the storage sites of catecholamines, known to be present in glomus cells by the use of formol-induced fluorescence methods, for example.

Some studies have suggested that the content of dense-core vesicles is released via exocytosis, although it was necessary either to incubate glomus cells in media containing both calcium and an ionophore[33] or to perfuse the carotid body with fixative containing a high concentration of potassium[34] to observe exocytotic profiles. It must be pointed out that these profiles occurred predominantly in nonsynaptic regions of glomus cells. It quickly appeared, on the one hand, that dense-core vesicles are of different sizes, and, on the other hand, that there are different catecholamines [mainly dopamine (DA) and norepinephrine or noradrenaline (NA)] in the carotid body. It was tempting, therefore to use the morphology of dense-core vesicles to distinguish different sub-types of glomus cells, storing different catecholamines. However, the literature is somewhat confusing on this subject, probably because several parameters interfere: the animal species, the method used to quantify, the size of samples used for quantification, the physiological state of the animal, etc. The large number of these interfering parameters probably explains why there are so many contradictory reports.

At first sight, it might seem unnecessary to come back to these problems which were considered in detail in previous reviews. However, some recent papers continue to describe glomus cell sub-types, according to the morphology of their dense-core vesicles. Since there are other criteria (both morphological and physiological), in favor of the existence of glomus cell sub-types, I shall discuss briefly the recent developments concerning this problem.

Identification of Glomus Cell Sub-types.

Catecholamines in glomus cells.

Classification of Glomus Cells According to the Morphology of their Dense-core Vesicles

In the rat carotid body, two glomus cell sub-types were described by McDonald and Mitchell[35] and Hellström.[36] Both of these papers described "small vesicle cells" (or type B cells) and "large vesicle cells" (or type A cells) although they disagree on numerical values, probably for methodological reasons. However, using larger samples and avoiding a prior selection, it was shown later by Pallot[20] that the vesicle diameters are, in fact, unimodally distributed between extreme values, suggesting a variability phenomenon within a unique cell type. However, Pequignot et al[37] again reported a bimodal distribution of dense-core vesicle diameters in control rats and, more recently, Kusakabe et al[38] also described two glomus cell sub-types in control rats, whereas four types were described by Morita et al[39] in the cat.

In the rabbit, I also observed, in control animals, glomus cells which differed by the diameter of their dense-core vesicles (by an order of magnitude !). However, by measuring all dense-core vesicles from 30 cells, selected at random, I obtained a unimodal distribution. Thus, although there are small and large vesicles as well as glomus cells containing predominantly small or large vesicles, these "kinds" of cells represented, actually, the extremes of a simple population.[40] Nevertheless, Xu et al[41,42] recently described three types of glomus cells in control rabbits: according to these authors 90% of glomus cells contain small dense-core vesicles of low electron density and the other cells were classified as cells with dense-core vesicles having the largest diameters and the highest electron density, and cells with dense-core vesicles having intermediate features. Information concerning other species (e.g. cat, dog, monkey, birds) may be found in previous reviews.[3,4]

What is the truth? In my opinion, it is clear that there exists, in all species, great variability of the diameter of dense-core vesicles. Similarly, glomus cells are characterized by a great variability of the mean diameter of their vesicles. Thus, I am convinced that there are "small vesicle cells" and "large vesicle cells" in all carotid bodies, and I have, in fact, observed them myself, both in the rabbit and in the rat. However, there is a methodological problem: if you preselect "small vesicle cells" on the one hand, and "large vesicle cells" on the other hand, to measure the diameter of their dense-core vesicles, you will, obviously, obtain a bimodal distribution of diameters. The real problem is to ascertain if intermediate cells exist. The former procedure will, of course, miss these cells. The recent papers on this subject[38,41,42] suffer from this methodological problem, as do some older ones.

In conclusion, I think that the sub-types of glomus cells described to date in control animals are in fact, arbitrary, and I suggest that "small vesicle cells" and "large vesicle cells" correspond to different functional states, and thus, not structurally different types of glomus cells.

If this interpretation is valid, one can suppose that different physiological conditions could influence the functional state of glomus cells and, therefore, their morphological aspect. This is precisely what happens after long-term hypoxia.

Effects of Long-term Hypoxia on Dense-core Vesicles/Glomus Cell Sub-types

The effects of long-term hypoxia on the morphology of dense-core vesicles were studied, in the rat, by Pequignot et al.[37] According to these authors the distribution of vesicle diameters (bimodal in controls) becomes unimodal after 1 to 3 weeks of hypoxia (10% O_2) because "small vesicle cells" transform into "large vesicle cells." The mean diameter of the total population is therefore increased (as reported by Laidler and Kay[43]) but within a unique cell type after hypoxia.

Unfortunately, a recent paper by Kusakabe et al[38] concluded in a very different manner: these authors, who also described two kinds of glomus cells in control animals (vesicle mean diameter: 40-60 nm versus 70-90 nm) reported the existence of four different types in chronically hypoxic animals (3 weeks): small vesicle cells (mean diameter of their dense-core vesicles: 50 nm); large vesicle cells (80 nm); dilated eccentric cells (400-800 nm) and mixed vesicle cells, containing large and eccentric vesicles.

Thus, although both studies conclude as to an overall increase in vesicle diameters, they disagree as regards the classification of glomus cells into different sub-types.

Correlations Between Dense-core Vesicle Morphometry and Catecholamine Content

Authors who distinguished between sub-types of glomus cells suspected, quite early, that these subtypes might store different catecholamines. However, to obtain conclusive evidence on this subject, it was necessary to use a method allowing the localization of catecholamines at the ultrastructural level. Using high resolution autoradiography, I demonstrated that a few glomus cells in the rabbit carotid body are able to take up ^3H-noradrenaline (^3H-NA).[44,45] Interestingly, these cells are characterized by the presence of dense-core vesicles which are larger than those of the other cells. Furthermore, using immunocytochemistry, it was demonstrated that a few glomus cells, in the rabbit, are positive for dopamine β-hydroxylase (DβH) and NA.[46] Again, these cells exhibited large dense-core vesicles (in addition to small ones) showing very dilated membrane and eccentric dense-cores (Fig. 1.7), as do the noradrenergic cells in the adrenal medulla. Thus, it seems that large dense-core vesicles are associated with NA content, at least in the rabbit.

On this subject, it must be noted that, in the rat, long-term hypoxia induces an increase in NA content,[47] an increase in the mean diameter of dense-core vesicles[37] and an increase in the number of NA-immunopositive glomus cells.[48,49] Although chronic hypoxia induces some mitoses among glomus cells,[50,51] their number cannot explain the dramatic increase in the number of NA-positive cells. This suggests that long-term hypoxia induces the ability to synthesize and store NA in cells previously devoid of this amine, in parallel with an increase in the diameter of their dense-core vesicles.

Is it thus possible to conclude as to the existence of distinct DA- and NA-storing glomus cells? If we consider the rabbit carotid body, the answer is yes, at least at first sight. Similarly, a few glomus cells, in control rats, are immunopositive for DβH[52] and for NA[49] whereas the others are not. Since all glomus cells contain catecholamines and since biochemical studies have shown that DA is predominant both in the rat and rabbit, it must be concluded that most glomus cells, in these species, store DA and a few store NA.

If we consider the cat carotid body, the situation is different: according to biochemical studies, the NA content is equivalent to or even superior to the DA content[53] and about 90% of glomus cells are immunopositive for DβH.[54] It must be concluded that most glomus cells, in the cat, store both DA and NA although the DA/NA ratio could vary from cell to cell. This leads us to reconsider the validity of the distinction between DA- and NA-storing cells, introduced above for the rabbit carotid body. The real question is to ascertain if, as for dense-core vesicle diameters, there are intermediates. In other words, are there glomus cells storing both DA and NA, in addition to cells storing only one of these amines? There is no conclusive evidence on this subject, although I remarked, using immunocytochemical detection of DβH and NA, that all intermediate cases between unlabeled and strongly labeled cells were present in the rabbit carotid body.

Classification of Glomus Cells According to Other Parameters

(a) Light/Dark Glomus Cells

Glomus cells, as for many other cells, appear more or less electron-dense in the electron microscope. This observation led some authors to use this parameter to discriminate between "light" and "dark" variants of glomus cells. This distinction was

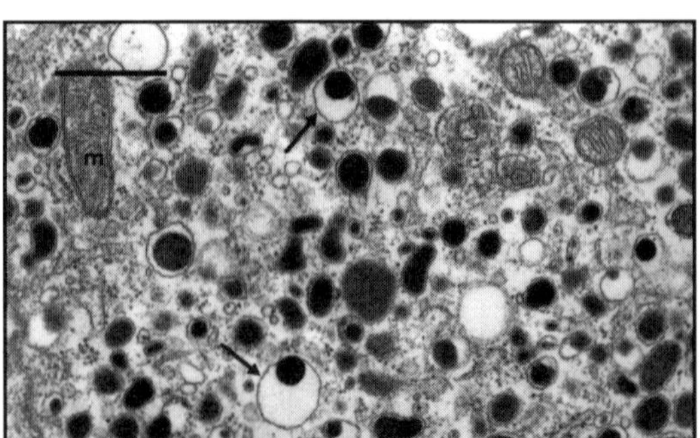

Fig. 1.7. Rabbit carotid body. Cytoplasm of a noradrenergic glomus cell. This kind of cell is characterized by very dense-core vesicles, some of them showing an eccentric dense core (arrows). Note that small dense-core vesicles are also present. M: mitochondria; Bar: 0.5 µm.

criticized by McDonald and Mitchell[35] who considered the light/dark aspect of glomus cells as a fixation artifact, more especially intense after immersion fixation. Although I concede that immersion fixation may artificially increase differences in electron density, I am not sure that all of these differences are due to fixation artefacts. Differences in protein content, for example, may induce, in my opinion, variations in electron density that I have frequently observed in glomus cells fixed by perfusion.

According to Heath and Smith[55] three distinct forms of glomus cells can be recognized in the human carotid body: light, dark and "pyknotic" cells. However, it was experimentally demonstrated that these aspects are postmortem changes due to the unavoidable delay (for human tissue) between circulatory arrest and fixation.[23]

(b) Chromaffinity

Some authors distinguished glomus cells sub-types according to criteria other than dense-core vesicles. For example, chromaffin and nonchromaffin glomus cells were identified in the dog by Kobayashi.[56] In the rabbit, I also observed chromaffin cells and I demonstrated that these cells have large dense-core vesicles and correspond to the cells which take up NA and are immunopositive for DβH and NA.[46] Thus, chromaffin glomus cells are, in fact, noradrenergic glomus cells.

(c) Pharmacological Criteria

Horseradish-conjugated alpha-bungarotoxin was used by Chen and Yates[57] to localize acetylcholine receptors in the rat carotid body. These authors distinguished A cells which lacked binding sites or were partly stained by the conjugate, and B cells which exhibited binding sites over their entire surface. Once distinguished by this labeling criteria, A and B cells were described as having morphological features (shape, volume density and mean diameter of dense-core vesicles) typical of A and B cells described by McDonald and Mitchell.[35] These morphological criteria were discussed above. Is alpha-bungarotoxin labeling more reliable? As reported by the authors themselves, all glomus cells exhibited reaction product to some extent and I am not sure that distinction between A and B glomus cells was so clear cut! Moreover, species differences may complicate the problem further, since muscarinic receptors appear to be dominant in the rabbit CB whereas nicotinic receptors are more abundant in the cat.[58]

The effects of reserpine on the electron density of dense-core vesicles (after chromate/dichromate treatment) were studied by Xu et al.[42] As reported above, these authors classified glomus cells into three subtypes (A, B, C) in control rabbits (note that A, B, and C cell types described by Xu et al,[42] refer to rabbit CB, while A and B types of McDonald and Mitchell[35] refer to rat CB). Xu et al[42] showed that reserpine treatment resulted in a marked decrease in electron density of dense-core vesicles in C cells, moderate in B cells whereas A cells were unmodified. Dense-core vesicles in A cells were characterized as having the highest electron density and largest diameters. These authors concluded that "the effects of reserpine offered morphofunctional evidence for the existence of sub-types of type I cells" and suggest that these different subtypes may store different catecholamines. Although I think that the subdivision of glomus cells into three categories is arbitrary, I agree with the final conclusion. As detailed above, I have good reasons to think that, in the rabbit, large dilated vesicles, with an eccentric dense-core characterize glomus cells storing NA. Furthermore, I noticed, many years ago, that a few glomus cells, in the rabbit, were still fluorescent (using the Falck-Hillarp method) 24 h after reserpine treatment. More recently, I demonstrated that these reserpine-resistant cells contain large dense-core vesicles (Schamel and Verna, unpublished observations). Thus, I agree with Xu et al[42] to say that there are reserpine-resistant glomus cells in the rabbit carotid body, but, in addition, I think that these cells are NA-storing cells. The reason why some glomus cells resist the depleting action of reserpine is unclear. Some morphological features (e.g. glycogen accumulation, chromatin alteration) which also characterize a few cells having very large dense-core[46] suggest that these cells may be metabolically inactive or even degenerating, and therefore less sensitive to reserpine.

Conclusion

To be concise, I propose the following assumptions:

1) There are "small vesicle cells" and "large vesicle cells" in the carotid body of many species, but all intermediates are also present.

2) The presence of "large" dense-core vesicle (more especially those showing a "dilated eccentric" morphology is associated with the ability to store NA (possibly in addition to DA).

3) The DA/NA ratio depends on (a) genetic factors: DA predominates in the rat and rabbit (for example) and the NA content may be equal or superior to the DA content in the cat (see Fig. 3.2). (b) physiological factors: long-term hypoxia increases the number of NA-storing cells, at least in the rat.

4) Dense-core vesicle sizes and catecholamine content are not sufficient parameters to unequivocally distinguish subtypes of glomus cells.

5) It seems more appropriate to consider the different aspects of glomus cells as functional states, not structural categories.

This conclusion is in keeping with the observations of Pérez-García et al[59] who reported a marked variability of electrophysiological properties of glomus cells but were unable to ascribe this variability to distinct subpopulations of glomus cells.

Glomus Cells and Neuropeptides

As in any research area, progress in the study of chemoreceptors is tightly bound to methodological improvements. In keeping with this notion, we can state that in the last ten years, most of new data concerning the structure of the carotid body were obtained by immunocytochemistry. The use of specific antibodies allowed, for example, to localize enzymes and neuropeptides in the organ. For functional aspects, see chapters 3 and 7 by González et al and Zapata, respectively.

Enkephalins

The occurrence of leu- and met-enkephalins in glomus cells was demonstrated immunocytochemically by Lundberg et al[60] and Wharton et al.[61] These light microscope studies were quickly followed by an electron immunocytochemical localization by Varndell et al.[62] Using an immunogold technique, these authors demonstrated that enkephalin-like immunoreactivity was localized to dense-core vesicles in glomus cells of the cat and piglet. Furthermore, they showed that enkephalin-like material was colocalized with DβH immunoreactivity. These results therefore suggested a colocalization of amines/peptides in glomus cells. Some years later, Kobayashi et al[63] also used an immunogold technique and demonstrated colocalization of NA and enkephalins in dense-core vesicles of the dog glomus cells. Although this study was not quantitative, the authors estimated that about 30% of glomus cells were immunoreactive for NA among which "a large proportion....were also positively immunostained for enkephalines." Enkephalins were also localized to the dense-core vesicles of glomus cells in the dog and monkey carotid body.[64] More recently, enkephalins were also localized in glomus cells of the human carotid body, but at the light microscope level, using necropsy material.[65] At last, Wang et al[54] demonstrated that most glomus cells of the cat CB are immunopositive for met-enkephalin, TH and DβH.

Thus, glomus cells store both enkephalins and amines, as do adrenal medulla cells. Recent experiments by González-Guerrero et al[66] showed that acute hypoxia induces a parallel decrease in the DA and enkephalin content of the rabbit CB, suggesting a corelease phenomenon, in agreement with the data in favor of costorage, reported above.

Neuropeptide Y (NPY)

This peptide does not seem to be abundant in glomus cells. However, a few NPY-immunoreactive cells were observed in the dog and monkey carotid body whereas glomus cells in the adult rat were found to be negative.[67,68] However, Oomori et al[69] observed a few NPY-positive glomus cells in colchicine-pretreated young rats (3 weeks of postnatal age). According to these authors, who used light and electron microscopy, the reaction product was mainly localized on the dense cores of granular vesicles.

Substance P (SP)

The occurrence of SP, reported first by Cuello and McQueen,[70] was investigated by Chen et al[71] with the light and electron microscope. They found some immuno-positive glomus cells in the cat carotid body, but none in the rat. In the cat, immunoreactivity resided primarily in the dense cores of vesicles, but with a very variable intensity. More recently, Scheibner et al[19] studied with the light microscope the distribution of SP in the developing cat. They reported that a large number of glomus cells acquire SP immunoreactivity between birth and six weeks of age, but suggested that this number may decrease by adulthood. The authors suggested that SP is involved in the carotid body resetting which occurs in the neonatal period. The presence of substance P in glomus cells was mentioned also by Prabhakar et al[72] and Wang et al[73] in the cat carotid body, and by Smith et al[65] in the human carotid body. However, no glomus cells with SP immunoreactivity were observed in the rabbit CB by Kusakabe et al.[74]

Using in situ hybridization, Gauda et al,[75] did not detect SP mRNA in the rat CB, an observation which seems to confirm the negative results of the immunocytochemical study of Cuello and McQueen,[70] concerning the same species.

Atrial Natriuretic Peptide (ANP)

A light microscope immunochemical study demonstrated that more than 80% of glomus cells, in the cat, contained immunoreactivity for ANP.[76] There is no electron microscope study to date. This study was extended to the rat carotid body with similar results.[77] Furthermore, the same study demonstrated that a peptide fragment (atriopeptin III) induced an increase in immunoreactivity for cGMP in glomus cells immunoreactive for ANP, suggesting that autoreceptors for ANP are present on glomus cells (see chapter 8).

Galanin

Galanin immunoreactivity was reported in glomus cells in the guinea pig and monkey carotid body.[68,78] On the contrary, Ichikawa and Helke[79] did not find glomus cells immunoreactive for galanin in control rats. However, immunoreactive cells appeared a few days after carotid sinus nerve section, but disappeared after one week. Furthermore, carotid sinus nerve section combined with superior cervical ganglionectomy resulted in the appearance of more numerous positive glomus cells than without ganglionectomy. The same authors reported the absence of any calcitonin gene-related peptide immunoreactivity in rat glomus cells.

Cholecystokinin/Calcitonin

Cholecystokinin (CCK) has been shown to be present in glomus cells of the dog and monkey by Heym and Kummer.[68] More recently, Wang et al,[80] using an immunogold procedure at the electron microscope level, also showed immunoreactivity for CCK in glomus cells of the human infant carotid body. Moreover, they showed that many cells were also positive for calcitonin. Labeling for both peptides was linked to the dense core of vesicles. In a more recent study, Wang et al[81] detected calcitonin mRNA in the human infant and monkey CB by an in situ hybridization method.

Vasointestinal Peptide (VIP) and Neurotensin

A light microscopic study on necropsy material allowed Smith et al[65] to observe, within the human carotid body, a positive immunoreaction of some glomus cells, for VIP and neurotensin. According to these authors, the immunoreaction for VIP was weak in most carotid bodies and absent in the others. The reactivity for neurotensin was observed in a minority of carotid bodies and was very weak. However, these results must be considered with caution since fixation conditions for necropsy material are not favorable. Electron microscopic data are lacking.

Calcitonin Gene-related Peptide (CGRP)

Although many CGRP-positive fibers were observed in the CB of laboratory animals, this peptide was not detected in glomus cells of these animals. However, CGRP immunoreactive dense-core vesicles were observed in a sub-population of glomus cells in the human CB by Kummer and Habeck.[82] This observation needs confirmation since the postmortem interval (3-12 h) between death and fixation may induce a redistribution of neuropeptides.

Glomus Cells and Serotonin/Acetylcholine

Although most studies were undertaken to localize catecholamines and neuropeptides, a few were devoted to other transmitters, among which, serotonin and acetylcholine (see chapters 3 and 7 for functional aspects).

Serotonin (5-HT)

The occurrence of 5-HT was mentioned several times in the past, but there were few attempts to localize this transmitter in the CB. Using an immunoperoxydase method, Perrin et al[83] reported 5-HT immunopositive glomus cells in the human infant CB. More recently, Habeck et al[84] reported that some glomus cells of the adult human CB are also immunopositive for 5-HT, many of them having close relationships with blood vessels. Wang et al[73] also demonstrated that most glomus cells in the cat CB are immunoreactive for 5-HT. Furthermore, using pairs of antibodies, these authors showed a high degree of co-ocurrence of 5-HT and neuropeptides (as well as chromogranin) in the same cells. At last, it was shown again by immunohistochemistry, that most glomus cells in the mouse CB contain 5-HT, which coexist with NA and gamma amino butyric acid (GABA).[85] Unfortunately, ultrastructural studies are lacking on this subject. It must be added that 5-HT is the predominant amine in glomus cells of the chicken CB.[86,87]

Choline Acetyltransferase

In the absence of any method allowing to localize acetylcholine itself, Wang et al[88] demonstrated, with the light microscope, that most glomus cells are immunopositive for choline acetyltransferase in the cat and the rabbit. These observations are to be added to others which demonstrated the occurrence of acetylcholinesterase at the level of glomus cells[89] as well as to autoradiographic and biochemical data showing the presence of muscarinic and nicotinic receptors on glomus cells.[57,90-93] However, once again, there are species differences since muscarinic receptors seem to predominate in the rabbit whereas nicotinic receptors are more abundant in the cat[58] (see Fig. 3.1).

Localization of Dopamine Receptors

While first results were obtained by binding experiments (see Dinger et al[94] for example), here again, new results have been obtained thanks to a new method: hybridization in situ. This technique, which allows us to link molecular biology and morphology, is very promising. The first attempts were devoted to the localization of mRNA coding for dopamine receptors. This is very important to identify the actual targets of dopamine within the CB. The conclusion of these studies are the following: mRNA coding for dopamine D2 receptors (D2R) is present in the glomus cells.[75,95-97] Furthermore, petrosal neurons projecting to the CB also express the D2R gene.[95] It can be concluded therefore that dopamine, released by glomus cells could act on glomus cells themselves, via autoreceptors, and on postsynaptic receptors located on the chemoafferent nerve endings. In addition, Verna et al[97] showed that long-term treatment with haloperidol increases the D2R mRNA level, suggesting a regulation phenomenon. Furthermore, Gauda et al[75] showed that D2R mRNA expression increased with age in the developing rat CB [whereas the tyrosine hydroxylase (TH) mRNA level decreases]. Similar results were obtained by Bairam et al[98] in the developing rabbit. It seems therefore, that regulation of gene expression for TH and D2R differs during development.

These results are very important for the interpretation of pharmacological and physiological experiments using dopamine or dopamine agonists/antagonists on chemoafferent activity (see chapter 3).

INNERVATION OF THE CAROTID BODY

The carotid body is innervated essentially by sensory nerve fibers having their soma in the petrosal ganglion and by postganglionic sympathetic fibers coming from the superior cervical ganglion. In addition, some neurones of the autonomic nervous system are often present at the CB periphery.

I do not consider necessary to re-draw, once again, the history of the different steps which led to the actual picture since many reviews have reported these events in detail. However, before considering nerve ending ultrastructure, I would like to mention a paradox: although I am a convinced microscopist, I must confess that about ten years of research were lost....because of electron microscopy! Indeed, the sensory nature of glomus cell innervation was demonstrated by de Castro[99] as early as 1928 and there was no problem until the middle 1960s, that is, when electron micrographs showed synaptic-like vesicles within nerve endings in contact with glomus cells. In other words, synaptic vesicles were found on the unexpected side of the junctions! What was wrong, in fact? The interpretation, not the observations! The model of the synapse which was current, at that time, was the neuromuscular junction and this led some people to consider every nerve ending containing synaptic vesicles as a motor one. After ten years of controversy and new experiments, it was finally demonstrated that glomus cells are actually innervated by sensory nerve endings, containing....synaptic-like vesicles! To end with this historical anecdote, I would conclude that the truth is in the electron micrographs...but is sometimes obscured by the a priori we have in mind!

I mean...do not reject electron microscopy, but, eventually, the microscopist!

Origin, Structure and Targets of Nerve Fibers

The carotid body innervation has three possible sources: the carotid sinus nerve, the ganglioglomerular nerve and intrinsic neurons.

Two kinds of nerve fibers coexist in the sinus nerve, and were studied in a very detailed way by McDonald[100,101] in the rat CB. There are, in this species, 450 to 750 axons, among which 86% are unmyelinated fibers of small diameter (about 0.8 µm in mean diameter) whereas the others are myelinated fibers (median diameter: 2.5 µm). The vast majority of fibers degenerate after sinus nerve section between the CB and the petrosal ganglion, but remain intact after section of central roots of the ninth cranial nerve. These fibers are, therefore, sensory axons and either chemo- or baroafferents. Chemoafferent fibers end on glomus cells whereas baroafferent fibers end in the carotid sinus wall, although a few of them may innervate small arteries within the CB. Early studies demonstrated that chemoafferents are more numerous than baroafferents. It must be remarked that most of available electrophysiological data come from myelinated chemoafferent fibers, that constitute a minority! Since there are about 10^4 glomus cells in the rat CB, most of them being innervated, it is obvious that sensory axons ramify upon entering the CB. It can be said, to simplify, that chemoafferent fibers originate in the petrosal ganglion, but there are, in fact, species differences: most chemoafferent neurons are located in the petrosal ganglion both in the rat and cat, but some are present in the jugular ganglion in the rat[102] whereas a few may occur in the nodose ganglion in the cat.[103,104]

In a very interesting paper, Torrealba and Alcayaga[105] described, in the cat CB, two kinds of terminal arborizations which differ by their size: the largest arborizations

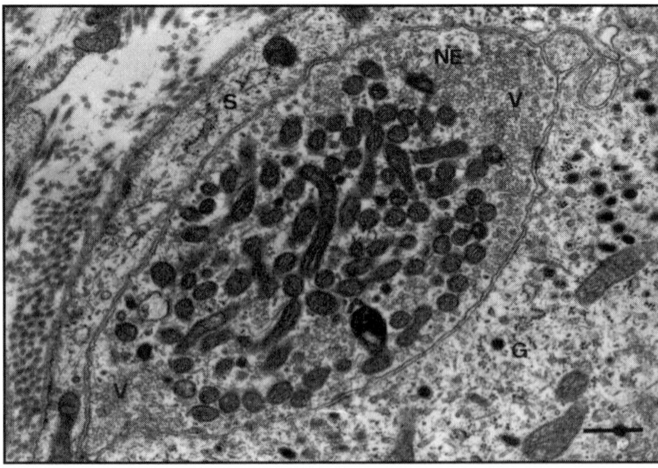

Fig. 1.8. Rabbit carotid body. A large nerve ending (NE) is in contact with a glomus cell (G). Note that the nerve ending contains numerous synaptic-like vesicles (V) dispersed in the axoplasm. The nerve ending also contains numerous mitochondria which differ from glomus cell mitochondria by their smaller size, darker matrix and longitudinally oriented cristae. S: Sustentacular cell. Bar: 0.5 µm.

consist of one or several clusters of polymorphous terminal swellings innervating 20 to 60 glomus cells. These arborizations probably arise from myelinated nerve fibers. The other type, called "sparsely branched axons," is less frequent and is characterized by a smaller domain (and concern less numerous glomus cells). The authors concluded as to the existence of two classes of sensory units, although they concede that intermediate forms also exist. If true, this distinction of two kinds of sensory units would have important functional implications.

The ganglioglomerular nerve links the superior cervical ganglion to the carotid body. It is made of very numerous unmyelinated nerve fibers (axons of sympathetic neurons) and a few myelinated ones (presumably preganglionic axons). Some postganglionic axons travel to the carotid body via the sinus nerve, at least in some species[106] (see Fig. 8.3). Postganglionic axons innervate blood vessels, but a notable proportion of noradrenergic varicosities are very close to glomus cell clusters and some of them are surrounded by sustentacular cells.[107] According to McDonald and Mitchell[35] a few preganglionic axons innervate some glomus cells.

Autonomic neurons may be present at the CB periphery. McDonald and Mitchell[35] identified two kinds of neurons in the rat: parasympathetic, receiving preganglionic fibers from the sinus nerve and sympathetic, innervated by preganglionic fibers from the ganglioglomerular nerve. It seems quite usual to find 10 to 20 neurons at the periphery of the rat CB whereas to find one in the rabbit CB is exceptional. It should be added that all along the carotid sinus nerve there are autonomic neurons which are positive for nitric oxide synthase and whose axons innervate blood vessels; these neurons appear to represent the elusive efferent pathway inhibiting chemosensory activity (see below; see also chapter 8).

Ultrastructure of Nerve Endings on Glomus Cells

The first ultrastructural studies showed nerve endings on glomus cells, as expected, but having very different sizes and shapes. The variability was so large that researchers quickly reported button-like, calyciform, "en passant" and basket-like endings. It was therefore tempting to ascribe different functions to these different morphological "types" of nerve endings. The occurrence of synaptic-like vesicles within some nerve profiles, but not all, substantiated a subdivision in "sensory" (devoid of vesicles) and "motor" (full of vesicles) nerve endings. In fact, the different aspects of nerve endings were due to their polymorphism, as demonstrated by favorable section planes showing different aspects along a same terminal[108] and by serial section reconstructions.[109-111]

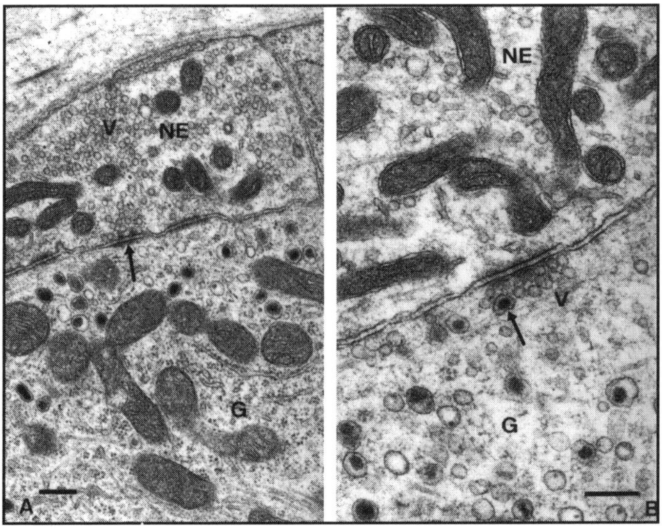

Fig. 1.9. Nerve ending-glomus cell junctions in the rabbit carotid body. (A) as in Fig. 1.8., the nerve ending (NE) contains numerous synaptic-like vesicles (V) but some of them are associated with an 'active zone' (arrow). Bar: 0.2 mm. (B) In this case, the nerve ending also contains some synaptic-like vesicles but they do not show any relationship with the nerve membrane. On the contrary, synaptic-like vesicles do not show any relationship with the nerve membrane. On the contrary, synaptic-like vesicles (V) (and a dense-core vesicle: arrow) are associated with an 'active zone' within the glomus cell (G). Bar: 0.2 μm.

The organelle content of nerve endings is well known: mitochondria, synaptic-like vesicles, some dense-cored vesicles, smooth reticulum, a few lysosomes and, eventually, glycogen particles. Neurotubules and neurofilaments may be present at preterminal levels but are usually absent in the endings. Mitochondria, with longitudinally oriented cristae, are generally smaller and show a darker matrix than glomus cell mitochondria (Fig. 1.8). These features, together with the absence of ribosomes, may help to distinguish nerve endings from glomus cell processes. Some nerve endings show impressive accumulations of mitochondria and/or glycogen particles,[108] but the functional significance of these accumulations is unknown (and not specific to the CB).

Dense-cored vesicles (around 90-100 nm in diameter) are occasionally present in nerve endings on glomus cells, but do not show any special relationships with membrane differentiations. Finally, the object of most investigations is a variable population of clear vesicles, about 60 nm in diameter. These vesicles may be dispersed within the ending (Fig. 1.8) or locally clustered, close to specialized zones of the membrane ("active zones") (Fig. 1.9A) or elsewhere in the neuroplasm. It was shown by McDonald,[4] in the rat, that ventilating the animal for 10 min with hypoxic or hypercapnic gas mixtures before fixation, decreased both the number and packing density of these clear vesicles in sensory nerve endings, whereas ventilation with 100% oxygen had the opposite effect. Furthermore, Morgan et al,[112] using cats, demonstrated that the effects of oxygen on vesicle concentration are dependent upon an intact sinus nerve. The authors claimed that these changes in the distribution of clear vesicles reflected transmitter release evoked by an "efferent" activity of sensory nerve fibers which develops in parallel with the chemoafferent activity (by an axon reflex mechanism, for example). Unfortunately, we do not know if clear vesicles really contain a neurotransmitter or something else. The morphological aspect and variations in number under the influence of nervous activity are insufficient, in my opinion, to conclude as to the release of a transmitter. Other mechanisms may be considered: for example, synaptic-like vesicles are supposed to control calcium homeostasis in neurosecretory terminals of the post-hypophysis.[113] I think we need new data such as the identification of the content of vesicles, by ultrastructural immunocytochemistry, for example.

According to McDonald and Mitchell,[35] the few sympathetic preganglionic axons which innervate some glomus cells in the rat, are characterized by closely packed clear vesicles which are slightly smaller than those in afferent endings and by more numerous dense-cored vesicles.

Structure of Junctions Between Nerve Terminals and Glomus Cells

Junctions between sensory nerve terminals and glomus cells look like chemical synapses between neurons, showing synaptic-like vesicles and membrane differentiations. However, a key-word must be added to the description: variability! Variability not only from species to species, but also from junction to junction in a given species. This variability affects the disposition of all components of the junctions (electron dense material, clear vesicles, dense-cored vesicles). In other words, it is possible to find dense projections (cone shaped dense material associated to the plasma membrane) on the glomus cell side, or on the nerve ending side, or both. It is possible to find clear vesicle accumulations on the glomus cell side, or the nerve ending side, or both (however, dense-cored vesicles may accumulate against the membrane in the glomus cell, but not in the nerve ending) (Fig. 1.9). This variability is quite confusing since the location of "membrane thickenings" (and more especially, dense projections) and clear vesicles is usually used to define the polarity of a chemical synapse!

This led many morphologists to distinguish synapses where the glomus cell is presynaptic, those where the glomus cell is postsynaptic and, of course, "reciprocal synapses," where dense projections and clear vesicles clusters are present on both sides! It must be added that the proportions of these different aspects vary from species to species; for example, junctions where the glomus cell is "presynaptic" are more frequent in the mouse CB than in the cat. The rabbit seems to be intermediate. Since all these animals have functional chemoreceptors, it could be said, (in a quite provocative way!)...that morphological variations are of little physiological significance!

I will not describe the junctions between glomus cells and nerve endings more extensively since very good descriptions may be found in previous reviews[3,25] and because there is nothing new, concerning their ultrastructure. However, I would like to make a comment: a chemical synapse is defined by its ultrastructure, and by a chemical transmitter which must satisfy well-known criteria: it should be present in the presynaptic compartment as well as the enzymes for its synthesis; inactivation processes (enzymatic or not) should operate in the synaptic region; the effects of the putative transmitter should mimic the effects of natural stimuli; substances which block synthesis, storage or release of the transmitter should block synaptic transmission; agents blocking the inactivation process should prolong transmitter action, etc. This list is "classical" and students must know it. Although this list may be considered obsolete in view of recent findings concerning corelease and cooperation of different transmitters, I wonder if it is possible to say that the existence of a chemical synapse between glomus cells and sensory nerve endings is really demonstrated! And what about the existence of a chemical synapse in the reverse direction? This problem will be considered in following chapters, but I would suggest the term "junction" rather than "synapse" to discuss the relationships between glomus cells and sensory nerve endings! Of course, I do not deny that glomus cells excite, in some way, sensory nerve endings; I am also ready to accept that sensory nerve endings exert some action on glomus cells, but the mechanisms may be quite different from those operating in "classical" synapses. The growing number of neuroactive substances discovered in glomus cells, as well as in sensory nerve fibers, suggest subtle interactions, which will be more difficult to understand than the effects of one neurotransmitter alone.

Furthermore, a temporal parameter must be introduced. Some neuroactive substances may act for a period of seconds, but others for minutes or hours. Trophic influences of nerve fibers on glomus cells were suggested by many authors and it is known that sections of the sinus nerve or of the sympathetic innervation modify the glomus cell metabolism.[47,114] Thus, I think that the relationships between glomus cells and sensory nerve fibers are probably more complex than previously expected.

Localization of Neurotransmitters in Sensory Nerve Fibers

As it is the case for glomus cells, new data in this area come mostly from immunocytochemistry. Most authors have focused particularly on the presence of neuropeptides.

Neuropeptides

Calcitonin-gene-related-peptide (CGRP)-immunoreactive nerve fibers were observed in the rat CB by Kondo and Yamamoto[115] who described these fibers as thin unmyelinated fibers coming mostly from the glossopharyngeal ganglia but also from vagal and spinal sensory ganglia. Most of these fibers were found in the interstitial spaces and only a few of them were observed in contact with glomus cells, although without membrane specializations. Interestingly, no CGRP-positive fibers were found in the CB of newborn rats: they first appear at postnatal day 3 and, thereafter, increased in number gradually. Since the CB is sensitive to blood gases at birth (and even before birth) Kondo and Yamamoto[115] suggested that CGRP-positive sensory fibers may subserve a special role or function in a way different from the typical sensory fibers which form specialized junctions with glomus cells. Finally, Kondo and Yamamoto[115] showed that section of one or two of the three possible sources of CGRP-positive fibers (glossopharyngeal nerve, vagal nerve or sympathetic trunk) induces a decrease in number of positive fibers for 2 days, followed by a progressive recovery up to control levels (after 4 weeks). The authors explained the recovery via proliferative sprouting from CGRP-containing fibers coming from the nonsevered nerves. The mechanism of this plasticity phenomenon is still unclear.

Torrealba and Correa[116] also described CGRP-immunoreactive unmyelinated axons in the cat CB. These axons were observed in the interstitial tissue sometimes very close to glomus cells, but never in contact with them. Using a sensitive immunocytochemical protocol at the ultrastructural level, the authors often observed reaction product in the extracellular space around labeled nerve endings and concluded that a "volume transmission" phenomenon takes place in the CB. Although such a phenomenon may actually occur in the CB as in other parts of the nervous system, a diffusion artefact of the reaction product cannot be ruled out.

Double-labeling experiments allowed Kummer[117] to demonstrate that substance P (SP) and CGRP coexist in nerve fibers of the guinea pig CB, as well as in sensory petrosal neurons retrogradely labeled from the carotid sinus nerve. With the electron microscope, Kummer et al[118] demonstrated that SP- and CGRP-reactive fibers were unmyelinated fibers of small diameter, containing dense-core vesicles positive for both antigens, suggesting costorage. Furthermore, these authors did not find "synaptic" contacts between SP/CGRP immunoreactive nerve fibers and glomus cells. They suggested these fibers to be a special class of chemoreceptor C-fibers or fibers having other functions such as polymodal nociception, local regulation of vascular tone and permeability or trophic functions.

Nerve fibers containing both SP and CGRP were also described in the human CB by Kummer and Habeck.[82] As in the guinea pig, these fibers are thin unmyelinated axons (0.1-1 mm) mostly located around glomus cells. Very few of them were found in contact with glomus cells, without junctional differentiations. Other CGRP-positive fibers were found around interlobular arteries. The authors concluded as to the existence of two different populations of SP/CGRP immunoreactive fibers: chemoafferent C-fibers and vascular sensory fibers.

An extensive study of the peptidergic innervation of the amphibian labyrinth (which corresponds to the mammalian CB and sinus) was undertaken by Kusakabe et al.[119] These authors reported the presence of nerve fibers containing almost all known neuropeptides. Interestingly, they noted that CGRP-positive fibers appear first during larval development, followed by SP fibers and then by VIP fibers. Coexistence of SP/CGRP was noted in many fibers and the authors even concluded with the possibility of coexistence of four different peptides in the same nerve fibers (SP, CGRP, VIP and NPY).

Nitric Oxide (NO)

The discovery of the neurotransmitter properties of the gas, NO, initiated many studies, concerning many organs, the CB included! Indeed, nitrergic structures have been found in the CB (I wonder if there exists any neuroactive substance which is not present in the CB!). Using the immunocytochemical detection of NO-synthase (NOS) or the histochemical detection of NADPH-diaphorase activity, Prabhakar et al,[120] Wang et al[121,122] and Tanaka and Chiba[123] observed a dense plexus of nitrergic nerve fibers in the rat, cat, and newborn guinea pig CB, respectively. Some of these fibers are axons from autonomic neurons in the CB and will be discussed later, but others are axons from sensory neurons located in the petrosal ganglion (or along the glossopharyngeal and sinus nerve) and are therefore of sensory nature. Hohler et al[124] also reported, again in the rat CB, NOS-containing fibers around arterial walls and (to a lesser extent) in the islands of glomus cells. These fibers persisted after carotid sinus nerve transection and were supposedly derived from intrinsic neurons.

According to Grimes et al[125] the NOS-positive innervation of the cat CB originates mainly from ganglion cells in and around the CB and from the glossopharyngeal nerve. The positive fibers were found around blood vessels and sometimes close to glomus cells. The authors concluded that the NOS-positive innervation of the cat CB is a parasympathetic autonomic supply, originating mainly from dispersed ganglion cells. In addition, some NOS-positive fibers were supposed to come from the superior cervical ganglion.

All these observations suggest that NO could have important vasomotor actions in the CB, and in addition, NO would act directly on glomus cells (or on glomus cell-sensory nerve ending complexes). This conclusion is in keeping with the physiological results of Wang et al,[122,126,127] and also with the immunocytochemical studies of the same authors[122] which showed that nitroglycerin (a NO donor) stimulates the formation of cGMP in both, glomus cells and blood vessels (see chapter 8 by Almaraz et al). It must be added, however, that a recent pharmacological study by Gozal et al[128] concluded that endothelial NOS provides the major source for NO within the CB and exerts a down regulatory effect upon chemoafferent activity.

It would be interesting to have more details on the relationship between NOS-positive nerve fibers and glomus cells, but ultrastructural data are still lacking.

Neurotransmitters in Petrosal Neurons

The neurochemical features of the chemoafferent pathway may be studied at one end (near glomus cells), or at the other, that is at the level of perikarya. Since most chemoafferent fibers come from neurons located in the petrosal ganglion, many authors have studied the distribution of neurotransmitters or neurotransmitter-related substances, in petrosal neurons.

Katz et al[129] were among the first to undertake this kind of study. They demonstrated that sensory neurons in the rat petrosal ganglion express catalytically active TH and exhibit catecholamine fluorescence. Some years later, Katz and Black[130] using retrograde labeling, showed that most of TH-immunoreactive neurons innervate the CB. Furthermore, these authors demonstrated that section of the carotid sinus nerve (or colchicine blockade) resulted in a marked and transient decrease in TH activity and immunoreactivity within a week. It was concluded that catecholaminergic characteristics expressed by sensory neurons which innervate the CB are regulated by mechanisms involving axonal transport. In a more recent study, Katz and Erb[131] showed that expression of TH immunoreactivity of petrosal neurons during embryological development is coincident with the innervation of glomus cells, and suggested that neuron-target interactions regulate the biochemical differentiation of petrosal neurons.

Following these studies on the rat petrosal ganglion, Kummer et al[106] investigated the guinea-pig sensory ganglia. They detected numerous TH-immunoreactive neurons in the petrosal/jugular ganglion and identified the CB as a target of these neurons. Double labeling experiments revealed that most TH-positive neurons were also immunoreactive for somatostatin but not for CGRP or SP. However, TH-positive neurons were neither immunoreactive for DOPA-decarboxylase or DbH, nor for dopamine or DOPA. They did not display glyoxylic acid-induced fluorescence. Kummer et al[106] concluded that, in the guinea-pig, TH-immunoreactive neurons do not synthesize dopamine. There is, therefore, a discrepancy between Katz and Black[130] working on the rat and Kummer et al[106] working on the guinea-pig. It is, of course, difficult to know if this discrepancy is due to methodological factors or to a species difference but, as usual in the CB world, there are also discrepancies between teams using the same animal model!

Finley et al[132] used retrograde labeling with fluorogold and immunocytochemistry to characterize sensory neurons which innervate the rat CB. They found that about 41% of these neurons express tyrosine hydroxylase. On the other hand, 7% of CB sensory neurons contained substance P. Furthermore, these two kinds of neurons differed by their size and location (15-20 μm and caudal part of the petrosal ganglion for TH-positive neurons; 20-30 μm and jugular ganglion/central part of the petrosal ganglion for SP-positive ones). An ultrastructural study showed that peripheral processes of TH-positive neurons were unmyelinated fibers forming endings apposed to glomus cells and containing clear and dense-cored vesicles. Membrane differentiations were not observed. Finley et al[132] concluded as to the existence of distinct subsets of chemoafferent neurons: catecholaminergic and peptidergic. Since 86% of TH-positive neurons were positive to DOPA-decarboxylase and negative to DβH, these authors suggested that these neurons are dopaminergic and constitute a morphologic substrate for the long debated "dopaminergic efferent inhibition" of chemoafferent activity. This conclusion is therefore in keeping with that of Katz et al.[129] Unfortunately, quite different results were obtained by another team: Ichikawa et al[133] also studied sensory neurons in the rat petrosal ganglion after immunocytochemistry and retrograde labeling with fluorogold (however, fluorogold was applied to the central cut end of the sinus nerve, a procedure which does not allow one to differentiate baro- from chemoafferents). Only 4% of fluorogold-labeled neurons were found to be immunopositive for TH (versus 41% for Finley et al[132]) and were located in the caudal part of the petrosal ganglion. The other neurons showed immunoreactivity for VIP (less than 1%), CGRP (25%), SP (17%) or galanin (43%). Many fluorogold-labeled petrosal neurons were positive for both CGRP and SP while some were positive for only one of these antigens.

More recently, Finley et al[134] demonstrated that in normal rats 3% of TH-containing petrosal neurons coexpress galanin but found that galanin expression was increased following fluorogold injection into the CB. There is, therefore, a phenotypic plasticity phenomenon which may explain, at least in part, some contradictory results reported in the literature (see chapter 9 by Katz et al).

In conclusion, the presence of TH-positive chemoafferent neurons in the rat petrosal ganglion may be considered demonstrated (and was recently confirmed by Massari et al),[135] but the numerical importance of these neurons remains to be established and, more importantly, the ability of these TH-positive neurons to synthesize dopamine remains controversial (but see Fig. 8.3).

The same kind of study was undertaken, also in the rat, by Okada and Miura,[136] using retrograde labeling with horseradish peroxidase (HRP) to identify neurons projecting in the carotid sinus nerve, and immunocytochemistry to localize glutamate (Glu), aspartate (Asp) and SP. Most of HRP-labeled neurons were positive for Glu and/or Asp. Since no significant difference was found in the diameter of these cells (around 25 mm), these authors suggested that Glu and Asp may coexist in the same neurons. A minority of neurons were positive for SP but were slightly larger (around 27 mm). Okada and Miura[136] speculated that Glu- and Asp-containing neurons were baroreceptors, while those containing SP were chemoreceptors.

Finally, NOS-positive (and/or NADPH diaphorase positive) neurons were observed by Wang et al[121,122] in the rat and cat petrosal ganglion. These neurons, of relatively small size (15-30 mm), are localized predominantly in the proximal (cranial) part of the petrosal ganglion. Colocalization studies showed that NOS-positive neurons were devoid of TH-immunoreactivity but were positive for SP. Wang et al[121,122] concluded from their morphological data and from physiological observations that NO released from sensory nerve endings could act in a retrograde fashion to interact with glomus cells. This mechanism (in addition to the effects of NO released by autonomic structures; see below) would explain the inhibitory role of NO on chemoreceptor activity reported by Prabhakar et al[120] and Wang et al.[122]

Autonomic Innervation

Although less studied than the sensory innervation, the autonomic nerve supply of the CB is important, morphologically and functionally. At first sight, it can be said, as already mentioned, that the CB is innervated by sympathetic neurons located in the superior cervical ganglion (SCG) which send their noradrenergic axons via the ganglioglomerular nerve (s) to innervate blood vessels. In fact, things are somewhat more complicated.

Autonomic Nerve Fibers

From a morphological point of view, the abundance of noradrenergic axons within the CB was clearly demonstrated via the use of the Falck-Hillarp method (formol-induced fluorescence). This method showed very numerous fluorescent varicose fibers all around CB blood vessels and cell clusters, which disappeared after removal of the SCG.[44] More recently, Claps and Torrealba[104] used a retrograde tracing method (in the rat) and found, after administration of the tracer in the CB, 3000 to 5000 labeled neurons in the ipsilateral SCG. In other words, efferent sympathetic neurons which project to the CB are much more numerous than sensory petrosal neurons which innervate glomus cells!

As indicated above, the vast majority of sympathetic axons reach the CB by the ganglioglomerular nerve(s), but it must be added that others travel through the carotid sinus nerve. Furthermore, among the latter, some go toward the CB and a few toward the petrosal ganglion, at least in the guinea-pig.[106]

The ultrastructure of postganglionic sympathetic axons is well known: they are unmyelinated fibers, more or less ensheathed by Schwann cells and characterized by varicosities containing mitochondria, large dense-core vesicles and small vesicles, either clear or containing a dense granule.[35,107] The presence of small (50-60 nm) granular vesicles is a sufficient index to identify a nerve profile as a noradrenergic one. Other methods allow one to demonstrate noradrenergic varicosities: chromaffin reaction (or variants for electron microscopy), autoradiography after tritiated noradrenaline administration, noradrenaline immunocytochemistry. Using some of these methods, I have confirmed, with the electron microscope, that noradrenergic axons are very numerous near blood vessels. On this subject, the number of noradrenergic varicosities which are close to capillaries is surprising. Usually, sympathetic axons innervate smooth muscle cells around arteries, not capillaries which are devoid of smooth muscle cells. If the function of the CB sympathetic supply is to control total blood flow, a few axons around arteries entering the organ would be sufficient. Why such a profuse sympathetic innervation of capillaries in the CB? To control local flow? This is a possibility but one may wonder why the nerve supply is not restricted to the arterio-venous shunts! However, if arterio-venous shunts play a minor role, local flow may be adjusted at the level of glomus cell clusters by the control of capillary diameters. It must be remarked that CB capillaries are characterized by an extensive layer of pericytes, which are considered as contractile cells. However, it remains to establish that pericytes contract effectively in response to sympathetic excitation. Other possibilities may be mentioned. I considered, above, short-term adjustments, but long-term effects are also possible. Does the vascular nerve supply of the CB play a role in the well known hypertrophy of blood vessels induced by long-term hypoxia? It may be recalled that Kondo et al[137] showed that CB postganglionic sympathetic axons contain NPY, a neuropeptide known to have mitogenic effects on vascular smooth muscle cells, in synergy with noradrenaline and ATP.[138]

Noradrenergic varicosities are numerous not only around blood vessels but also around glomus cells. In the rabbit CB, I showed[107] that about one third of noradrenergic varicosities are nearer to a glomus cell cluster than to a blood vessel (in a given plane of section) (Fig. 1.10). The mean distance between noradrenergic varicosities and cell clusters is about 2.7 μm, which compares with the mean distance between noradrenergic varicosities and blood vessels (2.2 μm). A direct action of sympathetic axons on glomus cells (or on sensory nerve endings, or both) is therefore morphologically possible. A consequence of this morphological relationship can be deduced: noradrenergic varicosities certainly participate in the inactivation of catecholamines released by glomus cells. It is well known that noradrenergic axons take up NA, DA and DOPA from their environment and I used this phenomenon to localize, autoradiographically, noradrenergic fibers within the rabbit CB.[44,107] It is obvious, therefore, that DA and/or NA released by glomus cells may be partly inactivated by uptake in sympathetic varicosities. This possibility must be taken into account by researchers studying catecholamine release from glomus cells, in vitro, for example: using CB containing an intact sympathetic innervation may lead to an underestimation of the amount of catecholamine actually released.

Parasympathetic (cholinergic) fibers are also present within the CB, but data on this subject are relatively few, probably because methods to identify cholinergic fibers are less numerous than methods showing catecholaminergic fibers. Using indirect evidence (presence of small clear synaptic vesicles) and denervation experiments, McDonald and Mitchell[35] identified parasympathetic nerve endings around blood vessels, in the rat CB. However, the exact destination of these fibers (arteries, capillaries, veins, arterio-venous shunts?) was not established. According to the same authors there are other cholinergic autonomic fibers in the CB, namely preganglionic sympathetic axons which end on intrinsic sympathetic neurons or directly on a few glomus cells. Such fibers could modulate the DA turnover during long-term hypoxia.[139]

Recent studies showed that the cat and rat CB contains nerve fibers which are able to synthesize NO.[120,122,126] Among these

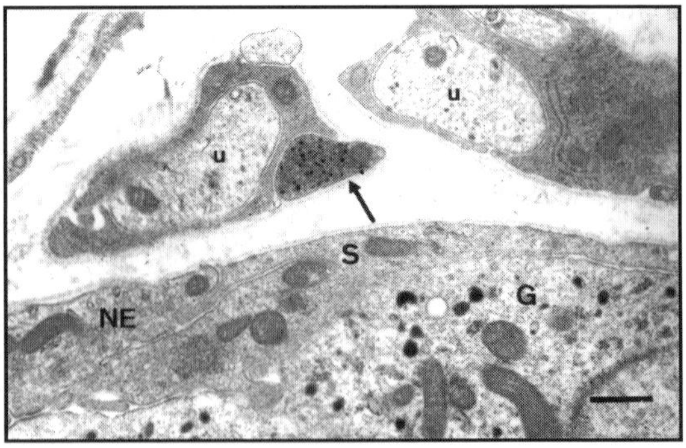

Fig. 1.10. Rabbit carotid body prepared with a variant of the chromaffin reaction to demonstrate noradrenergic structures. A sympathetic varicosity, containing chromaffin vesicles (arrow) is located close to a glomus cell cluster. G: glomus cell; S: sustentacular cell; NE; nerve ending (containing unlabeled synaptic-like vesicles), U: Unidentified nerve fibers. Bar: 0.5 μm.

fibers, some, as described above, are sensory axons from neurons located in the petrosal ganglion and do not belong to the autonomic innervation. However, other nitrergic fibers are axons from autonomic neurons located at the CB periphery or in the sinus nerve and glossopharyngeal nerve (see next section) and innervate both small and large arterial vessels, suggesting vasomotor influences. In other words, the autonomic innervation of the CB, introduced in a simple way at the beginning of this chapter, has recently gained a further degree of complexity.

Autonomic Neurons

Autonomic neurons are often present at the CB periphery, but, once again, their frequency seems to vary from species to species. Thus, although rare, they are usual in the cat and rat CB (1 to 8 neurons per rat CB according to Hess)[140] whereas they are exceptional in the rabbit CB. The ultrastructure of CB autonomic neurons was illustrated by McDonald and Mitchell[35] in the rat. These authors suggested that most of autonomic neurons are parasympathetic ones, innervated by preganglionic axons which travel in the glossopharyngeal nerve. The other neurons are of sympathetic nature and are innervated by preganglionic axons from the sympathetic trunk. It is generally admitted that CB autonomic neurons innervate blood vessels. In fact, these neurons, already observed by de Castro[141] have received little further attention. Recently, however, a special subclass of autonomic neurons was discovered in the CB: nitrergic neurons (Fig. 1.11). Wang et al,[121,122] looking at possible sources of NO in the CB, found NO-synthase immunopositive (and NADPH-diaphorase positive) neurons in the rat and cat CB. These neurons are relatively large (around 30 μm), show short dendrites and send varicose axons which contact blood vessels (mostly arterioles) into the central portions of the CB. Some of these neurons are located, in fact, in the sinus nerve and, preferentially, near the sinus nerve-glossopharyngeal nerve branch-point.[122] Colocalization studies[121] showed that NO-synthase and choline-acetyltransferase co-occur in the same neurons which were identified as parasympathetic ones. Thus, autonomic neurons in the CB may use NO, in addition to "classical" neurotransmitters, to regulate blood flow or other parameters (see chapter 8).

CONCLUSIONS

If we consider the results of the last ten years, it is clear that most of new data were obtained by immunocytochemistry. Thanks to this methodology, we have, now, an impressive list of neuroactive substances which are present somewhere in the CB. Do we have a better understanding of the CB physiology? I am not sure the answer is yes! It is quite funny to read the conclusions of papers reporting the occurrence of this or that neuropeptide in the CB: they all conclude "...this peptide could have a modulatory role on chemosensory activity"! But, finally, we have more "modulators" than actors! In fact, two keystones are still missing: the transduction mechanism, and the mechanism of excitation of sensory nerve endings. The morphological study alone cannot solve these problems and I think that a multidisciplinary approach is necessary. Recent studies based on new techniques such as in situ hybridization, appear promising. On this point, I hope that young people with a good formation in biochemistry and molecular biology will study arterial chemoreceptors with new eyes, and join the pieces of the puzzle...with the help of morphologists!

Acknowledgments

The author is deeply indebted to Mrs. C. Salat and Dr. T. Durkin for kind help.

References

1. Habeck J-O. A comparison of the blood supply of the carotid body in rats and rabbits. Anat Anz (Jena) 1987; 164: 313-322.
2. Adams WE. The Comparative Morphology of the Carotid Body and Carotid Sinus. Springfield:Thomas, 1958:272.
3. Verna A. Ultrastructure of the carotid body in the mammals. Int Rev Cytol 1979; 60:271-330.
4. McDonald D. Peripheral chemoreceptors. Structure-function relationships of the carotid body. In:Hornbein TF, ed. Regulation of Breathing, part 1. New York: Dekker, 1981:105-319.
5. Eyzaguirre C, Zapata P. Perspectives in carotid body research. J Appl Physiol 1984; 57:931-957.
6. González C, Almaraz L, Obeso A et al. Carotid body chemoreceptors:from natural stimuli to sensory discharges. Physiol Rev 1994; 74:829-898.
7. Seidl E, Schäefer D, Zierold K et al. Light-microscopic and electron-microscopic studies on the morphology of cat carotid body. In:Acker H, Fidone S, Pallot D et al, eds. Chemoreception in the Carotid Body. Berlin: Springer, 1977: 1-6.
8. Dhillon DP, Barer GR, Walsh M. The enlarged carotid body of the chronically hypoxic and chronically hypoxic and hypercapnic rat:a morphometric analysis. Q J Exp Physiol 1984; 69:301-317.
9. Clarke JA, de Burgh Daly M, Ead HW. Comparison of the size of the vascular compartment of the carotid body of the fetal, neonatal and adult cat. Acta Anat 1990; 138:166-174.
10. Daly M de B, Lambertsen CJ, Schweitzer A. Observations on the volume of blood flow and oxygen utilization of the carotid body in the cat. J Physiol (Lond.)1954; 125:67-89.
11. McDonald DM, Larue DT. The ultrastructure and connections of blood vessels supplying the rat carotid body and carotid sinus. J Neurocytol 1983; 12:117-153.
12. McDonald D. A morphometric analysis of blood vessels and perivascular nerves in the rat carotid body. J Neurocytol 1983; 12:155-199.
13. de Castro F. Nuevas observaciones sobre la inervacion de la region carotidea. Los quimio y pressoreceptores. Trab Lab Invest Biol Univ Madrid 1940; 32:297-384.
14. de Castro F, Rubio M. The anatomy and innervation of the blood vessels of the carotid body and the role of chemoreceptive reactions in the autoregulation of the blood flow. In: Torrance RW, ed. Arterial Chemoreceptors. Oxford: Blackwell 1968:267-277.
15. McDonald DM, Haskell A. Morphology of connections between arterioles and capillaries in the rat carotid body analyzed by reconstructing serial sections. In:Pallot DJ, ed. The Peripheral Arterial Chemoreceptors. London: Croom Helm, 1984:195-206.
16. Acker H, O'Regan RG. The effects of stimulation of autonomic nerves on carotid body blood flow in the cat. J Physiol 1981; 315:99-110.
17. Hilsmann J, Degner F, Acker H. Local flow velocities in the cat carotid body tissue. Pflügers Arch 1987; 410: 204-211.
18. Pequignot J-M, Hellström S. Intact and sympathectomized carotid bodies of long-term hypoxic rats. A morphometric light microscopical study. Virchows Arch (Pathol Anat) 1983; 400:235-243.
19. Scheibner T, Read DJC, Sullivan CE. Distribution of substance P-immunoreactive structures in the developing cat carotid body. Brain Res 1988; 453:72-78.
20. Pallot DJ. Relationship between ultrastructure and function in peripheral arterial chemoreceptors. In: Acker H, O'Regan RG, eds. Physiology of the Peripheral Arterial Chemoreceptors. Amsterdam: Elsevier, 1983:1-19.

21. Kondo H, Yamamoto M. Multi-unit compartmentation of the carotid body chemoreceptor by perineurial cell sheaths: immunohistochemistry and freeze-fracture study. Adv Exp Med Biol 1993; 337:61-66.
22. Abramovici A, Pallot DJ. An immunohistochemical approach to the study of the cat carotid body. Acta Anat 1990; 140:70-14.
22a. Kondo H, Iwanaga T, Nakajima T. Immunocytochemical study on the localization of neuron-specific enolase and S-100 protein in the carotid body of rats. Cell Tissue Res 1982; 227:291-295.
23. Pallot D, Seker M, Abramovici A. Postmortem changes in the normal rat carotid body: possible implications for human histopathology. Virchows Archiv. A Pathol Anat 1992; 420:31-35.
24. Woods RI. Penetration of horseradish peroxidase between all elements of the carotid body. In:Purves MJ, ed. The Peripheral Arterial Chemoreceptors. London: Cambridge University Press, 1975: 195-203.
25. McDonald D. Structure and function of reciprocal synapses interconnecting glomus cells and sensory nerve terminals in the rat carotid body. In: Coupland RE, Fujita T, eds. Chromaffin, Enterochromaffin and Related Cells. New York: Elsevier/North-Holland, 1976:375-394.
26. Baron M, Eyzaguirre C. Effects of temperature on some membrane characteristics of carotid body cells. Am J Physiol 1977; 233(Cell Physiol 2):C35-C46.
27. Abudara V, Eyzaguirre C. Electrical coupling between cultured glomus cells of the rat carotid body:observations with current and voltage clamping. Brain Res 1994; 664:257-265.
28. Eyzaguirre C, Abundara V. Possible role of coupling between glomus cells in carotid body chemoreception. Biol Signals 1995; 4:263-270.
29. Abudara V, Eyzaguirre C. Effects of calcium on the electric coupling of carotid body glomus cells. Brain Res 1996; 725: 125-131.
30. Eyzaguirre C, Abundara V. Reflections on the carotid nerve sensory discharge and coupling between glomus cells. Adv Exp Med Biol 1996; 41:159-168.
31. Monti-Bloch L, Eyzaguirre C. Effects of different stimuli and transmitters on glomus cell membranes and intercellular communications. In: Eyzaguirre C et al, eds. Arterial Chemoreception. New York: Springer-Verlag, 1990:157-167.
32. Kondo H, Iwasa H. Re-examination of the carotid body ultrastructure with special attention to intercellular membrane appositions. Adv Exp Med Biol 1996; 410:45-50.
33. Hansen JT. Morphological aspects of secretion in the glomus cell paraneurons of the carotid body:evidence for calcium-dependent exocytosis. Cytobios 1981; 32:79-88.
34. Grönblad M. Improved demonstration of exocytotic profiles in glomus cells of rat carotid body after perfusion with glutaraldehyde fixative containing a high concentration of potassium. Cell Tiss Res 1983; 229:627-637.
35. McDonald DM, Mitchell RA. The innervation of glomus cells, ganglion cells and blood vessels in the rat carotid body:a quantitative ultrastructural study. J Neurocytol 1975; 4:177-230.
36. Hellström S. Morphometric studies of dense-cored vesicles in type I cells of the rat carotid body. J Neurocytol 1975; 4:77-86.
37. Pequignot J-M, Hellström S, Johansson C. Intact and sympathectomized carotid bodies of long-term hypoxic rats:a morphometric ultrastructural study. J Neurocytol 1984; 13:481-493.
38. Kusakabe T, Powell FL, Ellisaman MH. Ultrastructure of the glomus cells in the carotid body of chronically hypoxic rats:with special reference to the similarity of amphibian glomus cells. Anat Record 1993; 237:220-227.
39. Morita E, Chiocchio SR, Tramezzani JH. Four types of main cells in the carotid body of the cat. J Ultrastruct Res 1969; 28:399-410.
40. Verna A. Dense-cored vesicles and cell types in the rabbit carotid body. In: Acker H, Fidone S, Pallot D et al, eds. Chemoreception in the carotid body. Berlin: Springer Verlag, 1977:216-220.
41. Xu GP, Ling YP, Zhong CS et al. Subtypes of type I cells and dense-cored

vesicles in the rabbit carotid body. Chin J Physiol Sci 1992; 8:234-241.
42. Xu GP, Ling YP, Zhong CS et al. Cytochemical demonstration of sub-types of type I cells in the rabbit carotid body chemoreceptor. Acta Histochem Cytochem 1994; 27:51-55.
43. Laidler P, Kay JM. A quantitative study of some ultrastructural features of the type I cells in the carotid bodies of rats living at a simulated altitude of 4300 meters. J Neurocytol 1978; 7:183-192.
44. Verna A. Observations on the innervation of the carotid body of the rabbit. In:Purves MJ, ed. The Peripheral Arterial Chemoreceptors. London: Cambridge University Press, 1975:75-99.
45. Schamel A, Verna A. Norepinephrine-containing glomus cells in the rabbit carotid body. I. Autoradiographic and morphometric study after tritiated norepinephrine uptake. J Neurocytol 1992; 21:341-352.
46. Schamel A, Verna A. Norepinephrine-containing glomus cells in the rabbit carotid body. II. Immunocytochemical evidence of dopamine-°-hydroxylase and norepinephrine. J Neurocytol 1992; 21: 353-362.
47. Pequignot J-M, Cottet-Emard JM, Dalmaz Y et al. Dopamine and norepinephrine dynamics in rat carotid body during long-term hypoxia. J Auton Nerv Syst 1987; 21:9-14.
48. Verna A, Schamel A, Pequignot J-M. Noradrenergic glomus cells in the rabbit carotid body:an autoradiographic and immunocytochemical study in the rabbit and rat. Adv Exp Med Biol 1993; 337:93-100.
49. Verna A, Schamel A, Pequignot J-M. Long-term hypoxia increases the number of norepinephrine-containing glomus cells in the rat carotid body: a correlative immunocytochemical and biochemical study. J Autonom Nerv Syst 1993; 44:171-177.
50. Bee D, Pallot DJ, Barer GR. Division of type I and endothelial cells in the hypoxic rat carotid body. Acta Anat 1986; 126:226-229.
51. Bee D, Pallot DJ. Acute hypoxic ventilation, carotid body cell division and dopamine content during early hypoxia in rats. J Appl Physiol 1995; 79: 1504-1511.
52. Chen IL, Hansen JT, Yates RD. Dopamine °-hydroxylase-like immunoreactivity in the rat and cat carotid body:a light and electron microscopic study. J Neurocytol 1985; 14:131-144.
53. Armengaud C, Leitner LM, Malber CH et al. Comparison of the monoamine and catabolite content in the cat and rabbit carotid bodies. Neurosci Lett 1988; 89: 153-157.
54. Wang Z-Z, Stensaas LJ, Dinger et al. Coexistence of tyrosine hydroxylase and dopamine β-hydroxylase immunoreactivity in glomus cells of the cat carotid body. J Autonom Nerv Syst 1991; 32: 259-264.
55. Heath D, Smith P. The Pathology of the Carotid Body and Sinus. London: Arnold, 1985:1-126.
56. Kobayashi S. Fine structure of the carotid body of the dog. Arch Histol Japn 1968; 30:95-120.
57. Chen IL, Yates RD. Two types of glomus cells in the rat carotid body as revealed by alpha-bungarotoxin binding. J Neurocytol 1984; 13:281-302.
58. Hirano T, Dinger B, Yoshizaki K et al. Nicotinic versus muscarinic binding sites in cat and rabbit carotid bodies. Biol Signals 1992; 1:143-149.
59. Pérez-García MT, Obeso A, López-López JR et al. Characterization of cultured chemoreceptor cells dissociated from adult rabbit carotid body. Amer J Physiol 1992; 263:C2-C1159.
60. Lundberg JM, Hökfelt T, Fahrenkrug J et al. Peptides in the cat carotid body (glomus caroticum):VIP-, enkephalin-, and substance P-like immunoreactivity. Acta Physiol Scand 1979; 107:279-281.
61. Wharton J, Polak JM, Pearse AGE et al. Enkephalin- VIP- and substance P-like immunoreactivity in the carotid body. Nature 1980; 284:269-271.
62. Varndell IM, Tapia FJ, De Mey J et al. Electron immunocytochemical localization of enkephalin-like material in catecholamine-containing cells of the carotid body, the adrenal medulla and in pheochromocytomas of man and other

mammals. J Histochem Cytochem 1982; 30:682-690.
63. Kobayashi S, Uchida T, Ohashi T et al. Immunocytochemical demonstration of the costorage of noradrenaline with met-enkephalin-arg6-phe7 and met-enkephalin-arg6-gly7-leu8 in the carotid body chief cells of the dog. Arch Histol Jap 1983; 46:713-722.
64. Kobayashi S, Uchida T, Ohashi T et al. Met-enkephalin-arg-gly-leu-like immunoreactivity in adrenal chromaffin cells and carotid body chief cells of the dog and monkey. Biomed Res 1983; 4: 201-210.
65. Smith P, Gosney J, Heath D et al. The occurrence and distribution of certain polypeptides within the human carotid body. Cell Tissue Res 1990; 261:565-571.
66. González-Guerrero PR, Rigual R, González C. Opioid peptides in the rabbit carotid body:identification and evidence for coutilization and interactions with dopamine. J Neurochem 1993; 60:1762-1768.
67. Heym C, Kummer W. Regulatory peptides in paraganglia. Prog Histochem Cytochem 1988; 18:1-95.
68. Heym C, Kummer W. Immunohistochemical distribution and colocalization of regulatory peptides in the carotid body. J Electron Microsc Tech 1989; 12:331-342.
69. Oomori Y, Ishikawa K, Satoh Y et al. Neuropeptide-Y-immunoreactive chief cells in the carotid body of young rats. Acta Anat 1991; 140:120-123.
70. Cuello AC, McQueen DS. Substance P: a carotid body peptide. Neurosci Lett 1980; 17:215-219.
71. Chen IL, Yates RD, Hansen JT. Substance P-like immunoreactivity in rat and cat carotid bodies:light and electron microscopic studies. Histol Histopath 1986; 1:203-212.
72. Prabhakar NR, Landis SC, Kumar et al. Substance P and neurokinin A in the cat carotid body: localization, exogenous effects and changes in content in response to arterial PO_2. Brain Res 1989; 481: 205-214.
73. Wang Z-Z, Stensaas LJ, Dinger et al. The coexistence of biogenic amines and neuropeptides in the type I cells of the cat carotid body. Neuroscience 1992; 47: 473-780.
74. Kusakabe T, Kawakami T, Tanabe Y et al. Distribution of substance P-containing and catecholaminergic nerve fibers in the rabbit carotid body: an immunohistochemical study in combination with catecholamine fluorescent histochemistry. Arch Histol Cytol 1994; 57:193-199.
75. Gauda EB, Bamford O, Gerfen CR. Developmental expression of tyrosine hydroxylase, D-2 dopamine receptor and substance P genes in the carotid body of the rat. Neuroscience 1996; 75:969-977.
76. Wang Z-Z, Stensaas LJ, Dinger et al. Localization and in vitro actions of atrial natriuretic peptide in the cat carotid body. J Appl Physiol 1991; 70:942-946.
77. Wang Z-Z, Stensaas LJ, Wang WJ et al. Atrial natriuretic peptide increases cyclic guanosine monophosphate immunoreactivity in the carotid body. Neuroscience 1992; 49:479-486.
78. Fried G, Meister B, Wikstrom et al. Galanin-, neuropeptide Y-, and enkephalin-like immunoreactivities in catecholamine-storing paraganglia of the fetal guinea pig and newborn pig. Cell Tissue Res 1989; 255:495-504.
79. Ichikawa H, Helke CJ. Distribution, origin and plasticity of galanin-immunoreactivity in the rat carotid body. Neuroscience 1993; 52:757-767.
80. Wang YY, Perrin DG, Cutz E. Localization of cholecystokinin-like and calcitonin-like peptides in infant carotid bodies: a light and electron-microscopic immunohistochemical study. Cell Tissue Res 1993a; 272:169-174.
81. Wang YY, Cutz E, Perrin DG. Detection of calcitonin gene expression in human infant and monkey carotid body chief cells by in situ hybridization. Cell Tiss Res 1994; 276:399-402.
82. Kummer W, Habeck J-O. Substance P- and calcitonin gene-related peptide-like immunoreactivities in the human carotid body studied at light and electron microscopical level. Brain Res 1991; 554: 286-292.
83. Perrin DG, Chan W, Cutz E et al. Serotonin in the human infant carotid body. Experientia 1986; 42:562-563.

84. Habeck J-O, Pallot DJ, Kummer W. Serotonin immunoreactivity in the carotid body of adult humans. Histol Histopath 1994; 9:227-232.
85. Oomori Y, Nakaya K, Tanaka H et al. Immunohistochemical and histochemical evidence for the presence of noradrenalin, serotonin and gamma amino butyric acid in chief cells of the mouse carotid body. Cell Tiss Res 1994; 278:249-254.
86. Le Douarin N, Le Lièvre C and Fontaine J. Recherches experimentales sur l'origine embryologique du corps carotidien chez les oiseaux. C R Acad Sci (D) Paris 1972; 275:583-586.
87. Kameda Y, Amano T, Tagawa T. Distribution and ontogeny of chromogranin A and tyrosine hydroxylase in the carotid body and glomus cells located in the wall of the common carotid artery and its branches in the chicken. Histochem 1990; 94:609-616.
88. Wang Z-Z, Stensaas LJ, Dinger et al. Immunocytochemical localization of choline acetyltransferase in the carotid body of the cat and rabbit. Brain Res 1989; 498:131-134.
89. Nurse CA. Localization of acetylcholinesterase in dissociated cell cultures of the carotid body of the rat. Cell Tiss Res 1987; 250:21-27.
90. Dinger B, González C, Yoshizaki K et al. Alpha-bungarotoxin binding in cat carotid body. Brain Res 1981; 205:187-193.
91. Dinger BG, Hirano T, Fidone SJ. Autoradiographic localization of muscarinic receptors in rabbit carotid body. Brain Res 1986; 367:328-331.
92. Dinger BG, Almaraz L, Hirano T et al. Muscarinic receptor localization and function in rabbit carotid body. Brain Res 1991; 562:190-198.
93. Chen IL, Mascorro JA, Yates RD. Autoradiographic localization of alpha-bungarotoxin-binding sites in the carotid body of the rat. Cell Tiss Res 1981; 219:609-618.
94. Dinger B, González C, Yoshizaki K et al. [3H] Spiroperidol binding in normal and denervated carotid bodies. Neurosci Lett 1981; 21:51-55.
95. Czyzyk-Krzeska MF, Lawson EE, Millhorn DE. Expression of D2 dopamine receptor mRNA in the arterial chemoreceptor afferent pathway. J Auton Nerv Syst 1992; 41:31-40.
96. Schamel A, Verna A. Localization of dopamine receptor mRNA in the rabbit carotid body and petrosal ganglion by in situ hybridization. Adv Exp Med Biol 1993; 337:85-92.
97. Verna A, Schamel A, Le Moine C et al. Localization of dopamine D2 R mRNA in glomus cells of the rabbit carotid body by in situ hybridization. J Neurocytol 1995; 24:265-270.
98. Bairam A, Dauphin C, Rousseau F et al. Expression of dopamine D-2 receptors mRNA isoforms at the peripheral chemoreflex afferent pathway in developing rabbits. Am J Resp Cell Mol Biol 1996; 15:374-381.
99. de Castro F. Sur la structure et l'innervation du sinus carotidien de l'homme et des mammifères. Nouveaux faits sur l'innervation et la fonction du glomus caroticum. Trab Lab Invest Biol Univ Madrid 1928; 25:331-380.
100. McDonald D. Morphology of the rat carotid sinus nerve: I. Course, connections, dimensions and ultrastructure. J Neurocytol 1983; 12:345-372.
101. McDonald D. Morphology of the rat carotid sinus nerve:II. Number and size of axons. J Neurocytol 1983; 12:373-392.
102. Finley JCW, Katz DM. The central organization of carotid body afferent projections to the brain stem of the rat. Brain Res 1992; 572:108-116.
103. Hess A, Zapata P. Innervation of the cat carotid body:nomal and experimental studies. Federation Proc 1972; 31: 1365-1382.
104. Claps A, Torrealba F. The carotid body connections:a WGA-HRP study in the cat. Brain Res 1988; 455:123-133.
105. Torrealba F, Alcayaga J. Nerve branching and terminal arborizations in the carotid body of the cat. A light microscopic study following anterograde injury filling of carotid nerve axons with horseradish peroxidase. Neurosci 1986; 19:581-595.
106. Kummer W, Gibbins IL, Stefan P et al. Catecholamines and catecholamine-synthesizing enzymes in guinea-pig sensory ganglia. Cell Tissue Res 1990; 261: 595-606.

107. Verna A, Barets A, Salat C. Distribution of sympathetic nerve endings within the rabbit carotid body:a histochemical and ultrastructural study. J Neurocytol 1984; 13:849-865.
108. Verna A. Terminaisons nerveuses afferentes et efferentes dans le glomus carotidien du lapin. J Microsc (Paris) 1973; 16:299-308.
109. Biscoe TJ, Pallot D. Serial reconstruction with the electron microscope of carotid body tissue. The type I cell nerve supply. Experientia 1972; 28:33-34.
110. Nishi K, Stensaas LJ. The ultrastructure and source of nerve endings in the carotid body. Cell Tissue Res 1974; 154: 303-319.
111. Kondo H. Innervation of the carotid body of the adult rat. A serial ultrathin section analysis. Cell Tissue Res 1976; 173:1-15.
112. Morgan SE, Pallot DJ, Willshaw P. The effect of ventilation with different concentrations of oxygen upon the synaptic vesicle density in nerve endings of the cat carotid body. Neuroscience 1981; 6: 1461-1467.
113. Nordmann JJ, Chevallier J. The role of microvesicles in buffering [Ca^{2+}] in the neurohypophysis. Nature 1980; 5777: 54-55.
114. Pequignot J-M, Hellström S, Forsgren S et al. Transection of carotid sinus nerve inhibits the turnover of dopamine and norepinephrine in long-term hypoxic carotid bodies:a biochemical and morphometric study. J Auton Nerv Syst 1991; 32:165-176.
115. Kondo H, Yamamoto M. Occurrence, ontogeny, ultrastructure and some plasticity of CGRP (calcitonin gene-related peptide)-immunoreactive nerves in the carotid body of rats. Brain Res 1988; 473:283-293.
116. Torrealba F, Correa R. Ultrastructure of calcitonin gene-related peptide- immunoreactive, unmyelinated afferents to the cat carotid body: a case of volume transmission. Neuroscience 1995; 64:777-785.
117. Kummer W. Retrograde neuronal labeling and double-staining immunocytochemistry of tachykinin- and calcitonin gene-related peptide immunoreactive pathways in the carotid sinus nerve of the guinea pig. J Auton Nerv Syst 1988; 23:131-141.
118. Kummer W, Fischer A, Heym C. Ultrastructure of calcitonin gene-related peptide- and substance P-like immunoreactive nerve fibers in the carotid body and carotid sinus of the guinea pig. Histochemistry 1989; 92:433-439.
119. Kusakabe T, Kawakami T, Takanka T. Peptidergic innervation in the amphibiam carotid labyrinth. Histol Histopathol 1995; 10:185-202.
120. Prabhakar NR, Kumar GK, Chang CH et al. Nitric oxide in the sensory function of the carotid body. Brain Res 1993; 625:16-22.
121. Wang Z-Z, Bredt DS, Fidone SJ et al. Neurons synthetisizing nitric oxide innervate the mammalian carotid body. J Comp Neurol 1993; 336:419-432.
122. Wang Z-Z, Stensaas LJ, Bredt DS et al. Localization and actions of nitric oxide in the cat carotid body. Neuroscience 1994; 60:275-286.
123. Tanaka K and Chiba T. Nitric oxide synthase containing neurons in the carotid body and sinus of the guinea pig. Microsc Res Tech 1994; 29:90-93.
124. Hohler B, Mayer B and Kummer W. Nitric oxide synthase in the rat carotid body and carotid sinus. Cell Tissue Res 1994; 276:559-564.
125. Grimes PA, Mokashi A, Stone RA, Lahiri S: Nitric oxide synthase in autonomic innervation of the cat carotid body. J Auton Nerv Syst 1995; 54:80-86.
126. Wang Z-Z, Dinger BG, Stensaas LJ, Fidone SJ. The role of nitric oxide in carotid chemoreception. Biol Signals 1995; 4:109-116.
127. Wang Z-Z, Stensaas LJ, Dinger BG, Fidone SJ. Nitric oxide mediates chemoreceptor inhibition in the cat carotid body. Neurosci 1995; 65:217-229
128. Gozal D, Gozal E, Gozal YM et al. Nitric oxide synthase isoforms and peripheral chemoreceptor stimulation in conscious rats. Neuroreport 1996; 7: 1145-1148.
129. Katz DM, Markey KA, Goldstein M et al. Expression of catecholaminergic characteristics by primary sensory neurons in

the normal adult rat in vivo. Proc Natl Acad Sci USA 1983; 80:3526-3530.

130. Katz DM, Black IB. Expression and regulation of catecholaminergic traits in primary sensory neurons:relationship to target innervation in vivo. J Neurosci 1986; 6:983-989.

131. Katz DM, Erb MJ. Developmental regulation of tyrosine hydroxylase expression in primary sensory neurons of the rat. Dev Biol 1990; 137:233-242.

132. Finley JC, Polak J, Katz DM. Transmitter diversity in carotid body afferent neurons:dopaminergic and peptidergic phenotypes. Neuroscience 1992; 51: 973-987.

133. Ichikawa H, Rabchevsky A, Helke C. Presence and coexistence of putative neurotransmitters in carotid sinus baro- and chemoreceptor afferent neurons. Brain Res 1993; 611:67-74.

134. Finley JCW, Erickson JT, Katz DM. Galanin expression in carotid body afferent neurons. Neuroscience 1995;68: 937-942.

135. Massari VJ, Shirahata M, Johnson TA et al. Carotid sinus nerve terminals which are tyrosine hydroxylase immunoreactive are found in the commissural nucleus of the tractus solitarius. J Neurocytol 1996; 25:197-208.

136. Okada J, Miura M. Transmitter substances contained in petrosal ganglion cells determined by a double-labeling method in the rat. Neurosci Lett 1992; 146:33-36.

137. Kondo H, Kuramoto H, Fujita T. Neuropeptide tyrosine-like immunoreactive nerve fibers in the carotid body chemoreceptor of rats. Brain Res 1986; 372: 353-356.

138. Erlinge D, Brunkwall J, Edvinsson L. Neuropeptide Y stimulates proliferation of human vascular muscle cells. Cooperation with noradrenaline and ATP. Regul Peptides 1994; 50:259-265.

139. Pequignot J-M, Dalmaz Y, Claustre J et al. Preganglionic sympathetic fibers modulate dopamine turnover in rat carotid body during long-term hypoxia. J Auton Nerv Syst 1991; 32:243-249.

140. Hess A. Chronically denervated rat carotid bodies. Acta Anat 1977; 97:307-316.

141. de Castro F. Sur la structure et l'innervation de la glande intercarotidienne (glomus caroticum) de l'homme et des mammifères et sur un nouveau systeme d'innervation autonome du nerf glossopharyngien. Trab Lab Invest Biol Univ Madrid 1926; 24:365-432.

CHAPTER 2

Oxygen Consumption and Energy Metabolism in the Carotid Body

Ana Obeso, Asunción Rocher, Benito Herreros and Constancio González

INTRODUCTION

In this chapter we will try to define the meaning of oxygen supply and energy metabolism in the carotid body (CB) in the frame of general concepts of metabolism. Energy metabolism has two purposes—one is to generate ATP from the oxidation of nutrients, and the other is to generate reduction equivalents (mostly in the form of NADPH) for the biosynthetic processes. ATP in turn is used for the performance of osmotic, mechanical and biosynthetic work, i.e., to maintain the functional and structural integrity of the cells.

The common intermediary in nutrient oxidation is acetyl-CoA. In the citric acid cycle the acetyl moiety is fully oxidized to CO_2 with the simultaneous reduction of the electron carriers NADH and $FADH_2$. These high potential electron carriers transfer the electrons to the respiratory chain, and ultimately to O_2 to form water. Coupled to this process, protons are pumped through the inner mitochondrial membrane, creating an electrochemical H^+ gradient with the mitochondrial interior alkaline and negatively charged with respect to the cell cytoplasm. This gradient of H^+ is used to drive the mitochondrial ATPase to synthesize ATP from ADP and P_i. Glucose can be converted to lactate with the genesis of only a small percentage of the ATP generated in the full oxidation to CO_2 (2 vs. 38 mol ATP/mol glucose).

In most biosynthetic processes the final products are more reduced than their precursors, and therefore they need, in addition to ATP, donors of reduction equivalents, namely NADPH obtained from the pentose cycle and from the mitochondrial citrate-pyruvate shuttle. Although we are not going to deal any further with the biosynthetic processes, it should be mentioned that the biosynthesis of cell constituents, as exemplified by the synthesis of proteins, are reduced in situations of compromise in the genesis of ATP, such as it occurs in hypoglycemia or hypoxia, leading for example to the well known muscle atrophy occurring

The Carotid Body Chemoreceptors,
edited by Constancio González.

at high altitude; even further, although hypoxia can induce the expression of certain specific proteins aimed to help cells coping with the hypoxic stress, there is an activation of proteolysis triggered at least in part by the concomitant increase in ACTH and glucocorticoids.

ENERGY METABOLISM AND O_2-SUPPLY TO TISSUES

As mentioned above, the oxidative phosphorylation, i.e., the synthesis of ATP coupled to the process of transference of electrons from NADH and $FADH_2$ to O_2 in the respiratory chain, is the main source of cellular ATP. Therefore there is a tight coupling between O_2 consumption (or cellular rate of respiration) and ATP synthesis. To fully substantiate this statement we should add that over 90% of the total O_2 consumption in the cell, in most of the cellular situations, occurs in the respiratory chain. In cells poisoned with cyanide, O_2 consumption declines to a very low level (< 10% of normal consumption), and in this circumstance the O_2 consumption of the cell occurs outside of the respiratory chain. On the contrary, O_2 consumption in the respiratory chain increases markedly in cells poisoned with dinitrophenol or other uncouplers; in this situation, the normal stoichiometry of O_2 reduction and ATP synthesis disappears and the percentage of O_2 consumption in the respiratory chain increases. In situations of shortage of O_2 supply to the cells (i.e., hypoxia) the extramitochondrial O_2 consumption decreases much earlier than the respiration of the cell; the reason being that the Km for O_2 of cytochrome oxidase is more than 100 times smaller than Km of the rest of the O_2-using enzymes.[1]

Since we are dealing with the energy metabolism of the CB, a chemoreceptor organ activated by decreases in arterial PO_2 (PaO_2), the discussion that follows will be centered on the dependence of cell respiration and oxidative phosphorylation on the availability of O_2 in tissues in general, and from there, we will consider the specific case of the CB itself. To best understand the availability of O_2 at the cellular level we will review first the O_2 supply to cells and its regulation, and the actual PO_2 at the cellular level (i.e., the tissue PO_2).

Oxygen Supply to Cells

Oxygen delivery to cells (FO_2) depends on the blood flow (Q) and the O_2-content of the arterial blood (CaO_2) according to the simple equation

$$FO_2 = Q \times CaO_2 \quad (1)$$

Referring to the oxygen delivery of the whole organism, Q represents cardiac output, and then inadequacy of FO_2 can result from either cardiovascular insufficiency or low CaO_2. We will leave out of consideration the cardiovascular causes (stagnant hypoxia) and the decrease in CaO_2 due to a decrease in the O_2-carrying capacity of the blood (anemic hypoxia), because they represent poor stimuli to the CB, and hypoventilation and impaired gas exchange, because they represent pathological processes causing hypoxic hypoxia; We will deal mostly with decreases in CaO_2 produced by environmental factors (decrease in ambient PO_2) causing physiological hypoxic hypoxia and representing the genuine physiological stimulus to the CB.[2-4] In turn, physiological or ambient-triggered hypoxic hypoxia can be acute or persistent, and the mechanisms that organisms put into play to solve the potential inadequacy of O_2 supply to cells in each case are different.

Acute Hypoxia

In acute hypoxia the first mechanism entering into play to solve the inadequate O_2 supply to cells is the CB-triggered hyperventilation. In fact, the CB plays an anticipatory hypoxic hypoxia-preventing mechanism in two regards: first, because it starts promoting hyperventilation at a PaO_2 of about 70 mmHg when the CaO_2 is approximately 94%, and second, because its response is instantaneous. In only a few seconds (equivalent to the circulation time from lung to the carotid artery) the CB-triggered hyperventilation starts fighting hypoxic hypoxia.[2,5] The CB function proceeds at higher intensities of hypoxia, in such a way that the more intense the hypoxia, the greater the hyperventilation. The function of the CB is best understood from two well known equations in respiratory physiology, the alveolar gas equation and the equation relating alveolar PCO_2 ($PACO_2$) and alveolar ventilation (VA). In the steady state, the alveolar gas equation can be approximated by the expression:

$$PAO_2 \approx PIO_2\text{-}1.2xPACO_2 \quad (2)$$

where PAO_2 and PIO_2 are the PO_2s in the alveolar and inspired gas, respectively, and the factor 1.2 comes from the assumption of a respiratory quotient of 0.8. On the other hand, in the steady state $PACO_2$ is directly proportional to CO_2 production (VCO_2) and inversely proportional to *VA*, according to the equation:

$$PACO_2 = Kx(VCO_2/VA) \quad (3)$$

From Equation 3 it follows that if *VA* doubles while VCO_2 is maintained constant, $PACO_2$ halves, and from Equation 2 it can be seen that PAO_2 will increase by approximately the same amount. Figure 2.1 shows ideal values for alveolar gas pressures at different altitudes before and after CB hyperventilation has driven them to a new steady state, as during acclimatization. As a reference value we would like to note that at about 5.8 Km of altitude, ventilation almost doubles and $PACO_2$ decreases from 40 to 24 mmHg allowing PAO_2 to rise from 25 to 45 mmHg; this in turn increases CaO_2 from just below 50% to near 80%.[6]

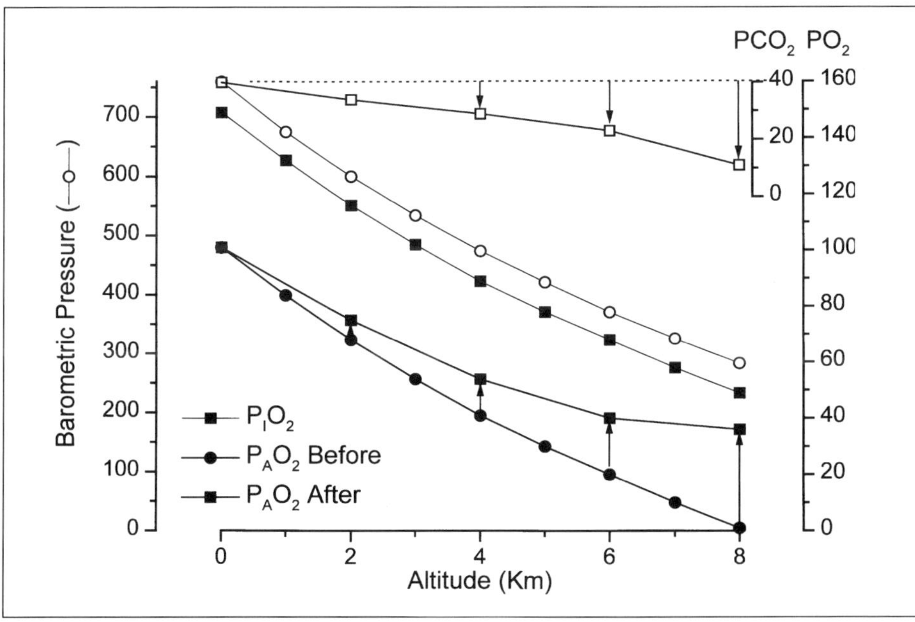

Fig. 2.1. Diagram illustrating the status of respiratory gases at different altitudes above sea level before and after the hyperventilatory compensation triggered by the CB chemoreceptors. The left y axis refers to the barometric pressures found at the different altitudes (x axis) and are labeled in the figure by empty circles. The filled symbols correspond to PO_2s (right y axis): in the inspired air after saturation with water vapor (filled squares and thin line; $P1O_2$); in the alveoli before any compensatory hyperventilation (i.e., as if ventilation remained at the sea level rate; filled circles; PAO_2 Before); and in the alveoli after the compensatory hyperventilation (filled squares and thick line; PAO_2 After). In the upper part of the figure the discontinuous line shows the $PACO_2$ before any compensation, and the empty square line shows the $PACO_2$ after the CB triggered hyperventilation is fully established. The vertical arrows in the lower and upper part of the figure show, respectively, the magnitude pf PAO_2 gain and $PACO_2$ loss as a result of the CB action. A respiratory quotient of 0.8 was assumed for the calculations.

The acute cardiovascular effects of hypoxia are multifactorial in their genesis and vary with the species and the intensity of hypoxia (see chapter 10). The consensus appears to be that acute hypoxic hypoxia in subprimate animals produces tachycardia, minor changes in blood pressure, increase in cardiac output and reduction of total peripheral resistances; in intense hypoxias, bradycardia and increase in peripheral resistances may appear. In primates and humans, tachycardia, increased cardiac output and peripheral vasodilatation are seen at all levels of hypoxia. Therefore, in short-term hypoxia the cardiac output/O_2 consumption ratio increases.

The most relevant response in the present context is the peripheral vasodilatation. The mechanisms involved in the genesis of vasodilatation produced by hypoxia are controversial. It seems well documented that whenever the O_2 uptake by the tissue starts to decline, responses are initiated to increase the O_2 supply. The decrease in O_2 uptake reflects a reduction in average tissue PO_2 below a critical level to maintain an adequate rate of the respiratory chain functioning and of oxidative phosphorylation, and it is coincident with an increase in lactate levels in tissues and in blood. The metabolic signals triggering local vasodilatation, and overriding the chemoreflex-induced sympathetically-mediated vasoconstriction, are not characterized in their quantitative importance, but lactic acid, H^+, and adenosine may interact to generate a vasodilatation adequate enough to compensate the decrease in CaO_2 (see ref. 7). In addition to these classical mediators of the hypoxic vasodilatation in the most distal parts of the arteriolar tree, it seems that shear-stress/hypoxia induced release of nitric oxide might contribute to the general vasodilatation of higher caliber arteries. Smooth muscle cells in some vascular beds possess K_{ATP} channels, and it has been suggested that they might contribute to the genesis of vasodilatation. However, the real significance of these channels could be questioned on the basis of the high PO_2 at the perivascular level and the inconsistency of findings with K_{ATP} channel blockers.[8] Quite recently it has been shown that arterial smooth muscle cells possess O_2-sensitive Ca^{2+} channels, that might participate in the hypoxic vasodilatation.[9,10] Finally, it has been shown in several vascular beds that there is an increase in the density of perfused capillaries. The degree of contraction of precapillary sphincters is controlled by the same metabolic signals controlling resistance vessels, allowing a coordinated response in the entire microcirculation during hypoxia. The very same factors, and probably some other tissue-specific factors, are responsible for the functional hyperemia occurring in all tissues during increased activity; an integration of neural and local mechanisms permits an intensification of the functional hyperemia during hypoxia.

Chronic Hypoxia

If hypoxia persists, second line mechanisms enter into play to secure an adequate CaO_2 and thereby an adequate FO_2 to tissues. mRNA for erythropoietin increases in the kidney within a few hours after the onset of hypoxia, and if hypoxia is intense, the increase is also observed in the liver, at least in the rat.[11,12] The response is proportional to the degree of hypoxia and is paralleled by changes in blood erythropoietin levels. The erythropoietin level in blood rises for 10-24 h, but if hypoxia is further prolonged it slowly returns to near-control values after 4-6 weeks.[13] Red cell count and Hb concentration increase with a slower time course, and remain elevated during the entire duration of hypoxia in spite of the decrease in erythropoietin levels. The increase in red blood cell mass and Hb concentration is such that it compensates, or even overcompensates for, the decreased O_2 saturation of Hb with the obvious result of normal or above normal CaO_2 (see ref. 14).

Within a few hours of continuous hypoxic exposure the sensitivity of the CB increases, and it continues to increase to reach a maximum in a few days (<1 week). This increase in hypoxic sensitivity is called hypoxic acclimatization and it is evidenced by a hyperventilation greater than expected for the actual hypoxic level.[6,15] It seems to be produced by changes in the proportions of neurotransmitters in chemoreceptor cells (see chapter 3 by González et al) and by an increase in the number of Na^+ and Ca^{2+} channels in the same cells.[16-18]

After hypoxic acclimatization, the cardiac output returns to near control values at sea level and the cardiac output/O_2 consumption ratio normalizes. The gain in the CB chemoreflex occurring during acclimatization could contribute to this resetting of the cardiac function, which has been interpreted by some as a protection of the heart in prolonged hypoxia by keeping its work at a normal level. Some authors stress the parallel time course for the increase red blood cell mass and the return of the cardiac index to prehypoxic levels.[6]

The increase in capillary density in tissues with sustained hypoxia has been a conflicting issue in the literature. Banchero[19] in his recent review concludes that "The bulk of evidence suggests that skeletal muscle capillarity does not respond to simple normothermic hypoxia even when the muscle is active...." The same conclusion is reached by Hudlicka et al[20] in a more recent review on skeletal and cardiac muscle.

Mitochondria represent the last link in the O_2 cascade. Possible changes in mitochondrial density as a response to prolonged hypoxic exposure, have been explored from two opposing rationales: on the one hand, it has been reasoned that a means to shorten diffusion distances and to facilitate oxidative metabolism would be to increase the density and/or distribution of mitochondria; on the other hand, it has been argued that a decrease in the number of mitochondria might well be related to the decreased maximal O_2 uptake evident in acclimatized humans above 3 Km of altitude. Whatever the rationale, it appears that only minor changes in the density of muscle mitochondria occur at high altitude, at least in humans, rabbits and guinea pigs.[6]

Finally, the enzymes involved in energy metabolism have also been investigated in skeletal muscle during prolonged hypoxia. The consensus in the findings is that in hypoxias of up to moderately high intensities (equivalent to altitudes of ≈5 Km) the activity of citric acid cycle and respiratory chain enzymes increases, albeit moderately, with no changes in glycolytic enzymes, while the opposite occurs at hypoxias of higher intensities. In this context it should be mentioned that Firth et al[21] (see also ref. 12) have described oxygen regulated control elements in the genes of phosphoglycerate kinase 1 and lactate dehydrogenase A which share structural and functional similarities with the 3' enhancer of the erythropoietin gene, also observing that hypoxia induced these glycolytic enzymes; the severe hypoxic conditions (1% O_2) used in their cultures correlate with the findings in intact organisms. The enzyme changes observed in up to moderately high hypoxias are the same as those seen after endurance training. This fact has been interpreted as evidence for an increased oxidative capacity, and the suggestion has been made that hypoxia itself might be the trigger for the changes in both situations.[22] In this regard it should be mentioned that cytochrome oxidase activity increases in brain tissue in response to sustained stimulation,[23] and then it might be suggested that increased metabolic demands produce an augmented oxidative capacity in all cell types.

Tissue PO_2

The final purpose of the adjustments just described is to provide an adequate amount of O_2 to allow a proper function of the cytochrome oxidase and to ensure a rate of oxidative phosphorylation according to cellular needs. In the paragraphs that follow, we will try to correlate the actual tissue PO_2 with the cellular performance. We discuss the metabolic processes regulated by O_2, and specifically consider the relationships between tissue PO_2 and cellular respiratory rate and oxidative phosphorylation.

At the outset of our discussion it might be useful to quote the conclusions of the review by Vanderkooi et al.[1] The authors state that there are not great differences in the PO_2 levels in tissues determined with different techniques, pointing out that the wide range of values provided by some of the methods reflect tissue inhomogeneities in O_2 tension distribution, which are adequately measured. They also state that the tissue O_2 measurements indicate that tissue PO_2 is lower than mixed venous PO_2. Finally, based on the comparison of tissues PO_2 with the Kms for O_2 of the O_2-utilizing enzymes, they conclude that the only enzyme with a Km for O_2 much smaller than the mean tissue PO_2 is cytochrome oxidase, implying that in normal conditions respiration rate is not limited by PO_2, but the rate of the rest of O_2-consuming reactions may be limited by O_2 availability (but see below).

There are, however, some comments pertinent to those conclusions. For example, in myoglobin-containing tissues there are important quantitative differences in histograms of tissue PO_2 distributions obtained with microelectrodes or with cryomicrospectroscopy of myoglobin O_2-saturation, with much lower values obtained with the latter method (see Table 1 in ref. 1). Regarding the relation between tissue PO_2 and mixed venous PO_2, other authors found a close agreement between both measurements in resting conditions; even more, an appropriate increase in functional capillary density may maintain a close agreement between both parameters during increased O_2 consumption by tissues or reduced CaO_2 in blood. It should be recalled, however, that high venous PO_2 in an organ may result from O_2-shunting via A-V anastomosis or countercurrent blood flow.[7]

Since there are two main sets of data on CB tissue PO_2 with great discrepancy among them (see below), it should be of interest to know the main determinants of tissue PO_2. All modellers of tissue PO_2 profiles include in their equations, albeit with different weights, the following parameters as determinants of tissue PO_2: organ blood flow and blood O_2 content (see Equation 1), organ O_2 consumption, capillarity of the tissue, and diffusivity of O_2 in the specific tissue. Other factors such as arteriovenous (A-V) O_2 shunting, capillary transit time, plasma skimming and clustering of mitochondria would certainly affect the profiles of tissue PO_2. Within the capillarity of the tissue the hyperemic responses observed during hypoxia and/or increased activity of the organ under study should be taken into account.

A detailed consideration of those factors is beyond the scope of this chapter, but for comparative purposes we will provide the reader with some data from other well studied tissues. Dog heart has a basal blood flow of around 90 ml x min^{-1} x 100 g^{-1}, an O_2 consumption of 10-12 ml x min^{-1} x 100 g^{-1} (ref. 24) and a mean tissue PO_2 averaging 30 mmHg (subepicardic), 17 mmHg (subendocardic) and 19 mmHg (2.5-9 mm depth)[1]. The capillarity of the dog heart is around 3000 capillaries/mm,[2] implying that around 10-15% of the surface area of a section is occupied by capillaries.[20] A-V O_2 difference in coronary circulation is near 11 ml O_2/100 ml of blood, implying that mixed coronary venous PO_2 is around 22-24 mmHg which is comparable to the average myocardial tissue PO_2. In striated muscle, and especially in heart muscle, most of extra O_2 consumption occurring during increased activity is the result of increased blood flow with much smaller contribution from an increase in O_2 extraction. In the rat brain the blood flow amounts to 120 ml x min^{-1} x 100 g^{-1}, the O_2 consumption is in the range of 8-10 ml x min^{-1} x 100 g^{-1} (ref. 25), and the PO_2 in the cerebral cortex is in the range of 20-40 mmHg[1]. The capillarity in rat brain cortex is near 600 capillaries/mm^2 (or below 5% of the surface area in a section.[26] The range of capillary density in the whole brain goes from above 850 in some nuclei to below 200 capillaries/mm^2 in the corpus callosum, showing a close correlation between capillary density and blood flow in the different brain regions.

The next point to consider is how those tissues PO_2 correlate with cell respiration and oxidative phosphorylation. Our understanding is that as far as tissue PO_2 is adequate to saturate cytochrome oxidase, the rate of respiration is unaffected and the availability of ATP is adequate. Owing to the low Km for O_2 cytochrome oxidase (below 0.3 mmHg) as obtained in mitochondria of many sources, tissues PO_2s in the range of

2-3 mmHg will maintain maximal or near maximal respiratory rate. A clear distinction should be made between systemic hypoxic hypoxia and increasing energy requirements, the two physiological situations that can result in tissue PO_2s below those required to saturate cytochrome oxidase. In the first case, the PO_2 gradient from the supplier capillaries to mitochondria is reduced, and as a consequence O_2 diffusion does not provide an adequate PO_2 for respiration at the mitochondrial level, and thereby oxidative phosphorylation cannot proceed at normal rates. In the second case, the O_2 sink effect that mitochondria represent increases, and even when the PO_2 gradient from capillaries to mitochondria augments, the rate of O_2 reduction and disappearance is so fast that not enough O_2 is delivered to build up an adequate PO_2. In both cases—hypoxia and increased energy requirements, a range of *intermediate* situations exists in which tissue PO_2s may not be high enough to saturate cytochrome oxidase (for example PO_2s between Km and x10 Km for cytochrome oxidase), yet biochemical regulatory mechanisms must enter into play to maintain respiratory and oxidative phosphorylation rates higher than those expected from the exclusive consideration of the actual PO_2s. Since data obtained in isolated mitochondria have shown that decreased external (cytoplasmic) [ATP]/[ADP][AMP][Pi] and increased mitochondrial [NADH]/[NAD^+] quotients increase respiration rates,[27-29] it is of great importance to know how these parameters are in those *intermediate* situations.

In relation to hypoxia, a first approach to characterize those *intermediate* situations can be obtained from consideration of high altitude physiology. At PaO_2 of 40 mmHg or slightly below, humans can perform adequately, and can increase their rate of cellular respiration such that their basal O_2 consumption can increase by a factor greater than 2-fold.[6] There are not, to our knowledge, measurements of tissue PO_2 in those conditions, but since the driving force for the diffusion of O_2 from capillaries to tissues drops from ≈90 mmHg in normal conditions to 40 mmHg, the actual tissue PO_2 would be more than halved. Data obtained in several species indicate that brain can maintain concentrations of ATP close to normal even at more severe levels of hypoxia. For example, in humans brain O_2 consumption is maintained at least down to a PaO_2 of 35 mmHg. In rats and mice brain O_2 consumption is maintained at PaO_2s down to 25-26 mmHg (cerebral venous PO_2 ≈8 mmHg,[30] and at the biochemical level in these conditions a notable decrease in P-creatine with minor changes in the levels of ATP is found.[30,31] However, because in most cells the concentrations of ATP, ADP, and AMP are in proportions 100:10:1, minor decreases in ATP will result in a large relative increase in ADP and will be even more pronounced in the relative concentration of AMP. This implies that minor decreases in ATP concentrations will result in significant decreases in the ratio [ATP]/[ADP][AMP][Pi]. Accompanying those changes is an increase in glycolysis with increasing production of lactate and an increase in the NADH/NAD ratio, and intracellular acidification.[30,31] Important modifications in the flow of metabolic intermediaries through the different metabolic pathways are well documented. After 30 min with those low levels of O_2, recovery of normal function is possible. However, concomitant alterations in the metabolism of neurotransmitters can trigger a rapid damage of brain cells. Unfortunately, most of the studies have been performed at these extreme hypoxic levels and more frequently in situations of ischemia, and therefore it can only be assumed that the same modifications outlined above will be found, albeit less pronounced, at less intense levels of hypoxia. Based on this assumption, it can be stated that moderate decreases in P-creatine and in [ATP]/[ADP][AMP][Pi] quotient, and moderate activations of glycolysis with increased [NADH]/[NAD^+] quotients maintain normal cell respiration, oxidative phosphorylation and ATP levels, and thereby a normal steady state in the ionic gradients across cell membranes.

Although mechanistically different, increased energy requirements associated with increased cellular activity cause a comparable picture. For example, at sustained 70% maximal capacity muscle work, a decrease in P-creatine, a minor change in the level of ATP and a relative larger increase in ADP and AMP, and an increase in lactate and in the [NADH]/[NAD^+] ratio has been observed.[7] As in the case of submaximal hypoxia, these biochemical modifications are regulatory and allow cells to respire at an adequate level for their increased activity, in spite of limited availability of O_2, and to maintain an ATP turnover according to needs. Even when the use of ATP during increased activity is different in muscle (myosin ATPase) than in neurons (ionic pumps), increased activity is associated with augmented cytoplasmic (and mitochondrial) [Ca^{2+}] which is known to activate pyruvate dehydrogenase and several dehydrogenases in the citric acid cycle.[32] Therefore, it is conceivable that the flow of NADH to the respiratory chain plays a quantitatively more important role in regulating cell respiration and oxidative phosphorylation during increased activity than during hypoxia.

A corollary of those findings, both in hypoxia and during increased metabolic activity, is that the mitochondrial [NADH]/[NAD^+] ratio increases, and that the electrochemical H^+ gradient across the inner mitochondrial membrane decreases. During submaximal increased activity, the exaggerated influx of H^+ to the mitochondria through the mitochondrial ATPase to maintain the increased turnover of ATP will be responsible for the decrease of the electrochemical H^+ gradient; during sustained maximal activity cells will enter into hypoxia. In hypoxia, the low O_2 levels will reduce the flow of electrons through the respiratory chain, and consequently the pumping rate of H^+ from the mitochondrial matrix to the cytoplasm. As the intensity of hypoxia increases the mitochondrial electrochemical H^+ gradient will progressively decrease and eventually collapse, and the synthesis of ATP will be reduced in parallel in spite of the increases in ADP and Pi.

ENERGY METABOLISM AND O_2-SUPPLY TO THE CAROTID BODY

Following the scheme used in the preceding section for the presentation of energy metabolism in tissues in general, we will review below the data available on CB oxygen supply in normoxia and hypoxia, and discuss the relation between tissue PO_2 and energy metabolism in the CB. In a final and separate subsection we will summarize the implications of those data for the O_2-sensing machinery in chemoreceptor cells; an ample discussion on O_2 sensing and transduction may be found in chapter 5.

OXYGEN SUPPLY TO THE CB

The CB blood flow is the greatest for any body organ. Initial measurements using gravidimetric methods indicated that the CB blood flow at normal blood gases and arterial pressure were close to 2,000 ml x min^{-1} x 100 g^{-1} (refs. 33, 34 and 35), and more recent measurements with the use of radioactive microspheres have yielded similarly high values of 1,417 ml x min^{-1} x 100 g^{-1} (ref. 36). O_2-consumption rates derived from A-V O_2 differences were in the range of 9 ml x min^{-1} x 100 g^{-1} (ref. 33, 34 and 35), but as pointed out by other researchers[37] the A-V difference for O_2 was so small that analytical methods produced unreliable results. O_2-consumption rates measured in vitro using confinement methods oscillate between 0.6 and 2 ml x min^{-1} x 100 g^{-1} (see ref. 2), and measurements derived from O_2-disappearance curves in CBs impaled with oxygen-microelectrodes after stopping the flow have yielded rates of O_2 consumption in the range of 1-1.5 ml x min^{-1} x 100 g^{-1}. It is estimated that the "true" O_2 consumption rate is near 1.3 ml x min^{-1} x100 g^{-1} in basal conditions, i.e., with perfusion pressures close to 100 mmHg and with PO_2 of the perfusates (either blood or saline) of 100 mmHg.[38] Comparable values for O_2 consumption have been derived based on the rate of glucose consumption.[39] Using standard figures it can be easily calculated that the A-V difference for O_2 in blood perfused CBs is 1 ml x l^{-1} of blood, and thereby the PO_2 in the venous blood of the CB should be ≈90 mmHg. An inference from these data is that at an arterial PO_2 below 60 mmHg, the A-V difference for PO_2 in the CB would decrease due to the change in the slope of the dissociation curve of HbO_2, which by releasing O_2 would maintain a PO_2 in the CB tissue closer to that of arterial blood.

Consistent with the high blood flow, the capillarity of the CB is very high, being occupied by capillaries 25-33% of the CB volume.[40,41] The distance from the center of most glomus cells to capillaries is between 10 and 20 μm in young rat CBs, and a median distance of 15.77 μm from the center of CB cell clusters to the nearest capillary has been obtained in the adult cat CB.[42]

During acute hypoxia (PaO_2 of 30-40 mmHg) there is an increase in CB blood flow of about 35%, as determined gravidimetrically, and morphologically several authors have reported marked increases in the volume of blood vessels.[41] Mechanistically this hyperemic response should correspond to a sum of hypoxic and functional hyperemia, being conceivable that in addition to the general metabolic factors involved in the response in other tissues, some neurotransmitters released from chemoreceptor cells (e.g., dopamine;[43] see chapter 3 by González et al) and nitric oxide released from nerve fibers[44] (see chapter 8) might be involved in the vasodilatation. There is a marked increase in the volume of the CB during chronic or persistent hypoxia. Many authors have shown that the enlargement of the CB is the result of increased capillarity[45-48] (see Heath and Smith).[49] Thus, prolonged hypoxic exposure at different simulated altitudes (4.3 to 7.5 Km) is accompanied by a marked increase in CB capillaries, with an increase of up to 10 times the control capillary volume, and a decrease from 3 to 1.8 μm in the mean distance from capillaries to the border of chemoreceptor cells.[48] The increase in capillary volume is due to engorgement of preexisting capillaries and to proliferation or formation of new capillaries; the increase in capillarity was partially reversible, and was only 1.5 times above controls 1-2 months after the hypoxic exposures. There are opposing views in relation to the density of mitochondria in the CB chemoreceptor cells during persistent hypoxia. Some authors have found conspicuous increases in the number of mitochondria and others have found no clear increase in the number of mitochondria.

Carotid Body Tissue PO_2

As summarized in Table 2.1, the reported values for CB tissue PO_2 cover an unexpectedly broad range. From the data discussed above for other tissues it appears that the data of Whalen and coworkers are in agreement with the rates of delivery and consumption of O_2 in the CB. In fact Lubbërs et al,[42] after a thorough analysis of the capillary distances to chemoreceptor cells, concluded that only about 4% of the tissue PO_2 values should be below 40 mmHg. In order to explain the low PO_2 values found in his measurements, Acker has successively postulated the occurrence of massive plasma skimming or A-V blood shunting (up to 90% of the blood flow) as possible peculiarities of the CB circulation. However, the occurrence of massive plasma skimming in the CB seems unlikely since it was shown that the CB capillaries were full of red blood cells after ultrarapid freezing of the CB in situ;[50] on the other hand, after a careful analysis of the vasculature of the CB it was found that only two out of fourteen arterioles reconstructed (i.e., 14%) and having a diameter similar to the others (about 10 μm in diameter) were directly connected by an end-to-end anastomosis to thin walled vessels considered to be venules.[51] The double set of intravascular PO_2 values reported by Rumsey and coworkers are difficult to explain taking into consideration that perfusing pressures and other experimental variables were similar in both studies (see Table 2.1).

Following the studies of Whalen and associates,[38] other data of interest in relation to the CB tissue PO_2 include: (a) the threshold PO_2 for carotid sinus nerve (CSN) discharge to increase oscillates between 50 and 65 mmHg; (b) the tissue P_{50} for CSN

Table. 2.1. Cat carotid body tissue PO_2 according to different authors

CB Perfusate	Perfusate pressure	Perfusate PO_2	CB tissue PO_2	Author
Saline	80	111 ± 15	23 ± 3[a]	Rumsey et al 1991[52]
Saline	80	131 ± 12	74 ± 11[a]	Rumsey et al 1991[52]
Saline	80	109 ± 5	59 ± 13[a]	Rumsey et al 1992[53]
Blood	100	91	49 ± 3[a]	Rumsey et al 1992[53]
Blood	120	95-113	25[b]	Acker et al 1971[54]
Blood	>70	84	>65[c]	Whalen and Nair 1983[38]
Blood	>70	39	20[d]	Whalen and Nair 1976[55]

[a]Intravascular PO_2, mostly microvascular PO_2 values measured with a phosphorescent dye. [b]Fifty-two percent of the PO_2 values measured with microelectrodes were below 20 mmHg, and 79% were below 40 mmHg. In a different article the same group reported a mean tissue PO_2 of 7 mmHg in the rabbit CB. [c]The mean CB tissue PO_2 value shown here represents a mean of means from several works. In some of these works very few values were below 10 mmHg, and in one of them no value below 40 mmHg was recorded. d In these series of experiments CB tissue PO_2 was measured with microelectrodes at different PO_2 in the superfusing blood; in the table it is shown the mean CB tissue PO_2 when perfusing with blood at PO_2 in the range of 30-49 mmHg; in these conditions very few values were below 5 mmHg. In other works the authors measured CB tissue PO_2 while perfusing the organ with air equilibrated saline, and obtained PO_2 in the range 62-160, with a mean value of 133 mmHg.

discharges is around 10 mmHg in some studies and 32 mmHg in others, and; (c) the peak CSN discharge is reached at tissues PO_2*s* of 3-5 mmHg. It should be recalled that the values of arterial blood PO_2 corresponding to these values are: 70-75 mmHg for the threshold, 40 mmHg for the P_{50}, and 10 mmHg for the maximum CSN discharges.[2] As predicted, these values of PaO_2 and CB tissue PO_2 indicate that there is a drop in PO_2 from capillaries to tissue of around 15-20 mmHg at blood PO_2*s* corresponding to the flat part of HbO_2 dissociation curve, and a smaller drop at blood PO_2*s* falling in the steepest part of the HbO_2 curve.

Energy metabolism in the CB has not been studied in detail, and therefore the available data are fragmentary and difficult to relate to precise values of tissue PO_2. It has been found that ATP levels were reduced by 19% in CBs incubated with air-equilibrated solutions (10 min) when compared with controls incubated with 100% O_2-equilibrated solutions.[56] In other study using superfusates equilibrated with air as control solutions and with 10% O_2 as hypoxic solutions, no significant change was observed in ATP or ADP levels at either 4 or 30 min, and while at 4 min there was an increase in AMP by a factor of 10 in the hypoxic CBs, no differences were observed at 30 min.[57] Glucose consumption, measured as the rate of 2-deoxyglucose phosphorylation, was reduced by 20-25% in the presence of 1 mM ouabain in CBs incubated with 100% O_2-equilibrated solutions; in air-equilibrated solutions glucose consumption increased by 45%, and ouabain completely abolished this increase.[39] It should be noted that the release of dopamine in CBs incubated with air-equilibrated solution in the identical conditions is 2- to 3-fold greater than that shown in organs incubated with 100% O_2, and, that the ouabain sensitive glucose uptake in the CB is lower than that of brain tissue (40-50%), but much higher than that of the heart (5-10%).

In recent years Biscoe and coworkers[58,59] (for additional references, see González et al[2]) using microfluorometric methods have measured the redox state of the mitochondria of isolated chemoreceptor cells (as NADH autofluorescence) and the mitochondrial inner membrane potential with rhodamine 123. They found that in mitochondria of chemoreceptor cells these two parameters exhibited a unique PO_2 dependence, such that with a threshold of about 60 mmHg (bath PO_2) there was an increase in NADH autofluorescence and a decrease in mitochondrial membrane potential as PO_2 decreased. Since in adrenomedullary cells and neurons from sensory ganglia used as control cells, either NADH autofluorescence or mitochondrial membrane potential did not change until PO_2 in the bath was lower than 10 mmHg, they proposed that mitochondria of chemoreceptor cells had a unique sensitivity to hypoxia. However, there is no need to invoke any special property for chemoreceptor cell mitochondria, because, as discussed above, these changes are the expected ones for the mitochondria of any activated cell, and certainly hypoxia activates chemoreceptor cells, precisely with a threshold in the range of 60 mmHg, and not adrenomedullary cells or sensory neurons.

Speculations on the O_2-Sensing Mechanisms

From the behavior of the CB in vivo, and of the entire CB or isolated chemoreceptor cells in vitro, it is evident that chemoreceptor cells are activated with a PO_2 threshold in their surroundings of 50-60 mmHg. At these tissue PO_2s, CSN discharges start to increase, isolated chemoreceptor cells start to release dopamine, and their mitochondrial redox state and membrane potential start to be modified. Comparing this PO_2 threshold for chemoreceptor cell activation with the much lower Km values of cytochrome oxidase for O_2, well below tissues PO_2 (see above), it would appear that this enzyme is not well suited for PO_2 signaling.

However, it might be argued that regional differences in CB tissue PO_2 (CB tissue PO_2 histograms cover the almost entire range of PO_2 from 0 to 100 mmHg) would allow the redox state of cytochrome oxidase to be the signal for O_2 chemoreception: different chemoreceptor cell-CSN units would be recruited at every single arterial blood PO_2, with specific units being recruited alternatively and setting the basal CSN discharge, and with progressively more units being recruited as arterial PO_2 decreases. The data obtained in isolated cells on mitochondrial redox state/membrane potential[58,59] or dopamine secretion[10,60] cannot be explained with this model.

Recently it has also been suggested that an NADPH oxidase, like that present in phagocytes, could be a key element in the O_2-sensing machinery, or even the O_2-sensor itself.[61] From a kinetic point of view this enzyme is reasonably well suited to act as an O_2 sensor because its Km for O_2 oscillates between 5 and 30 mM (3-18 mmHg).[62] There are, however, many facts that do not fit the proposal. First, cytochrome b_{-245} (also known as cytochrome b_{558} because of the absorption maximum of its a-band), which is the last element in the electron transport mechanism of this enzymatic complex, does not bind CO at all,[63,64] and yet CO interferes with the O_2-sensing machinery[65,66] (see chapter 5).

Then, what is the O_2 sensor and where is it located? The honest answer is that we do not know. However, the fact that CO prevents the production of erythropoietin induced by hypoxia in hepatoma cells,[67] as well as the inhibition of K^+ currents produced by hypoxia in chemoreceptor cells,[65] strongly suggest that the O_2 sensor could be a hemoprotein. This notion is strengthened by the fact that prokaryotic cells sensitive to environmental PO_2 express a membrane hemoprotein named FixL which is the O_2 sensor triggering the activation of the transcription of several genes and the expression of an entire family of proteins needed by the bacteria to cope with the low PO_2 in their habitat (see Bunn and Poyton).[68]

CONCLUDING REMARKS AND PERSPECTIVES

We have given in this chapter a brief account of the principles operating in tissues directed to assure an O_2 supply according to needs in spite of increased demands or reduced O_2 availability. We also give an overview on O_2 metabolism and ATP genesis in normal situations, and discuss cellular mechanisms regulating cell respiration and oxidative phosphorylation; these regulating mechanisms allow cells to maintain adequate levels of ATP for cell function in spite of augmented needs or reduced O_2 supply. Tissue capillarity and the regulation of capillary density in tissues in response to sustained O_2 demands or reduced availability, tissue PO_2 and the uncertainties of tissue PO_2 measurements, $[NADH]/[NAD^+]$ and $[ATP]/[ADP][AMP][Pi]$ quotients and their regulatory significance are also discussed.

These topics are presented in a wide context, in reference to several tissues but with more emphasis on muscle and nervous tissue where the information is most abundant, and they are used to frame the scarce information existing in the CB. Even though extrapolations involve an unknown degree of uncertainty, it appears that the regulation of O_2 metabolism in the CB follows the same basic principles encountered in other tissues. The uniqueness of the CB resides in the fact that reduced O_2 availability and increased demands are always concurrent in this chemoreceptor organ. The concurrence of both factors, i.e., hypoxia and increased activity, is imposed by the unique function of the CB which needs to be activated in direct proportion to the decrease in arterial PO_2, which has not always been appreciated by researchers in the field. The great vascular density of the CB, its high blood flow, and the increased number of capillaries during sustained hypoxia represent specific features of the CB which support the increased activity during hypoxia. Probably, some enzymes of intermediary metabolism and the respiratory chain also are constitutively overexpressed or are more amenable to upregulation during hypoxia, because hypoxia in the CB also implies "endurance"; however, direct information on this is missing.

Studies on energy metabolism in the CB are needed to fill the existing gaps. From those studies we will learn how the CB manages to cope with the increased energy demands in acute and chronic hypoxia. Already de Castro in his classical works emphasized the importance of the study of the CB vasculature to understand the functioning of the organ; we will add to that message the need to know and understand the factors regulating the proliferation of capillaries in the CB in sustained hypoxia. Finally, considering actual trends in O_2-sensing research and the importance given to the changes in the redox state of the cells as possible triggers of hypoxic responses (see chapter 5), a detailed definition of those changes eill be needed in terms of their magnitude and the redox pairs affected in the entire range of PO_2 activating the CB chemoreceptors.

Acknowledgments

This work has been supported by the Spanish DGICYT grant PB92/0267.

References

1. Vanderkooi JM, Erecinska M, Silver IA. Oxygen in mammalian tissue:methods of measurement and affinities of various reactions. Am J Physiol 1991; 260: C1131-C1150.
2. González C, Almaraz L, Obeso A, Rigual R. Carotid body chemoreceptors: from natural stimuli to sensory discharges. Physiol Rev 1994; 74:829-898.
3. González C, López-López JR, Pérez-García MT, Obeso A, Rocher A. Cellular mechanisms of carotid body chemoreception. Respir Physiol 1995; 102: 137-147.
4. González C. Sensitivity to physiological hypoxia. In: Weir EK, Lopez-Barneo J, eds. Oxygen Regulation of Ion Channels and Gene Expression. Armonk NY: Futura Press, 1997: (in press).
5. Fidone SJ, González C. Initiation and control of chemoreceptor activity in the carotid body. In: Fishman AP, ed. Handbook of Physiology. The Respiratory System. Bethesda, MD: Amer Physiol Soc, 1986:247-312.
6. Ward PW, Milledge JS, West JB. High Altitude Medicine and Physiology. 2nd ed. London: Chapman & Hall, 1995:618.

7. Crystal RG, West JB, eds. The Lung. Scientific Foundations. New York: Raven Press, 1991:1445-1551.
8. Bolton TB, Beech DJ. Smooth muscle potassium channels: their electrophysiology and function. In: Weston AH, Hamilton TC, eds. Potassium Channel Modulators. Oxford: Blackwell Scientific Publications, 1992:144-180.
9. Franco-Obregon A, Ureña J, Lopez-Barneo J. Oxygen-sensitive calcium channels in vascular smooth muscle and their possible role in hypoxic arterial relaxation. Proc Natl Acad Sci USA 1995; 92: 4715-4719.
10. Lopez-Barneo J. Oxygen-sensing by ion channels and the regulation of cellular functions. Trends Neurosci 1996; 19: 435-440.
11. Chorh CT, Eckardt KU, Firth JD, Ratcliffe PJ. Feedback modulation of renal and hepatic erythropoietin mRNA in response to graded anemia and hypoxia. Am J Physiol 1992; 263:F474-F481.
12. Ratcliffe PJ, Ebert BL, Ferguson DJP, Firth JD, Gleadle JM, Maxwell PH, Pugh CW. Regulation of the erythropoietin gene. Nephrol Dial Transplant 1995; 10:18-27.
13. Abbrecht PH, Littell JK. Plasma erythropoietin in men and mice during acclimatization to different altitudes. J Appl Physiol 1972; 32:54-58.
14. Monge C, Leon-Valverde F. Physiological adaptation to high altitude: oxygen transport in mammals and birds. Physiol Rev 1992; 71:1135-1172.
15. Weil JV. Ventilatory control at high altitude. In: Fishman AP, ed. Handbook of Physiology. The Respiratory System. Bethesda: Am Physiol Soc, 1986:703-727.
16. Stea A, Jackson A, Nurse CA. Hypoxia and N6, O2-digutyryladenosine 3', 5'-cyclic monophosphate, but not nerve growth factor, induce Na^+ channels and hypertrophy in chromaffin-like arterial chemoreceptors. Proc Natl Acad Sci USA 1992; 82:9469-9473.
17. Stea A, Jackson A, Macintyre L, Nurse A. Long-term modulation of inward currents in O_2 chemoreceptors by chronic hypoxia and cyclic AMP in vitro. J Neurosci 1995; 15:2192-2202.
18. Nurse CA. Carotid body adaptation to hypoxia: cellular and molecular mechanisms in vitro. Biol Signals 1995; 4: 286-291.
19. Banchero N. Cardiovascular responses to chronic hypoxia. Ann Rev Physiol 1987; 49:465-476.
20. Hudlicka O, Brown M, Egginton S. Angiogenesis in skeletal and cardiac muscle. Physiol Rev 1992; 72(2):369-417.
21. Firth JD, Ebert BL, Pugh CW, Ratcliffe PJ. Oxygen-regulated control elements in the phosphoglycerate kinase 1 and lactate dehydrogenase A genes: similarities with the erythropoietin 3' enhancer. Proc Natl Acad Sci USA 1994; 91:6496-6500.
22. Cerretelli P, Kayser B, Hoppeler H, Pette D. Muscle morphometry and enzymes with acclimatization. In: Sutton JR, Coates G, Remmers JE, eds. Hypoxia: The Adaptations. Toronto: BC Decker Inc, 1990: 220-224.
23. Wong-Riley MTT. Cytochrome oxidase: an endogenous metabolic marker for neuronal activity. Trends Neurosci 1989; 12:94-101.
24. Feigl EO. Coronary physiology. Physiol Rev 1983; 63:1-205.
25. Ghajar JBG, Plum F, Duffy TE. Cerebral oxidative metabolism and blood flow during acute hypoglycemia and recovery in unanaesthetized rats. J Neurochem 1982; 38:397-409.
26. Hunziker O, Frey H, Schulz U. Morphometric investigations of capillaries in the brain cortex of the cat. Brain Res 1974; 65:1-11.
27. Erecinska M, Silver IA. ATP and brain function. J Cereb Blood Flow Metab 1989; 9:2-19.
28. Erecinska M, Wilson DF. Regulation of cellular energy metabolism. J Memb Biol 1982; 70:1-14.
29. Wilson DF. Oxygen dependence of neuronal metabolism. In: Bazan NG, Braquet P, Ginsberg MD, eds. Neurochemical Correlates of Cerebral Ischemia. New York: Plenum Press, 1992:85-101.
30. Bachelard HS, Lewis LD, Ponten U, Siesjo BK. Mechanisms activating glycolysis in the brain in arterial hypoxia. J Neurochem 1974; 22:395-401.

31. Duffy TE, Nelson SR, Lowry OH. Cerebral carbohydrate metabolism during acute hypoxia and recovery. J Neurochem 1972;19:959-977.
32. McCormack JG, Halestrap AP, Denton RM. Role of calcium ions in regulation of mammalian intramitochondrial metabolism. Physiol Rev 1990; 70:391-425.
33. Daly M de B, Lambertsen CJ, Schweitzer A. Observations on the volume of blood flow and oxygen utilization of the carotid body in the cat. J Physiol Lond 1954; 125:67-89.
34. Purves MJ. The role of the cervical sympathetic nerve in the regulation of oxygen consumption of the carotid body of the cat. J Physiol Lond 1970; 209: 417-431.
35. Purves MJ. The effect of hypoxia, hypercapnia and hypotension upon carotid body blood flow and oxygen consumption in the cat. J Physiol Lond 1970; 209:395-416.
36. Barnett S, Mulligan E, Wagerle LC, Lahiri S. Measurement of carotid body blood flow in cats by use of radioactive microspheres. J Appl Physiol 1988; 65: 2484-2489.
37. Whalen WJ, Nair P. Tissue PO2 in the cat carotid body and related functions. Adv Exp Med Biol 1977; 78:225-232.
38. Whalen WJ, Nair P. Oxidative metabolism and tissue PO_2 of the carotid body. In: Acker H. and O'Regan RG, eds. Physiology of the Peripheral Arterial Chemoreceptors. Amsterdam: Elsevier, 1983:117-132.
39. Obeso A, González C, Rigual R, Dinger B, Fidone S. Effect of low O_2 on glucose uptake in rabbit carotid body. J Appl Physiol 1993; 74:2387-2393.
40. de Castro F, Rubio M. The anatomy and innervation of the blood vessels of the carotid body and the role of chemoreceptive reactions in the autoregulation of the blood flow. In: Torrance RW, ed. Arterial Chemoreceptors. Oxford, UK: Blackwell Scientific Publications, 1968: 267-277.
41. McDonald DM. Peripheral chemoreceptors. Structure-function relationships of the carotid body. In: Hornbein TF, ed. Regulation of Breathing. Part I. New York: Marcel Dekker, Inc., 1981:105-319.
42. Lubbërs DW, Teckhaus L, Seidl E. Capillary distances and oxygen supply to the specific tissue of the carotid body. In: Acker H, Fidone S, Eyzaguirre C, Lübbers DW, Torrance RW, eds. Chemoreception in the Carotid Body. Berlin: Springer-Verlag, 1977:62-68.
43. Almaraz L, Perez-Garcia MT, González C. Presence of D_1 receptors in the rabbit carotid body. Neurosci Lett 1991; 132: 259-262.
44. Wang ZZ, Stensaas JJ, Bredt DS, Dinger B, Fidone SJ. Localization and actions of nitric oxide in sensory function of the carotid body. Neuroscience 1994; 60: 275-286.
45. Heath D, Edwards C, Winson M, Smith P. Effects on the right ventricle, pulmonary vasculature, and carotid bodies of the rat of exposure to, and recovery from, simulated high altitude. Thorax 1973; 28:24-28.
46. Laidler P, Kay JM. A quantitative morphological study of the carotid bodies of rats living at a simulated altitude of 4300 metres. J Pathol 1975; 117:183-191.
47. Laidler P, Kay JM. The effect of chronic hypoxia on the number and nuclear diameter of type I cells in the carotid bodies of rats. Am J Pathol 1975; 79:311-320.
48. Dhillon DP, Barer GR, Walsh M. The enlarged carotid body of the chronically hypoxic and chronically hypoxic and hypercapnic rat: a morphometric study. QJ Exp Physiol 1984; 69:301-317.
49. Heath D, Smith P. Diseases of the Human Carotid Body. London, UK: Springer-Verlag, 1992:73-79.
50. Verna A. The carotid body blood supply: evidence against plasma skimming. In: Belmonte C, Pallot DJ, Acker H, Fidone S, eds. Arterial Chemoreceptors. Leicester, UK: Leicester University Press, 1981:336-343.
51. McDonald DM, Haskell A. Morphology of connections between arterioles and capillaries in the rat carotid body analyzed by reconstructing serial sections. In: Pallot DJ, ed. The Peripheral Arterial Chemoreceptors. London: Croom Helm, 1984:195-206.
52. Rumsey WL, Iturriaga R, Spergel D, Lahiri S, Wilson DF. Optical measurements of the dependence of chemorecep-

tion on oxygen pressure in the cat carotid body. Am J Physiol 1991; 261: C614-C622.
53. Rumsey WL, Lahiri, S, Iturriaga R, Mokashi A, Spergel D, Wilson DF. Optical measurements of oxygen and electrical measurements of oxygen chemoreception in the cat carotid body. Adv Exp Med Biol 1992; 317:387-395.
54. Acker H, Lübbers DW, Purves MJ. Local oxygen tension field in the glomus caroticum of the cat and its change at changing arterial PO_2. Pflügers Arch 1971; 329:136-155.
55. Whalen WJ, Nair P. Factors affecting the tissue PO_2 in the carotid body of the cat. In: Paintal AS, ed. Morphology and Mechanisms of Chemoreceptors. Delhi: Navchetan Press, 1976:91-102.
56. Obeso A, Almaraz L, González C. Correlation between adenosine triphosphate levels, dopamine release and electrical activity in the carotid body: support for the metabolic hypothesis of chemoreception. Brain Res 1985; 348:64-68.
57. Verna A, Talib N, Roumy M, Pradet A. Effects of metabolic inhibitors and hypoxia on the ATP, ADP and AMP content of the rabbit carotid body in vitro: the metabolic hypothesis in question. Neurosci Lett 1990; 116:156-161.
58. Duchen MR, Biscoe TJ. Relative mitochondrial membrane potential and $(Ca^{2+})_i$ in type I cells isolated from the rabbit carotid body. J Physiol Lond 1992; 450:33-61.
59. Duchen MR, Biscoe TJ. Mitocondrial function in type I cells isolated from rabbit arterial chemoreceptors. J Physiol Lond 1992; 450:13-31.
60. Montoro RJ, Ureña J, Fernandez Chacon R, Alvarez de Toledo G, Lopez Barneo J. Oxygen sensing by ion channels and chemotransduction in single glomus cells. J Gen Physiol 1996; 107:133-143.
61. Acker H, Xue D. Mechanisms of O2 sensing in the carotid body in comparison with other O_2-sensing cells. News Physiol Sci 1995; 10:211-215.
62. Cross AR, Jones OTG. Enzymic mechanisms of superoxide production. Biochim Biophys Acta 1991; 1057:281-298.
63. Iizuka T, Kanegasaki S, Makino R, Tanaka T, Ishimura Y. Studies on neutrophil b-type cytochrome in situ by low temperature absorption spectroscopy. J Biol Chem 1985; 260:12049-12053.
64. Parkos CA, Dinauer MC, Walker LE, Allen RA, Jesaitis AJ, Orkin SH. Primary structure and unique expression of the 22-kilodalton light chain of human neutrophil cytochrome b. Proc Natl Acad Sci USA 1988; 85:3319-3323.
65. Lopez-Lopez JR, González C. Time course of K+ current inhibition by low oxygen in chemoreceptor cells of adult rabbit carotid body: effects of carbon monoxide. FEBS Lett 1992; 299:251-254.
66. Lahiri S, Iturriaga R, Mokashi A, Ray DK, Chugh D. CO reveals dual mechanisms of chemoreception in the cat carotid body. Res Physiol 1993; 94:227-240.
67. Goldberg M, Dunning SP, Bunn HF. Regulation of the erythropoietin gene: evidence that the oxygen sensor is a heme protein. Science 1988; 242: 1412-1415.
68. Bunn HF, Poyton RO. Oxygen sensing and molecular adaptation to hypoxia. Physiol Rev 1996; 76:839-885.

CHAPTER 3

Functional Significance of Chemoreceptor Cell Neurotransmitters

Constancio González, Bruce Dinger and Salvatore J. Fidone

INTRODUCTION

In the first chapter of this book, Alain Verna presents a clear overview of the neurotransmitters present in the mammalian carotid body (CB). Verna emphasizes that although histochemical, immunohistochemical, and in some cases biochemical data have succeeded in demonstrating a great variety of putative neurotransmitters in the CB, it is perhaps still premature to unequivocally accept as fact the notion of sensory neurotransmission in this chemoreceptor organ. At the same time, the structural and functional arrangement of CB elements is consistent with these chemoreceptors being secondary sensory receptors, in which chemoreceptor cells detect changes in blood PO_2 and PCO_2/pH, and signal these changes via chemical synapses with the sensory terminals of the carotid sinus nerve (CSN). As stated in chapter 5 by Pérez-García and González, the experimental data supporting neurotransmission between the receptor cells and the sensory terminals include: 1) the demonstrated neurosecretory sensitivity of chemoreceptor cells to blood gases; 2) the requirement for structurally intact synaptic contacts between chemoreceptor cells and sensory nerve endings in order for the CB to exhibit chemoreceptor activity; and 3) the lack of hypoxic sensitivity of regenerated CSN fibers following ischemic or cryogenic destruction of the CB. Consistent with these concepts, and clearly summarized in chapter 7 by Patricio Zapata, there exists a wealth of pharmacological data that allows one to readily envision a synaptic relationship between the chemoreceptor type I cells and the sensory nerve endings of the CNS. However, the uncertainty of the site(s) of action of neurotransmitter agonists and antagonists, together with the variable results observed as a function of dose, animal species and preparation (e.g., in vivo vs. in vitro), as well as other experimental variables, renders the concept of

The Carotid Body Chemoreceptors,
edited by Constancio González. © 1997 Landes Bioscience.

neurotransmission in the CB, a difficult and unsettled topic of CB physiology.

The definitive solution of this neurotransmission issue ultimately rests upon studies of the microelectrophysiological and pharmacological characterization of the appositional/synaptic-like contacts between chemoreceptor cells and their sensory nerve endings. In this regard, the experimental endeavors recently initiated by Nurse and coworkers[1] coculturing chemoreceptor cells and petrosal ganglion neurons, may help resolve the issue of neurotransmission in the CB. These authors obtained electrophysiological evidence for excitatory postsynaptic potentials preceding the genesis of propagated electrical activity. It should also be recalled that Hayashida et al[2] obtained similar data in blind intracellular recordings from intact CBs. However, a clear understanding of the direction, sign and intensity of trans-junctional activity requires knowledge of the biochemical features of the putative neurotransmitter(s), including their metabolism and the unambiguous localization of their receptors. Unfortunately, the biochemical data to date have often been fragmentary, and alternative interpretations are frequently invoked, according to personal bias and experimental preferences.

In the following sections, we summarize the currently available data regarding the metabolism of putative chemoreceptor neurotransmitters, but emphasize in particular the effects of CB stimulation on these metabolic processes. Attention is also given to identifying the location of the neurotransmitter receptors, as a means of determining the direction(s) of the transmitter-mediated signal. Similar considerations related to neurotransmitters associated with the sensory and autonomic innervation of the CB are reviewed in a later chapter by Almaraz, Dinger and Fidone.

ACETYLCHOLINE

Acetylcholine (ACh) Metabolism

ACh was the first substance proposed as neurotransmitter between the chemoreceptor (type I) cells and the sensory nerve endings.[3] This proposal was based on the observation that ACh[4] and inhibitors of ACh-esterase[3] increased ventilation in a manner similar to that produced by low PO_2. The earliest studies (see Fidone and González,[5] for references), which focused on the pharmacology of cholinergic transmission in the CB, proved to be largely inconclusive, and a role for ACh in the genesis of CSN activity was sometimes defended and frequently denied (see also chapter 7 by P. Zapata).

A quantum leap in the study of the role of CB ACh was begun in the 1960s by Eyzaguirre and his coworkers (reviewed by Eyzaguirre and Zapata).[6] Using bioassays, these authors found an ACh content in the cat CB of 20-30 mg/g tissue; a similar value (23 mg/g tissue) was found by Jones[7] also using bioassays. Somewhat later, using the newly available gas chromatography-mass fragmentography technique, Fidone et al[8] and Hellstrom[9] in the cat and rat CBs, respectively, confirmed with this analytical method the presence of ACh in the CB, but reported much lower (10%) values than earlier found with bioassays. ACh in the CB could be localized in type I cells, based on the presence of a high affinity uptake for choline and immunoreactivity for choline acetyltransferase[10,11] in these cells. Fidone and coworkers[12] also reported that the CB could synthesize in 90 min an amount of ACh equivalent to the endogenous stores. No other data are available on ACh metabolism, except for the observation made by Eyzaguirre and coworkers in Loewi-type experiments showing that anoxic cat CBs located upstream release a substance capable of exciteingthe downstream normoxic organs; this excitation was blocked by nicotinic antagonists, potentiated by ACh-esterase inhibitors and prevented by the addition of ACh-esterase to flowing saline. Numerous other studies in the cat demonstrating that cholinergic blockers reduce, and ACh-esterase inhibitors augment hypoxic chemosensory discharge would seem to clearly suggest that ACh is released from the type I cells as a chemoexcitatory agent (see Fitzgerald et al;[13,14] but see also McQueen).[15]

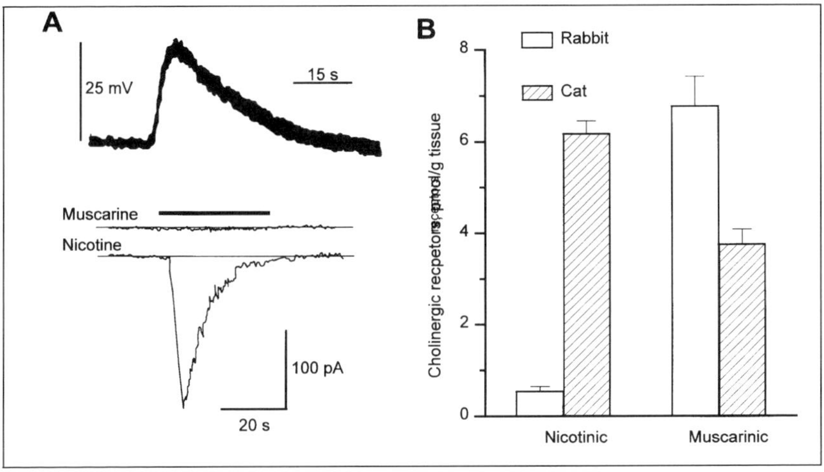

Fig. 3.1. Biochemical and electrophysiological assessment of cholinergic receptors in the carotid body. (A) Top, change in membrane potential elicited by a bolus injection in the superfusion system of 50 mg of ACh in a chemoreceptor cell recorded in the intact cat CB; and (bottom) whole-cell ionic currents elicited by muscarine and nicotine at concentrations of 100 μM in isolated rat chemoreceptor cells recorded at a membrane potential of -70 mV. (B) Bmax for ^{125}I-α-bungarotoxin and ^{3}H-quinucludinyl benzilate specific binding in the rabbit and cat CBs. The binding capacity of the tissue indicates density of nicotine receptors (^{125}I-α-bungarotoxin binding sites) in the cat CB. This figure has been drawn with data from Hayashida and Eyzaguirre, 1979; and Wyatt and Peers, 1993 and Hirano et al, 1992 (references 2, 21 and 18, respectively).

Acetylcholine Receptors

It is well established that chemoreceptor cells possess cholinergic receptors. Ligand binding studies performed in the rabbit and cat CBs using α-bungarotoxin and quinuclidinyl benzilate as nicotinic and muscarinic radioligands, respectively, have shown that in both species the number of binding sites were unchanged following chronic CSN denervation; autoradiography localized the binding sites to type I cells.[16-18] Further studies demonstrated that muscarinic receptors predominated in the rabbit, whereas nicotinic receptors were more abundant in the cat CB (see González et al[19] for references; Fig. 3.1). Consistent with the binding studies, Hayashida and Eyzaguirre[20] and Wyatt and Peers[21] demonstrated electrophysiologically the presence of nicotinic receptors in cat and rat type I cells, respectively (Fig. 3.1), while Gomez-Niño et al[22] showed that nicotinic agonists release catecholamines (preferentially norepinephrine) from normal and chronically sympathectomized rabbit CBs. Quite recently, Dasso et al[23] have shown that both nicotinic and muscarinic agonists produce large transients in Ca_i levels in rat chemoreceptor cells, indicating that both types of cholinergic receptors are also present in these species. However, recent neurochemical findings obtained from the cat CB show that concentrations of α-bungarotoxin near 20 times higher than its binding Kd reduced by only 56% the release of CA elicited by nicotine, while the classical nicotinic blocker, mecamylamine, abolished that release completely.[24] These findings imply that a set of nicotinic receptors located on the chemoreceptor cells is not labeled or blocked by the snake toxin, and consequently the possibility that there are nicotinic receptors located on the sensory nerve endings which are also insensitive to α-bungarotoxin must be considered.

Conclusions

It is evident that ACh is present in type I cells and may be released from these cells during chemostimulation of the CB. The evidence suggests that ACh excites chemosensory discharge via nicotinic receptors and depresses discharge via muscarinic receptors.[25] Cholinergic receptors are present on type I cells, and their possible location in the sensory nerve endings cannot be ruled out. These observations indicate that the effects of ACh on chemosensory activity are mediated through autoreceptors located on type I cells, which likely modulate release of other chemoactive substances, such as the catecholamines DA and NE. Consistent with this notion is the important observation (see Eyzaguirre et al[26]) that the excitatory action of ACh could be markedly reduced or even abolished in CBs superfused with Ca^{2+}-free/Mg^{2+}-rich solutions. However, it is possible that some direct actions of ACh on the sensory nerve endings also contribute to the overall effects of ACh on CSN activity. In regards to the diverse mechanisms of ACh action in the CB, it should be pointed out that nicotinic receptors evoke cell depolarization, which Wyatt and Peers[21] showed leads to Ca^{2+} channel activation. Muscarinic receptors, on the other hand, reduce cAMP levels in the rabbit CB,[27] and because a positive correlation exists between cAMP and catecholamine release/chemosensory discharge (see chapter 5 by Pérez-García and González), it might be suggested that the muscarinic effect of ACh results from adenylate cyclase inhibition.

CATECHOLAMINES

Catecholamine Metabolism

Although a few publications appeared prior to 1957 dealing with the effects of catecholaminergic agents on respiration or CSN discharge and with the histochemical demonstration of CA in the organ, it was in this year that Lever and Boyd[28] first showed that type I cells possess dense-cored granules similar to those found in adrenal medulla chromaffin cells. There quickly followed numerous publications demonstrating the presence of CA in these cells using formaldehyde-induced fluorescence (FIF) and quantifying tissue CA levels biochemically (see Fidone and González for references);[5] in recent years, refined techniques for the measurement of dopamine (DA) and norepinephrine (NE) have significantly re-

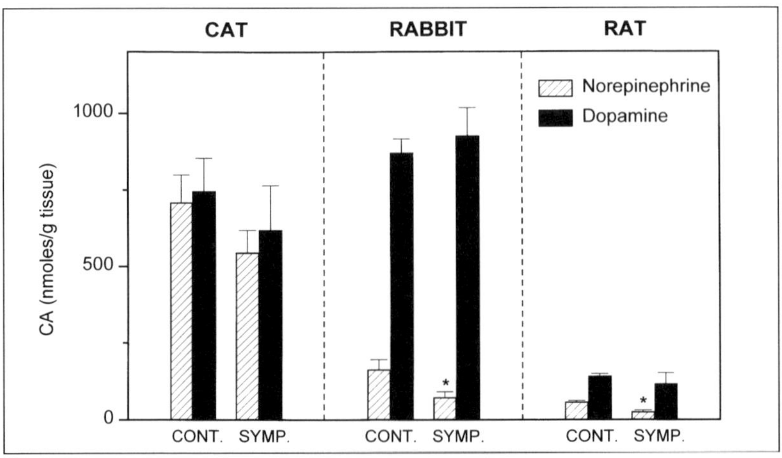

Fig. 3.2. Catecholamine levels in control and chronically (7-15 days prior) superior cervical ganglionectomized cat, rabbit and rat carotid bodies. Note that the rat and rabbit CBs are predominantly dopaminergic organs, while the cat CB exhibits similar levels of dopamine and norepinephrine. Also note that sympathectomy reduces by nearly 50% the norepinephrine content in the rat and rabbit CBs and does not alter the norepinephrine levels in the cat organ. Finally, note that the absolute levels of DA are nearly 5 times lower in the rat than in the rabbit and cat CBs. Drawn from González-Guerro et al, 1993[48] and with unpublished data.

duced the dispersion for reported CA values in the CB (cf. González et al;[19] Fig. 3.2). In a general sense, the rabbit CB can be considered as primarily a dopaminergic organ (DA, 500-700 nmol/g tissue; NE, 100-200 nmol/g tissue; sympathectomy further reduces NE by nearly 50% without affecting DA content). In the cat CB, DA and NE levels are similar (600-800 nmol/g tissue; sympathectomy only marginally reduces NE content). In the rat CB, CA levels are lower (DA, 120-150; NE, 50-60 nmol/g tissue; sympathectomy reduces NE levels by 50% without altering DA levels).

The enzymes tyrosine hydroxylase (TH) and dopamine-β-hydroxylase (DβH) involved in the biosynthesis of CB CA have also been measured in the rat, rabbit and cat. The enzyme levels in all cases are sufficiently high to explain a high turnover rate for DA and a lower turnover for NE. Additionally, it could be shown that TH, but not DβH, is inducible by hypoxic stimulation (see González et al for references[19]). Estimated turnover times for DA and NE vary with the different techniques employed for these determinations; reported DA turnover times vary from 5 and nearly 80 hr for rabbit and cat, and approximately 3 hr for rat CB; NE turnover times are nearly double these values for the respective species (see González et al[19]). Despite the variability, there is general agreement that turnover rates for DA increase with acute hypoxic stimulation, and that both DA and NE turnover rates (and tissue CA levels) increase with chronic hypoxic stimulation. These increased turnover rates imply that hypoxia increases both DA and NE release, although in the case of NE this occurs with an apparently slower time course or higher threshold.[29,30] Acute acidic/hypercapnic stimulation also increases the rate of DA and NE synthesis in the in vitro cat CB preparation, and chronic hypercapnic stimulation produces an increase in DA, NE and dihydroxyphenylacetic acid (DOPAC; the principal DA catabolite) in the rat CB, suggesting increased turnover of CA during hypercapnia.

Consistent with the above findings, many laboratories have measured the actual release of CAs during hypoxic and acidic stimulation, using for this purpose a variety of techniques, including radioisotopic and amperometric methods applied to intact CBs in vitro or to isolated chemoreceptor cells. These studies have clearly demonstrated in both the rabbit and cat CBs that a close correlation exists between the intensity of hypoxic or acid/hypercapnic stimulation on the one hand, and the amount of DA release and action potential frequency, on the other;[29,31,32] Figs. 3.3A and B). A similar relationship has been found for a number of pharmacological chemoexcitatory agents, including CN^-, dinitrophenol and 2-deoxyglucose;[33,34] Fig. 3.3C). In all cases, the stimulus-induced release of DA exhibited a marked dependency on extracellular Ca^{2+}, which was >95% for hypoxia and high external K^+, and ≈80% for acidic stimuli.[35] More recent studies using the amperometric technique have provided further information on the dynamics of this release process. Donnelly[36] showed that the low PO_2 and CN-induced DA release preceded the neural discharge, and he confirmed the Ca^{2+}-dependency of the release process. In a more recent study, Buerk et al[37] used rapid kinetic measurements to show that the onset of DA release in response to hypoxia or stagnant hypoxia preceded by a few seconds the chemosensory discharge (Fig. 3.3D). This group also showed in one experiment that nicotine increased the discharge without an accompanying proportional increase in DA release. This is an intriguing finding because Gomez-Niño et al[22] had previously shown that nicotine, in the predominantly "muscarinic" rabbit CB (see earlier), increased CA release 10-fold above basal levels. However, as previously described most of the released CA was in the form of NE (NE release increased 15x, DA release 2.5x), and therefore the possibility exists that the amperometric technique did not detect NE.

Two important studies by Donnelly and Doyle[38] and Donnelly[39] merit description here. In the first study, these investigators

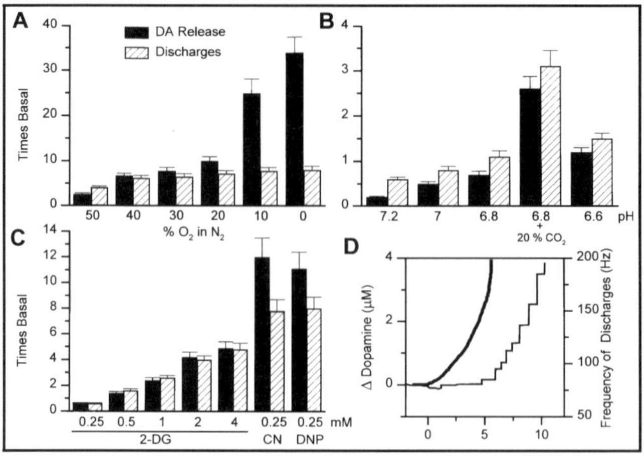

Fig. 3.3. Release of dopamine and carotid sinus nerve action potential frequency increase elicited by different types of stimulation of the cat CB, and time course of both, the secretory and neural responses to a hypoxic/asphyctic stimulus. (A) Hypoxic stimuli of different intensities (superfusion of the carotid bodies with solutions equilibrated with gas mixtures containing the percentages of O_2 shown, balance N_2) were applied for 10 minutes; control conditions, superfusion with 100% O_2-equilibrated solutions. The low rate of superfusion in these experiments determined that the threshold for hypoxic stimulus corresponded to solutions equilibrated with 50-60% O_2. (B) Bicarbonate/CO_2-free solutions of different pH were used to superfuse (stimulate) the CB for periods of 10 min. Note the greater responses when the superfusing solution contained bicarbonate and CO_2. Control conditions, superfusion with 100% O_2-equilibrated solutions, pH 7.40, except for the high PCO_2/low pH (95% O_2/5% CO_2; pH 7.40). (C) Metabolic poisons at the concentrations shown were included in the superfusing solutions during 10 min to stimulate the CB. Control conditions, as in A. (D) Onset of the increase in the release of DA and CSN discharges in response to flow interruption. Parts A and B of the figure were drawn with data from Rigual et al 1986, 1991;[31-32] part C with data from Obeso et al 1986, 1989;[33-34] and part D with data from Buerk et al, 1995.[37]

showed in newborn rats up to 30 days postnatal that there is a progressive age-dependent increase in basal and hypoxia-evoked release of DA (e.g., between days 10-30, basal release doubled and low PO_2-induced release increased by 30%); comparable results have recently been reported for developing rabbits.[40] In the second study,[39] the author claims to have demonstrated an independence between CA secretion and chemosensory nerve activity. This assertion is based on two principal observations: first, that in response to a repeated hypoxic stimulus, the chemosensory neural discharge is maintained while there is progressive reduction in the secretory response; and second, that in response to hypoxia reserpinized rats exhibit near normal levels of chemosensory discharge, while CA release is reduced to 5-8% of control values. In respect to the first observation, it should be pointed out that this is not an uncommon finding. In fact, we have previously reported this phenomenon for the CB.[41,29] It has also been described in the adrenal medulla, using nicotine as the secretagogue,[42] in the sympathetic endings of cat spleen, using high external K^+ as the stimulus,[43] and in the sympathetic endings of the isolated heart, using electrical stimulation.[44] In this latter preparation, it was also shown that despite the reduction in NE release (67% decrease at the third consecutive stimulus), the heart rate and the auricular and ventricular tension attained were identical in response to the first and third stimulus. Surely, the cause-effect relationship between NE release and increase in heart rate and tension is not in doubt. Regarding the second observation, i.e., near normal levels of chemosensory discharge, and marked reduction of CA release after reserpinization, we have again already reported and discussed a comparable situation while perfusing the CB with Ca^{2+}-free solutions[29] (see also González et al).[19] Leitner et al[45] reported some modifications in CSN discharge in reserpinized rabbit and cat CBs, including a decrease in basal normoxic action potential frequency, as well as a sluggish onset and reduction in the maximum CSN discharge elicited by hypoxic and hypercapnic stimulation. In general, following reserpine treatment of sympathetically innervated organs, there is a marked (greater than 90%) reduction in CA content and release with only moderately reduced contractile responses (≈ 30%; see González et al[19] for a further discussion). Thus, in respect to the loss of parallelism between the release of DA and the response of the CSN, it should be noted that the CB behaves as do other catecholaminergic organs when subjected to similar experimental protocols, i.e., repeated stimulation and reserpinization produce a marked decrease in the release of CA and only minor changes in the neurotransmitter-mediated responses (see also below).

The hypoxia-evoked release of DA from type I cells is modulated by several neurotransmitters known to be present in these cells. D2-DA receptors located on type I cells (see below) are activated by endogenously released DA, resulting in feedback inhibition of DA release. Thus, it is observed that dopaminergic blockers increase basal and low PO_2-induced release of DA,[46] and that bromocryptine and quinpirole (D2 agonists) inhibit this release (González et al, unpublished). Isoproterenol, a nonselective β-adrenergic agonist, was found to augment the low PO_2-induced release of DA, and selective α_2-adrenergic agents also modified release, specifically, selective α_2-antagonists augmented and α_2-agonists inhibited the low PO_2-induced release of CA. The effects of α_2-antagonists imply that NE is released by hypoxia and, acting via α_2-receptors feedback controlling the release of CA. Adrenergic effects are mediated, at least in part, by cAMP, but α_2-agonists also inhibited Ca^{2+} currents in type I cells.[47] Opioid peptides inhibit the low PO_2-induced release of DA in the rabbit CB acting on δ-opioid receptors, because δ-agonists inhibit and the antagonist, naloxone, augment release.[48] Prostaglandin E_2, which itself exhibits increased release during hypoxia, is also a negative modulator of low PO_2-induced DA release; a close correspondence exists between the dose-response curves for prostaglandin E_2 inhibition of low PO_2-induced DA release and Ca^{2+} currents in type I cells.[49] As mentioned earlier, cholinergic agents also modulate the release of CA from type I cells in both a positive (nicotinic) and negative (muscarinic) manner. Finally, it should be emphasized that there exists also a close correspondence between the action of these neuroactive agents on chemosensory discharge and CA release from type I cells (see González et al).[19]

Inactivation of DA released from the CB has been studied by González et al.[50] They showed that rabbit type I cells do not possess a high affinity uptake system for DA, a finding which likely explains the lack of toxicity of 6-hydroxydopamine on these cells.[51,52] Low affinity uptake followed by oxidation and to a lesser extent methylation, together with wash-out of the amines, effectively terminates the action of released CAs. It has recently been shown that the sympathetic innervation of the CB exhibits a high affinity uptake for NE.[47] It is conceivable that the increased sympathetic activity that accompanies hypoxic stimulation increases the release of NE from sympathetic endings, while low PO_2 in vitro acting directly on sympathetic endings does not augment the normoxic rate of NE release. High external K^+-induced release of the accumulated NE by sympathetic endings is also controlled by presynaptic α_2-adrenergic receptors.[47]

Catecholamine Receptors

There have been several studies describing the localization of DA receptors in the CB. Ligand binding studies using spiroperidol in the rabbit CB[53] and domperidone in the rat CB[54] showed that the Bmax for D2 DA receptors in these organs was significantly reduced (≈40%) following chronic CSN denervation. Consistent with these earlier studies, three more recent investigations employed in situ hybridization techniques in the rat,[55] rabbit[56] and cat CBs,[57] and identified D2 receptor mRNA in type I cells and subpopulations of petrossal ganglion neurons, thus confirming the dual localization (type I cells and CSN) of D2 receptors in the CB. The effect of dopaminergic agonists on CA release from type I cells (see above) constitutes a functional assessment of DA autoreceptors on these cells.

The CB also possesses pharmacologically demonstrable D1 DA receptors. Thus, DA and the selective D1 agonist, SKF 38393, increases cAMP levels in the CB, while the selective D1 antagonist, SCH 23390, completely blocks this effect.[58] Because these D1 dopaminergic agents did not affect CA release, whilst the remaining test stimuli affecting cAMP did alter release, it was suggested that D1 DA receptors may be located on the CB vasculature. The possibility also remains that the CB expresses some other type of DA receptor, because we have observed that selected dopaminergic agents exhibit paradoxical effects on type I cell metabolism (DA synthesis and release, and cAMP levels; González et al, unpublished observations; see also Bairam et al).[59]

Pharmacological Actions of DA in the CB

The role of DA in the CB remains a controversial and unsettled issue in the field of arterial chemoreception. A coherent view of DA actions in the CB must account for the observed effects of dopaminergic agents on CSN activity (see González et al[19] for a comprehensive review; see also chapter 7 of this book by P. Zapata). In the cat CB, both in vivo and in vitro, DA produces inhibition of CSN discharge at low doses, a transient inhibition followed by excitation at intermediate doses, and a marked excitation at high doses.[60-62] Reserpinization abolishes the inhibitory effects of DA. Dopaminergic blockers with preferential D2 blocking activity augment CSN discharge at low doses, tend to inhibit at intermediate doses, and are clearly inhibitory at high doses. Another common observation is that after administration of D2 blocking agents, the inhibitory action of DA is transformed into one of excitation. In the rabbit, DA is an excitatory agent in vitro at all concentrations, while in vivo the dual excitatory and inhibitory actions of DA are manifest, suggesting that a vascular component of DA action may be responsible for the inhibitory effect.

When these data are interpreted in light of DA metabolism and receptor localization in the CB, the pharmacological actions of DA may be explained as follows. Endogenously released DA acts on both sets of D2 receptors at any rate of release; DA action at the presynaptic level would modulate the rate of release, while DA action on the endings of the CSN would set the chemosensory action potential frequency. At the basal normoxic rate of DA release, the low affinity of postsynaptic receptors would determine the low frequency of CSN discharge. When chemoreceptor cells are activated by low PO_2 or increased $PCO_2/[H^+]$, the release of DA increases, leading to an augmentation in the action potential frequency in the CSN. At the same time, the increased levels of DA in the extracellular space produce a negative modulation of the release through action on the high affinity presynaptic receptors, thereby acting to limit the rate of release; this negative modulation helps maintain adequate neurotransmitter levels in these "slowly-adapting" chemoreceptor cells in spite of prolonged periods of stimulation. As the stimulus strength increases, both the intensity of chemoreceptor cell activation and the negative modulation via presynaptic receptors are likewise increased, thus setting levels of release and CSN discharge which are proportional to stimulus intensity. The concept of differential affinities of presynaptic vs. postsynaptic DA receptors is essential to this schema.[63,64]

To understand the pharmacological effects of dopaminergic agents it should be considered that exogenous dopaminergic agonists produce an imbalance in the actions of endogenous DA due to the different affinities of presynaptic vs. postsynaptic receptors, and probably also due to the different accessibility of the drug to both set of receptors. Thus, the inhibition of CSN discharge produced by low doses of exogenously-administered DA would result from the preferential activation of high affinity presynaptic receptors, thereby inhibiting the ongoing release of DA, and reducing DA concentration at the level of the postsynaptic receptors; at high doses, exogenous DA would directly activate the sensory nerve endings and an increase in CSN discharge would follow in spite of the inhibition of the endogenous release. The vascularly-mediated inhibitory component of exogenous DA action might result from vasodilatation effected through D1-DA receptors which have been tentatively localized to vascular smooth muscle cells;[58] this vascular component would accommodate the differences in the action of DA in in vitro vs. in vivo preparations. The attenuation or reversal of the inhibitory action of exogenous DA in reserpinized animals should result from two concomitant effects: 1) a reduction of the presynaptic effects of DA due to the low levels of endogenous DA available for release; and 2) a postsynaptic supersensitivity to DA produced by reserpine itself (see Trendelenburg[65] for a discussion on this topic). A similar phenomenon might also account for the maintained CSN discharge under the condition of low-level DA release in Ca^{2+}-free solutions; in this situation the affinity of receptors for neurotransmitters tends to increase,[66] and the efficacy of neurotransmitter action on postsynaptic receptors also increases.[67,68] Finally, an interpretation of the action of D2 blockers on CSN discharge is also possible under this same schema. At low doses, these agents would act preferentially at presynaptic receptors, blocking the negative modulation exerted by endogenously-released DA, and thereby augmenting DA release and the effective DA concentration at postsynaptic receptors. At sufficiently high doses, D_2 antagonists would also block postsynaptic receptors, inhibiting CSN discharge. Although as pointed out by McQueen,[69] most studies with dopaminergic blockers have utilized single-dose protocols, in those studies where dose-response curves have been generated,[70] the effects of dopaminergic blockers are similar to those described above.

OPIOID PEPTIDES

Opioid Peptide Metabolism

The presence of opioid peptides (OP) in the CB of several species and their costorage with CA in dense-core vesicles of type I cells has been well documented by several groups using immunohistochemical techniques (for review, see González et al;[19] see also chapter 1 by A. Verna). While the literature on OP metabolism is not abundant, OP levels have been measured by four different laboratories,[48,71-73] and despite some variation in absolute values, there is unanimous agreement that pentapeptides predominate over higher molecular weight forms by a factor nearly 5x. Met-enkephalin and leu-enkephalin sequences are expressed in a ratio of 5 to 1 (see González et al).[19] In one study,[48] it was observed that OP levels in the CB (248 equivalent pmole Leu-enkephalin/mg protein) were not affected by 7-15 days prior sympathectomy or CSN denervation. A 3 hr hypoxic episode in vivo (8% O_2; PaO_2 = 40 mmHg) reduced DA, low molecular weight (pentapeptides, native opioid peptides), and high molecular weight forms of OP in identical proportion (≈ 40%). This observation is consistent with the costorage of OP and DA, and indicates corelease of both these neurotransmitters (Fig. 3.4A). These same authors[74] exposed animals to an eight-day hypoxic episode (normobaric atmosphere of 11% O_2), which was followed by a recovery period of another eight days. They observed an initial decrease in OP levels (≈35%; at day 2 of hypoxia), followed by a slow increase which reached normal, prehypoxic levels by the end of the hypoxic exposure period. During the subsequent recovery period, low molecular weight forms remained at prehypoxic values while the high molecular weight forms continued to increase well above prehypoxic levels (at days 10 and 12) before returning to control values at the end of the experiment (day 16).

Fig. 3.4B summarizes the changes in OP and CA levels during the 16 days of the experiment, and emphasizes that during the hypoxia and recovery periods there was an increase in the ratio of DA/low molecular weight OP.

Opioid Receptors

There have been no studies which directly assessed the localization and characterization of OP receptors in the CB. However, Kirby and McQueen[75] recorded CSN discharge from the cat CB in vivo and concluded that OP acted at δ-opioid receptors to produce inhibition of sensory discharge. This finding is consistent with the fact that met-enkephalin, the preferential natural ligand to δ-opioid receptors, is the more abundant opioid in the type I cells. As mentioned earlier, selective δ-opioid agonists (but not μ-opioid agonists) inhibit the low PO_2-induced release of DA.[48] The results of this study agree with that of Kirby and McQueen, and in addition, demonstrate that type I cells possess δ-opioid receptors. However, they do not exclude other possible locations for this or other types of opioid receptors in the CB.

It would thus appear that OP are inhibitory modulators of DA release and CSN discharge. A causal link between these two actions, namely, that OP inhibit CSN discharge by reducing DA release, remains to be demonstrated. However, it is tempting to speculate from the study of OP during long-term hypoxic exposure, that the decrease in DA/OP ratios during hypoxia and the first few days of the recovery period, might contribute to the *increased reactivity* of the chronically hypoxic CB.[76,77] It is likely that other cellular mechanisms as well contribute to the hyper-reactivity of the chronically hypoxic CB, including increases in the density of Na^+ channels[78] and probably also Ca^{2+} channels.[74]

SUBSTANCE P

Substance P Metabolism

The presence of substance P (SP) in the CB is well documented immunohistochemically, but there remains some disagreement regarding the precise identity of the immunoreactive elements in the organ and degree of positiveness to SP antibodies. Cuello and McQueen[79] found that ≈20% of cat CB type I cells were immunopositive for SP, but Wharton et al[73] and Lundberg et al[80] reported for the same species that type I cells were negative and that SP was limited to the nerve fibers in the organ. Chen et al[81] found some immunopositive type I cells in the cat CB, none in the rat. Scheibner et al[82] reported that type I cells were negative to SP at birth, then acquired the neuropeptide during the first six weeks of postnatal life, but decreased in immunopositivity thereafter. Prabhakar et al[83] found that most type I cells in the cat were immunoreactive to SP and neurokinin (NK) A, and Heath and Smith[72] reported faint SP immunoreactivity of type I cells in only 16 of 24 human CBs. Wang et al[10] observed that over 70% of type I cells in the cat were immunostained for SP. More recently, Kusakabe et al[84] showed that while rabbit type I cells were negative to SP, many nerve fibers surrounding the cell clusters were clearly immunopositive for this peptide; Pizarro et al[85] found a comparable distribution of SP in the goat CB, also reporting SP-positive baroreceptor fibers and endings in the carotid sinus.

The reported SP levels in the CB are: in the cat, 54 and 57 pmol/g tissue;[83,73] in the human, 16 pmol/g tissue;[72] and in the rabbit, ≈295 pmol/g tissue.[71] Neurokinin A levels in the cat CB are 85 pmol/g tissue. SP levels in the rabbit CB decreased nearly 40% following hypoxic stimulation,[71] but were increased three-fold in the cat following a similar hypoxic episode.[83] In this latter study, neurokinin A levels were not affected by hypoxia, but were reduced by ≈60% after 1 hr of breathing 100% O_2.

Agreement has also been lacking in respect to the effects of SP antagonists on CSN discharge. Use of the same antagonists at similar doses has resulted in near blockage of hypoxia-evoked discharge,[86] or no effect.[87] More recently, Prabhakar and coworkers[88] reported that CP-96,345, a nonpeptide

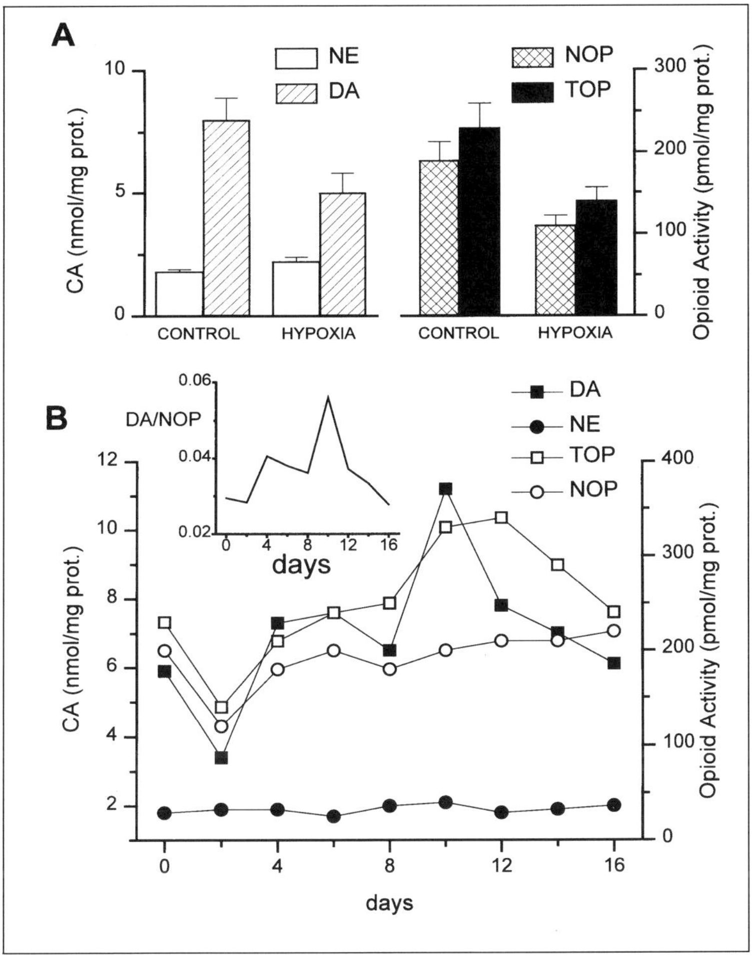

Fig. 3.4. Effects of acute and chronic hypoxia on catecholamine and opioid peptide levels in the rabbit CB. (A) Groups of 4-6 rabbits were placed during 3 h in a plastic chamber continuously flushed with compressed air (control) or 8% O_2 balanced N_2 (hypoxia), and immediately thereafter the CBs were removed and used to assay CA and opioid peptide activity. CA were determined by HPLC and opioid peptide activity was measured with a radioreceptor assay. NOP refers to native opioid peptide (pentapeptides) and TOP refers to total opioid active (pentapeptides plus high molecular weight opioid peptides). Note that the hypoxic episode decreased in the same proportion DA and NOP/TOP and did not affect NE levels, indicating co-storage of DA and opioid peptides and co-release of both transmitters. (B) Groups of four rabbits were exposed to an 11% O_2 normobaric atmosphere and sacrificed at days 2-8; an identical number of animals were exposed to the hypoxic atmosphere for 8 days and sacrificed after different periods of recovery in a normoxic atmosphere. Upon sacrifice the CBs were removed and used to assay CA and opioid peptide levels. Note the progressive increase of the DA/NOP ratio (inset) all along the hypoxic episode and its return to control prehypoxic values during the recovery period. Drawn with data from González-Guerrero et al, 1993.[48, 74]

NK-1 blocker, reduced in a dose-dependent manner the low PO_2-induced chemosensory discharge of the cat CB, reaching the maximal inhibition of 73% at a dose of 0.3-0.6 mg/Kg; the same dose did not affect CO_2-induced chemosensory activity. DeSanctis et al,[89] on the other hand, reported that the maximal level of inhibition of the low PO_2-induced hyperventilation obtained in the rat was approx. 22% using doses of CP-96,345 up to 10 mg/Kg. It should also be mentioned that this NK-1 antagonist is not free of side effects, in particular its significant action as a Ca^{2+} channel antagonist.[90]

Substance P Receptors

Based on pharmacological studies of the effects of SP agonists and antagonists on CSN discharge, it is generally agreed that the receptors which mediate the response to SP are of the NK-1 subtype,[86,87] but their intraglomic localization is unknown.

From these data it is not possible to attain meaningful conclusions on the physiological significance of SP in the chemoreception process.

OTHER NEUROTRANSMITTERS

Chemoreceptor type I cells contain in addition a number of other putative neurotransmitters (see González et al;[19] see also chapters 1 and 7). Among these, serotonin (5-HT) has been demonstrated immunohistochemically and biochemically in the CB of several species, including rat, cat and humans; there are at present little data describing the metabolic fate of this biogenic amine. Qualitative autoradiographic studies have revealed binding of specific ligands for different 5-HT receptor subtypes, and have shown that ^{3}H-5-HT binding in the CB is increased after chronic CSN denervation. The reported pharmacological effects of serotonin on ventilation and CSN discharge are highly variable. 5-HT injections produce either marked hyperventilation or apnea, and this response either disappeared or persisted after CSN denervation; likewise, the excitation, or inhibition, of CSN discharge produced by 5-HT was either sensitive to or unaffected by 5-HT receptor blockers (see González et al[19] for references). In a recent study it was concluded that 5-HT does not play a significant role in the chemoreception process.[91]

Other putative neurotransmitters reported to be present in the type I cells include neuropeptide Y, galanin, cholecystokinin, vasoactive intestinal peptide (VIP), calcitonin gene-related peptide (CGRP), atrial natriuretic peptide (ANP) and endothelin. There are some interesting findings regarding ANP which are reviewed in detail in chapter 8 by Almaraz et al. Endothelin has been localized in the rat and cat CB, being demonstrated by binding and functional studies that chemoreceptor cells possess receptors for the peptide.[92-94] Endothelin would represent the prototype modulator of chemoreceptor activity: endothelin levels are modified by acute and chronic hypoxia, when pharmacologically injected potentiates CSN discharges and ventilation and endothelin actions are blocked by specific antagonists, but the same antagonists do not alter the responses to hypoxia. It has also been reported recently that mouse CB type I cells are positive for glutamate decarboxylase and its product GABA.[95] It is possible that all these substances play some role in fine-tuning the traffic of signal transduction information exchanged between type I cells and CSN sensory endings. Essential to understanding this process will be the mapping of receptor populations for these substances, as well as the thorough study of their metabolism and pharmacological actions.

CONCLUDING REMARKS AND PERSPECTIVES

The CB is a secondary sensory receptor in which the sensory chemoreceptor cells are connected with the sensory nerve endings by chemical synapses. The study of this chemical synapse has been, historically speaking, full of controversies and plagued of experimental data of doubtful significance. Amongst the controversies it should be underlined the proposal of hypothesis of chemoreception as if the CB chemoreceptors were primary sensory receptors, and therefore denying the existence of a synapse between chemoreceptor cells and sensory nerve endings. These hypotheses slowed dramatically the advance of the study of chemical transmission, as they forced many laboratories to repeat experiments that ultimately reinstated neurotransmission as a necessary step for chemoreception. Among the data of doubtful significance, it should be mentioned, following McQueen,[69] the great number of single or few doses pharmacological experiments that lead to questionable conclusions which require a great deal of effort to demonstrate their rightness or wrongness. It should be added that in the field of the CB there has been a great inertia, or even resistance, to accept genuine progresses; the case of the in vitro preparation comes to mind. However, in spite of this inertia, we have been forced to the main stream of current trends in biology, and it is gratifying to read articles on CB physiology in general, and CB neurotransmission in particular, involving the use of the most modern techniques of molecular biology or cell imaging.

The experimentally supported body of doctrine on neurotransmission in the CB, we believe, lags behind general knowledge on CB physiology. The field has not attracted enough neurochemists or electrophysiologists devoted to the study of synapses. On the other hand, so many neurotransmitters have appeared in the last 15 years that the groups working in the CB chemoreceptors have been unable of satisfactorily digest such abundant banquet. Many of us have been trying bits of this or the other neurotransmitter as a means to have a personal opinion on the particular. Obviously, this is the frame in which our chapter has been written, and fairness forces to say that at the present moment it is not known how the chemoreceptor cell/sensory nerve ending synapse works, mostly because the identity of the primary neurotransmitter conveyor of the information from cells to nerve endings is not known.

Surely readers have noticed that the authors make a case for DA as a plausible candidate for that role. Our personal bias has two simple reasons: first, DA is the only chemoreceptor cell neurotransmitter with identified receptors in the postsynaptic element of the synapse, and second, the many years of research in our laboratories devoted to the study of DA in the CB have generated a wealth of data which can readily be interpreted considering that DA is the primary neurotransmitter. Additionally, most, if not all, data present in the literature and used as arguments against the primary role of DA at the chemosensory synapse can be satisfactorily explained within the dopaminergic hypothesis. However, if somebody would ask if we are sure that DA is the main neurotransmitter, the answer must be no, we are not sure. There are other potential candidates for such a role, but the lack of data on their metabolism or on the location of their receptors, added to unsolved controversies in the description of their pharmacological actions, faint those potential candidates. The possibility exists that the primary neurotransmitter in the CB is not yet discovered. Sooner or later researchers in the CB field will have preparations suitable for the study of the microphysiology and micropharmacology of the sensory synapse; only then, the answers would have the possibility of being unequivocal. In the meantime, neurochemical studies characterizing the metabolism of neurotransmitters as a function of the activity of the organ, and receptor binding studies for the known neurotransmitters, coupled to in situ hybridization or to immuno-histochemical location of the receptors, would allow us to envision the direction(s) of the information flowing in the synaptic complexes formed by chemoreceptor cells and the sensory nerve endings of the CSN. Whatever the neurotransmitter chosen to our study, experimental designs and data interpretations should follow the rules of the general field of neurotransmission, and we should be skeptical when our findings do not fit the general doctrine on neurotransmission. A special attention should be paid to the interpretation of any possible finding in the context of the organ and system physiology. To gain power in the analysis of unitary physiological and/or biophysical data, we are forced to use simplified preparations; the tribute to that can be that we are generating very interesting information, but letting out of consideration the important issues of the CB physiology. Finally, we should always keep in mind, in interpreting our findings, that the CB is the origin of chemoreflexes which have different properties along the life-span of individuals.

Acknowledgments

This work was supported by Spanish DGICYT grant PB92/0267 and by U.S. NIH grants NS07938 and NS12636.

References

1. Zhong H, Nurse C. Co-cultures of rat petrosal neurons and carotid body type I cells: A model for studying chemosensory mechanisms. Adv Exp Med Biol 1996; 410:189-193.
2. Hayashida Y, Koyano H, Eyzaguirre C. An intracellular study of chemosensory fibers and endings. J Neurophysiol 1980; 44:1077-1088.
3. Schweitzer A, Wright S. Action of prostigmine and acetylcholine on respiration. Q J Exp Physiol 1938; 28:33-47.
4. Heymans C, Bouckaert JJ, Farber S, Hsu FJ. Influence réflexogène de l'acétylcholine sur les terminaisons nerveuses chimio-sensitives du sinus carotidien. Arch Int Pharmacodyn Ther 1936; 54: 129-135.
5. Fidone SJ, González C. Initiation and control of chemoreceptor activity in the carotid body. In: Fishman AP, ed. Handbook of Physiology. The Respiratoy System. Bethesda: Amer Physiol Soc, 1986: 247-312.
6. Eyzaguirre C, Zapata P. A discussion of possible transmitter or generator substances in carotid body chemoreceptors. In: Torrance RW, ed. Arterial Chemoreceptors. Oxford, UK: Blackwell Scientific Publications, 1968:213-251.
7. Jones JV. Localization and quantitation of the carotid body enzymes: their relevance to the cholinergic transmitter hypothesis. In: Purves MJ, ed. The Peripheral Arterial Chemoreceptors. London, UK: Cambridge University Press, 1975: 143-162.
8. Fidone SJ, Weintraub ST, Stavinoha WB. Acetylcholine content of normal and denervated cat carotid bodies measured by pyrolysis gas chromatography/mass fragmentometry. J Neurochem 1976; 26:1047-1049.
9. Hellstrom S. Putative neurotransmitters in the carotid body. Mass fragmentographic studies. Adv Biochem Psychopharmacol 1977; 16:257-263.
10. Wang ZZ, Stensaas LJ, Dinger B, Fidone S. The co-existence of biogenic amines and neuropeptides in the type I cells of the cat carotid body. Neuroscience 1992; 47:473-480.
11. Wang ZZ, Stensaas LJ, Dinger B, Fidone SJ. Immunocytochemical localization of choline acetyltransferase in the carotid body of the cat and rabbit. Brain Res 1989; 498:131-134.
12. Fidone S, Weintraub S, Stavinoha W, Stirling C, Jones L. Endogenous acetylcholine levels in cat carotid body and the autoradiographic localization of a high affinity component of choline uptake. In: Acker H, Fidone S, Pallot D, Eyzaguirre C, Lübbers DW, Torrance RW, eds. Chemoreception in the Carotid Body. Berlin: Springer-Verlag, 1977:106-113.
13. Fitzgerald RS, Shirahata M. Acetylcholine and carotid body excitation during hypoxia in the cat. J Appl Physiol 1994; 76(4):1566-1574.
14. Fitzgerald RS, Shirahata M, Ide T, Lydic R. The cholinergic hypothesis revisited—an unfinished story. Biol Signals 1995; 4:298-303.
15. McQueen DS. A quantitative study of the effects of cholinergic drugs on carotid chemoreceptors in the cat. J Physiol Lond 1977; 273:515-532.
16. Dinger B, González C, Yoshizaki K, Fidone S. Localization and function of cat carotid body nicotinic receptors. Brain Res 1985; 339:295-304.
17. Dinger BG, Almaraz L, Hirano T, et al. Muscarinic receptor localization and function in rabbit carotid body. Brain Res 1991; 562:190-198.
18. Hirano T, Dinger B, Yoshizaki K, González C, Fidone S. Nicotinic versus muscarinic binding sites in cat and rabbit carotid bodies. Biol Signals 1992; 1: 143-149.

19. González C, Almaraz L, Obeso A, Rigual R. Carotid body chemoreceptors: from natural stimuli to sensory discharges. Physiol Rev 1994; 74:829-898
20. Hayashida Y, Eyzaguirre C. Voltage noise of carotid body type I cells. Brain Res 1979; 167:189-194.
21. Wyatt CN, Peers C. Nicotinic acetylcholine receptors in isolated type I cells of the neonatal rat carotid body. Neuroscience 1993; 54:275-281.
22. Gomez-Niño A, Dinger B, González C, Fidone SJ. Differential stimulus coupling to dopamine and norepinephrine stores in rabbit carotid body type I cells. Brain Res 1990; 525:160-164.
23. Dasso LLT, Buckler KJ, Vaughan-Jones RD. Muscarinic and nicotinic receptors rise intracellular Ca^{2+} in rat carotid body type I cells. J Physiol 1997; 498:327-338.
24. Obeso A, Gomez-Niño A, Almaraz L, Dinger B, Fidone S, González C. Evidence for two types of nicotinic receptors in the cat carotid body chemoreceptor cells. Brain Res 1997; 754:298-302.
25. Monti Bloch L, Eyzaguirre C. A comparative physiological and pharmacological study of cat and rabbit carotid body chemoreceptors. Brain Res 1980; 193: 449-470.
26. Eyzaguirre C, Fidone S, Nishi K. Recent studies on the generation of chemoreceptor impulses. In: Purves MJ, ed. The Peripheral Arterial Chemoreceptors. London, UK: Cambridge University Press, 1975:175-194.
27. Perez-Garcia MT, Gómez-Niño A, Almaraz L, González C. Neurotransmitters and second messenger systems in the carotid body. Adv Exp Med Biol 1993; 337:279-287.
28. Lever JD, Boyd JD. Osmiophile granules in glomus cells of the rabbit carotid body. Nature London 1957; 179: 1082-1083.
29. Fidone S, González C, Yoshizaki K. Effects of low oxygen on the release of dopamine from the rabbit carotid body in vitro. J Physiol Lond 1982; 333:93-110.
30. Pequignot JM, Cottet Emard JM, Dalmaz Y, Peyrin L. Dopamine and norepinephrine dynamics in rat carotid body during long-term hypoxia. J Auton Nerv Syst 1987; 21:9-14.
31. Rigual R, González E, González C, Fidone S. Synthesis and release of catecholamines by the cat carotid body in vitro: effects of hypoxic stimulation. Brain Res 1986; 374:101-109.
32. Rigual R, Lopez-Lopez JR, González C. Release of dopamine and chemoreceptor discharge induced by low pH and high PCO_2 stimulation of the cat carotid body. J Physiol Lond 1991; 433:519-531.
33. Obeso A, Almaraz L, González C. Effects of 2-deoxy-D-glucose on in vitro cat carotid body. Brain Res 1986; 371:25-36.
34. Obeso A, Almaraz L, González C. Effects of cyanide and uncouplers on chemoreceptor activity and ATP content of the cat carotid body. Brain Res 1989; 481: 250-257.
35. Obeso A, Rocher A, Fidone S, González C. The role of dihydropyridine-sensitive Ca^{2+} channels in stimulus-evoked catecholamine release from chemoreceptor cells of the carotid body. Neuroscience 1992; 47:463-472.
36. Donnelly DF. Electrochemical detection of catecholamine release from rat carotid body in vitro. J Appl Physiol 1993; 74:2330-2337.
37. Buerk DG, Lahiri S, Chugh D, Mokashi A. Electrochemical detection of rapid DA release kinetics during hypoxia in perfused superfused cat CB. J Appl Physiol 1995; 78(3):830-837.
38. Donnelly DF, Doyle TP. Developmental changes in hypoxia induced catecholamine release from rat carotid body in vitro. J Physiol 1994; 475(2):267-275.
39. Donnelly DF. Does catecholamine secretion mediate the hypoxia-induced increase in nerve activity? Biol Signals 1995; 4:304-309.
40. Bairam A, Basson H, Marchal F et al. Effects of hypoxia on carotid body dopamine content and release in developing rabbits. J Appl Physiol 1996; 80:20-24.
41. Almaraz L, González C, Obeso A. Effects of high potassium on the release of [3H]dopamine from the cat carotid body in vitro. J Physiol Lond 1986; 379: 293-307.
42. Artalejo AR, Garcia AG, Montiel C, Sanchez-Garcia P. A dopaminergic receptor modulates catecholamine release

from the cat adrenal gland. J Physiol 1985; 362:359-368.
43. Garcia AG, Kirpekar SM, Sanchez-Garcia P. Release of noradrenaline from the cat spleen by nerve stimulation and potassium. J Physiol 1976; 261:301-317.
44. Fuder H, Muscholl E, Wegwart R. The effects of methacholine and calcium deprivation on the release of the false transmitter alfa-methyladrenaline from the isolated rabbit heart. Naunyn-Schmiedeberg's Arch Pharmacol 1976; 293: 225-234.
45. Leitner LM, Roumy M. Chemoreceptor response to hypoxia and hypercapnia in catecholamine depleted rabbit and cat carotid bodies in vitro. Pflugers Arch 1986; 406:419-423.
46. Fidone S, González C, Dinger B, Gomez-Niño A, Obeso A, Yoshizaki K. Cellular aspects of peripheral chemoreceptor function. In: Crystal RG, West JB, eds. The Lung. Scientific Foundations. New York: Raven Press, 1991:1319-1332.
47. Almaraz L, Perez Garcia MT, Gomez-Niño A, González C. Mechanisms of alfa-2 adrenoceptor-mediated inhibition in rabbit carotid body. Am J Physiol 1997; 272:C628-C637.
48. González-Guerrero PR, Rigual R, González C. Opioid peptides in the rabbit carotid body: Identification and evidence for co-utilization and interactions with dopamine. J Neurochem 1993; 60:1762-1768.
49. Gomez-Niño A, Lopez-Lopez JR, Almaraz L, González C. Inhibition of ^{3}H-catecholamine release and Ca^{2+} currents by prostaglandin E_2 in the rabbit carotid body chemoreceptor cells. J Physiol Lond 1994; 476:269-277.
50. González E, Rigual R, Fidone SJ, González C. Mechanisms for termination of the action of dopamine in carotid body chemoreceptors. J Auton Nerv Syst 1987; 18:249-259.
51. Hess A. The effects of 6-hydroxydopamine on the appearance of granulated vesicles in glomus cells of the rat carotid body. Tissue Cell 1976; 8:381-387.
52. Zuazo A, Zapata P. Effects of 6-hydroxy-dopamine on carotid body chemosensory activity. Neurosci Lett 1978; 9:323-328.
53. Dinger B, González C, Yoshizaki K, Fidone S. [^{3}H]Spiroperidol binding in normal and denervated carotid bodies. Neurosci Lett 1981; 21:51-55.
54. Mir AK, McQueen DS, Pallot DJ, Nahorski SR. Direct biochemical and neuropharmacological identification of dopamine D2-receptors in the rabbit carotid body. Brain Res 1984; 291:273-283.
55. Czyzyk-Krseska MF, Lawson EE, Millhorn DE. Expression of D_2 dopamine receptor mRNA in the arterial chemoreceptor afferent pathway. J Auton Nerv Syst 1992; 41:31-40.
56. Verna A, Schamel A, Le Moine C, Bloch B. Localization of dopamine D_2 receptor mRNA in glomus cells of the rabbit carotid body by in situ hybridization. J Neurocytol 1995; 24:265-270.
57. Gauda EB, Shirahata M, Fitzgerald RS. D2-dopamine receptor mRNA in the carotid body and petrosal ganglia in the developing cat. Adv Exp Med Biol 1994; 360:317-319.
58. Almaraz L, Perez-Garcia MT, González C. Presence of D1 receptors in the rabbit carotid body. Neurosci Lett 1991; 132:259-262.
59. Bairam A, Dauphin C, Rousseau F, Khandjian EW. Expression of dopamine D2-receptor mRNA isoforms at the peripheral chemoreflex afferent pathway in developing rabbits. Am J Respir Cell Mol Biol 1996; 15:374-381.
60. Docherty RJ, McQueen DS. Inhibitory action of dopamine on cat carotid chemoreceptors. J Physiol Lond 1978; 279:425-436.
61. Llados F, Zapata P. Effects of dopamine analogues and antagonists on carotid body chemosensors in situ. J Physiol Lond 1978; 274:487-499.
62. Zapata P. Effects of dopamine on carotid chemo- and baroreceptors in vitro. J Physiol Lond 1975; 244:235-251.
63. Lehmann J, Briley M, Langer SZ. Characterization of dopamine autoreceptor and [^{3}H]-spiperone binding sites in vitro with classical and novel dopamine receptor agonists. Eur J Pharmacol 1983; 88:11-26.
64. Siggins GR. Monoamines and message transduction in central neurons. In: Magistretti PJ, Morrison JH, Reisine TD,

eds. Transduction of Neuronal Signals. Geneva: FESN, 1986:61-68.

65. Trendelenburg U. Factors Influencing the concentration of catecholamines at the receptors. In: Blaschko H, Muscholl E, eds. Handbook of Pharmacology vol. XXXIII: Catecholamines. Berlin: Springer-Verlag, 1972:726-761.
66. Van Buskirk R, Dowling JE. Calcium alters the sensitivity of intact horizontal cells to dopamine antagonist. Proc Natl Acad Sci USA 1982; 79:3350-3354.
67. Kato E, Narahashi T. Characteristics of the electrical response to dopamine in neuroblastoma cells. J Physiol Lond 1982; 333:213-236.
68. Kuffler S. The effect of calcium on the neuromuscular junction. J Neurophysiol 1944; 7:17-31.
69. McQueen DS. Pharmacological aspects of putative transmitters in the carotid body. In: Acker H, O'Regan RG, eds. Physiology of the Peripheral Arterial Chemoreceptors. Amsterdam: Elsevier Science Publishers, 1983:149-195.
70. Aminoff MJ, Jaffe RA, Sampson SR, Vidruk EH. Effects of droperidol on activity of carotid body chemoreceptors in cat. Br J Pharmacol 1978; 63:245-250.
71. Hanson G, Jones L, Fidone S. Physiological chemoreceptor stimulation decreases enkephalin and substance P in the carotid body. Peptides 1986; 7:767-769.
72. Heath D, Smith P. Diseases of the Human Carotid Body. London, UK: Springer-Verlag, 1992:63-72.
73. Wharton J, Polak JM, Pearse AG, et al. Enkephalin-, VIP- and substance P-like immunoreactivity in the carotid body. Nature 1980; 284:269-271.
74. González-Guerrero PR, Rigual R, González C. Effects of chronic hypoxia on opioid peptide and catecholamine levels and on the release of dopamine in the rabbit carotid body. J Neurochem 1993; 60:1769-1776.
75. Kirby GC, McQueen DS. Characterization of opioid receptors in the cat carotid body involved in chemosensory depression in vivo. Br J Pharmacol 1986; 88: 889-898.
76. Ward PW, Milledge JS, West JB, eds. High Altitude Medicine and Physiology. 2nd ed. London: Chapman & Hall, 1995:69-97.
77. Weil JV. Ventilatory control at high altitude. In: Fishman AP, ed. Handbook of Physiology. The Respiratory System. Bethesda: Am Physiol Soc, 1986:703-727.
78. Stea A, Jackson A, Nurse CA. Hypoxia and N6,O2-dibutyryladenosine 3', 5'-cyclic monophosphate, but not nerve growth factor, induce Na^+ channels and hypertrophy in chromaffin-like arterial chemoreceptors. Proc Natl Acad Sci USA 1992; 82:9469-9473.
79. Cuello AC, McQueen DS. Substance P: a carotid body peptide. Neurosci Lett 1980; 17:215-219.
80. Lundberg JM, Hokfelt T, Fahrenkrug J, Nilsson G, Terenius L. Peptides in the cat carotid body (glomus caroticum): VIP-, enkephalin-, and substance P-like immunoreactivity. Acta Physiol Scand 1979; 107:279-281.
81. Chen IV, Yates RD, Hanse JT. Substance P-like immunoreactivity in rat and cat carotid body. Histol Histopathol 1986; 1:203-212.
82. Scheibner T, Read DJ, Sullivan CE. Distribution of substance P-immunoreactive structures in the developing cat carotid body. Brain Res 1988; 453:72-78.
83. Prabhakar NR, Landis SC, Kumar GK, Mullikin Kilpatrick D, Cherniack NS, Leeman S. Substance P and neurokinin A in the cat carotid body: localization, exogenous effects and changes in content in response to arterial pO_2. Brain Res 1989; 481:205-214.
84. Kusakabe T, Kawakami T, Tanabe Y, Fujii S, Takenaka T. Distribution of substance P containing and catecholaminergic nerve fibers in the rabbit carotid body: an immunohistochemical study in combination with catecholamine fluorescent histochemistry. Arch Histol Cytol 1994; 57(2):193-199.
85. Pizarro J, Ryan ML, Hedrick MS, Xue DH, Keith IM, Bisgard GE. Intracarotid substance P infusion inhibits ventilation in the goat. Respir Physiol 1995; 101: 11-22.
86. Prabhakar NR, Gauda E, Cherniack NS. The mechanism of action of tachykinins in the carotid body. In: Eyzaguirre C, Fidone SJ, Fitzgerald RS, Lahiri S,

McDonald DM, eds. Arterial Chemoreception. New York, N.Y: Springer Verlag, 1990:192-198.

87. McQueen DS, Evrard Y. Use of selective antagonists for studying the role of putative transmitters in chemoreception. In: Eyzaguirre C, Fidone SJ, Fitzgerald RS, Lahiri S, McDonald DM, eds. Arterial Chemoreception. New York, NY: Springer-Verlag, 1990:168-173.
88. Prabhakar NR, Cao H, Lowe III JA, Snider RM. Selective inhibition of the carotid body sensory response to hypoxia by the substance P receptor antagonist CP-96,345. Proc Natl Acad Sci USA 1993; 90:10041-10045.
89. De-Sanctis GT, Green FH, Jiang X, King M, Remmers JE. Ventilatory responses to hypoxia in rats pretreated with nonpeptide NK1 receptor antagonist CP-96345. J Appl Physiol 1994; 76(4): 1528-1532.
90. Schmidt AW, McLean S, Heym J. The substance P receptor antagonist CP-96345 interacts with Ca^{2+} channels. Eur J Pharmacol 1992; 219:491-492.
91. Yoshioka M. Effect of a novel 5-hydroxytryptamine3-antagonist, GR38032F, on the 5-hydroxytryptamine-induced increase in carotid sinus nerve activity in rats. J Pharmacol Exp Ther 1989; 250: 637-641.
92. Dashwood MR, McQueen DS, Sykes RM, et al. The effects of almitrine on (^{3}H)5HT and (^{125}I) endothelin binding to central and peripheral receptors: an in vitro autoradiographic study in the cat. Adv Exp Med Biol 1993; 337:17-23.
93. He L, Chen J, Dinger B, Fidone S. Endothelin modulates chemoreceptor cell function in mammalian carotid body. Adv Exp Med Biol 1996; 410:305-311
94. McQueen DS, Dashwood MR, Cobb VJ, Bond SM, Marr CG, Spyer KM. Endothelins and rat carotid body: autoradiographic and functional pharmacological studies. J Auton Nerv Syst 1995; 53: 115-125.
95. Oomori Y, Nakaya K, Iuchi H, Ishikawa K, Satoh Y, Ono K. Immunohistochemical and histochemical evidence for the presence of noradrenaline, serotonin and gamma-aminobutyric acid in chief cells of the mouse carotid body. Cell Tissue Res 1994; 278(2):249-254.

CHAPTER 4

Electrical Properties of Chemoreceptor Cells

José Ramón López-López and Chris Peers

INTRODUCTION

Carotid body (CB) chemoreceptor cells, in spite of their neural origin, were considered nonexcitable until the late 1980s. The remarkable complexity of the organ, together with the small size of type I cells, represented a limitation for conventional intracellular microelectrode recordings, making a definitive electrophysiological study problematic. The neurochemical approach used during the early 1980s, following the stimulus-secretion model established in other neurosecretory systems, suggested an important role for the plasma membrane of type I cells in the hypoxic chemotransduction process. Development of isolated type I cell cultures, together with the use of the patch-clamp technique, have brought direct evidence in support of this idea.[1,2] We now have a general picture about the electrical properties of these cells, and their excitable character is unequivocally established; they possess voltage-dependent ion channels and they are capable of firing action potentials. Although there is a general agreement in the literature about the basic facts, the details are far from clear. The role of ionic currents in the transduction process by type I cells has been a matter of discussion, and differences in the results reported by different laboratories are evident. In most of the cases the differences could be interpreted on basis of the fact that either cells from different species or at different stages of development have been studied, but in some cases, the differences have led to the proposal of different hypotheses about the mechanisms of chemotransduction.

This chapter will present an overview of the ionic currents present in type I cells, and will especially on those differences. All patch-clamp data available so far have been obtained from rabbit or rat type I cells isolated either from adult or neonatal animals. When physiological intra- and extracellular solutions are used, chemoreceptor cells exhibit, on step depolarization, inward currents due to Na^+ and/or Ca^{2+} channels, and outward currents due to

The Carotid Body Chemoreceptors,
edited by Constancio González. © 1997 Landes Bioscience.

multiple types of K^+ channels. Below, we consider the separate ionic currents of type I cells, and compare results obtained from different preparations in different laboratories.

Na^+ CURRENTS

Using standard procedures for blocking K^+ currents (i.e., intracellular Cs^+) and Ca^{2+} currents (i.e., extracellular Cd^{2+}), Na^+ currents (I_{Na}) can be routinely recorded in isolation in adult rabbit type I cells[3,4] (Fig. 4.1A). I_{Na} is sensitive to tetrodotoxin (TTX), has an apparent activation threshold around -40 mV and a fast activation time course, reaching its peak in less than 1 ms. The peak amplitude at 0 mV is approximately 0.4 nA on average. The half steady-state inactivation occurs at a membrane potential of -50 mV. Inactivation follows a monoexponential time course, with a time constant of 0.67 ms at 0 mV. All these characteristics are typical of Na^+ currents found in other neurosecretory cells.

Na^+ currents have not been found in rabbit embryos[5] and their presence is not ubiquitously reported in rat type I cells. Some groups have reported a lack of Na^+ currents in freshly dissociated type I cells from adult[6] and young rats.[7] However, other groups have reported rapidly activating and inactivating TTX-sensitive Na^+ currents present in cells from young rats maintained in long-term cultures[8] or in freshly dissociated cells from adult[9] and neonatal rats.[10] The wide range of reported percentages of cells having Na^+

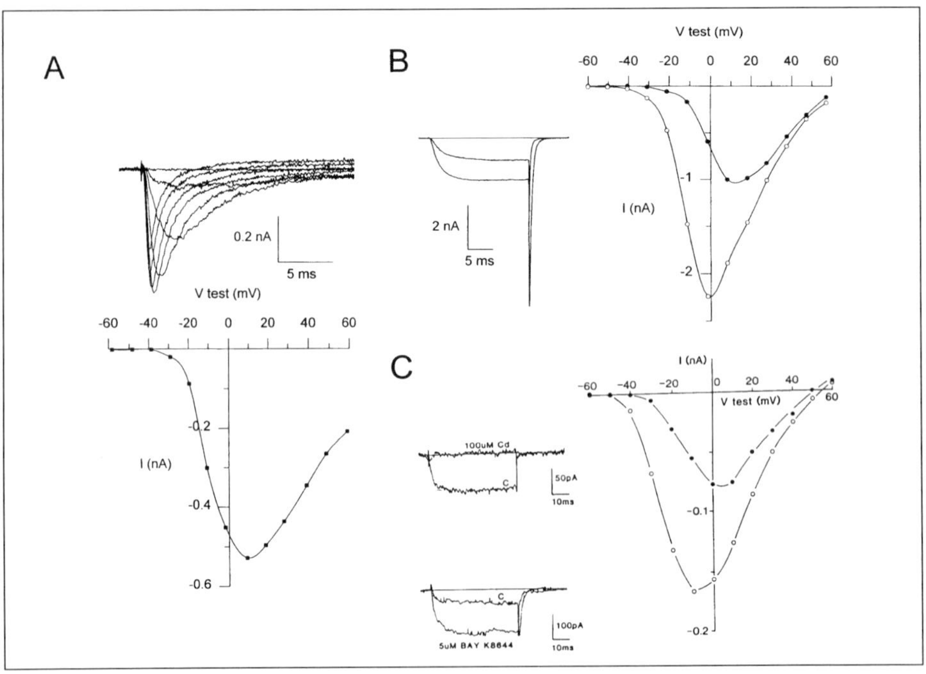

Fig. 4.1. Whole-cell inward currents recorded in adult rabbit (A & B) and neonatal rat (C) cells. (A) Family of Na^+ currents recorded in the presence of 0.1 mM Cd^{2+}. The I-V relationship of the peak current is also shown. (B) I-V relationship for Ca^{2+} currents obtained in an adult rabbit chemoreceptor cell using 10 mM Ca^{2+} (filled circles) or 10 mM Ba^{2+} (open circles) as charge carriers. Na^+ currents are blocked with 0.1 mM TTX. The currents obtained with Ca^{2+} and Ba^{2+} at +10 mV are shown superimposed. (C) Ca^{2+} channel currents recorded in a neonatal rat type I cell using 10 mM Ba^{2+} as charge carrier. Note the lack of rapidly activating and inactivating Na^+ current, despite the fact that TTX was not present. Ca^{2+} channel currents could be fully blocked by 100 mM Cd^{2+} and enhanced by the DHP agonist Bay K 8644 (5 mM). The I-V relationship from the same cell is shown in the absence (filled circles) and presence (open circles) of Bay K 8644.

currents in rat cells (from none[6,7] to 46% [10]) may reflect age-related differences or more likely, an heterogeneous expression of Na^+ channels in type I cells, as has been proposed with respect to the different types of Ca^{2+} channels (see below).

Ca^{2+} CURRENTS

Neurochemical studies of dopamine release from intact carotid bodies implicated L-type (dihydropyridine (DHP)-sensitive) Ca^{2+} channels as being involved in hypoxic chemotransduction before their presence was confirmed with the patch-clamp technique.[11,12] Typically, Ca^{2+} currents (I_{Ca}) can be recorded in isolated type I cells when K^+ currents are blocked with internal Cs^+, and TTX is present in the bath solution. I_{Ca} is present in both rabbit and rat cells, and it appears to be mainly due to L-type Ca^{2+} channels (Figs. 4.1B and C).

Kinetic properties of I_{Ca} have been studied thoroughly in rabbit cells using both Ca^{2+} and Ba^{2+} as charge carriers[3,4] (Fig. 4.1B). The apparent activation threshold is about -40 mV, and the peak current is obtained at +10 to +20 mV. I_{Ca} inactivation is very slow, and 200 ms after the onset of depolarization the current amplitude is still about 70% of the peak current. When I_{Ca} is elicited with a depolarizing pulse, the relatively small current is followed by a much larger inward tail current, the time course of which reflects the closing of Ca^{2+} channels and has been used to define the type of Ca^{2+} channels present in type I cells. Tail currents can be fitted by the sum of two exponential functions, suggesting that I_{Ca} is carried through more than one type of Ca^{2+} channel. The biggest component has a time constant typical of the fast deactivating or L-type currents (160 ms). The other component (20 times smaller) could reflect the slow deactivating or T-type current, although its presence has not been confirmed using different voltage protocols. I_{Ca} shows also the phenomenon of wash out or run down. Wash out is use- and ATP-dependent, as happens typically with L-type Ca^{2+} currents.[3,4]

In the last few years the classification of Ca^{2+} channels in different cells has been made mainly through pharmacological criteria, using different peptide toxins. At present, there is little available evidence in the literature concerning the use of toxins to further characterize I_{Ca} in rabbit type I cells. However, a recent brief report[13] has indicated that I_{Ca} in adult rabbit type I cells is sensitive to ω-conotoxin GVIA and to ω-agatoxin IVA as well as to nifedipine, indicating the possible presence, in addition to L-type channels, of N- and P-type. This finding supports the idea that multiple Ca^{2+} channel types coexist in adult rabbit type I cells.

Rabbit embryo type I cells also have Ca^{2+} currents with properties similar to those of the adult animals, which are activated by the DHP agonist Bay K8644 and blocked by D600, as expected for L-type Ca^{2+} channels.[5] However, blockade of I_{Ca} is incomplete even when high (10 mM) concentrations of organic blockers are used, which may suggest that these cells also possess non-L-type Ca^{2+} channels.[5]

Whole-cell patch-clamp recordings from neonatal (as well as adult) rat type I cells have confirmed the presence of L-type channels, since whole-cell Ca^{2+} channel currents can be enhanced by Bay K 8644, and can be suppressed by DHP blockers[7,14,15] (Fig. 4.1C). However, as for adult rabbit cells (see above), L-type channels do not account for all of the Ca^{2+} channel current: maximal or supramaximal concentrations of DHP blockers do not completely inhibit Ca^{2+} currents,[15-17] nor do they fully prevent the voltage-dependent rise of $[Ca^{2+}]_i$ seen in response to high K^+-containing solutions.[18,19] The remaining, non-L-type current has yet to be fully characterized, but there is evidence for a heterogeneous distribution of N-type channels in some type I cells from young and adult rats. Fieber and McCleskey found the N-type channel blocker ω-conotoxin GVIA (ω-CgTx) to partially inhibit currents in one of four cells,[6] and studies in 10 day old rat type I cells have shown partial inhibition by ω-CgTx in two out of eight cells.[16] Stea et al reported a lack of effect of ω-CgTx,[14] but its effects were only tested in four cells. The possibility that N-type channels exist in some but not all type I cells would suggest that the cells themselves are heterogeneous (although Silva and Lewis have reported a 40% inhibition of peak Ca^{2+} current by ω-CgTx in all the cells they have tested, when recording in type I cells from adult rats).[15] These findings also suggest that type I cells from young and also adult rats possess a type or types of Ca^{2+} channel which are not L- or N-type.

Despite the similar, heterogeneous nature of Ca^{2+} channels in rabbit and rat type I cells, the difference in size of whole cell currents is quite remarkable. Using Ba^{2+} as the charge carrier, the peak amplitude is about 50 pA in rat type I cells, more than 10 times smaller than the Ca^{2+} currents in adult rabbit cells (typically ranging between 0.4 and 1 nA); if we take into account the fact that the size of the cells are similar, the density of channels per unit of membrane surface area has to be much bigger in the adult rabbit type I cells.

K^+ CURRENTS

When type I cells are dialyzed with a solution containing high [K^+], and are perfused with a solution of physiological composition, the dominant currents elicited upon membrane depolarization are outward currents that exhibit a voltage dependence and a sensitivity to blockers such as tetraethylammonium (TEA) and 4-aminopyridine (4-AP), characteristic of K^+ currents (IK).[3-5,20,21]

IK from rabbit type I cells can be divided into at least three different components.[20] If IK is recorded in the absence of Ca^{2+} channels blockers, the current-voltage (I-V) relationship exhibits a typical outward shoulder at voltages between 0 and +40 mV (the potential range at which the Ca^{2+} current is predominant). This shoulder disappears either after Ca^{2+} channel currents wash out or after application of Ca^{2+} channel blockers (Fig. 4.2A). Therefore this component of IK

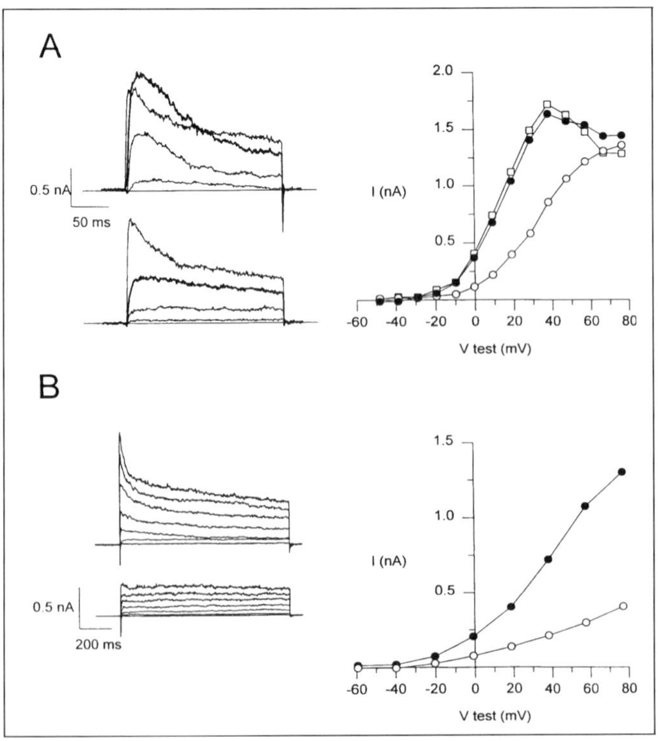

Fig. 4.2. Whole-cell K^+ currents recorded in adult rabbit chemoreceptor cells. (A) I-V relationship for IK obtained in solution control (open squares), in the presence of 1 mM Co^{2+} (open circles) and after washing the solution with Co^{2+} (filled circles). The typical shoulder in the I-V curve, due to the Ca^{2+}-dependent K^+ channels, is clearly inhibited by the Ca^{2+} channel blocker Co^{2+}. The currents shown are those elicited at -10, +10, +30 (thicker trace) and +70 mV, both in solution control (up) and in the presence of Co^{2+} (down). (B) I-V relationship of IK_V obtained (after Ca^{2+} currents washed out) in a physiological solution (filled circles) and in the presence of 1 mM 4-AP. The original traces are also shown. Note how in the presence of 4-AP (down), the inactivating component of the current is not present.

is clearly due to Ca^{2+}-dependent K^+ channels, the presence of which has been confirmed using single channel recordings.[22] Although only a 210 pS Ca^{2+}-dependent K^+ channel (maxi-K or BK) has been recorded at the single channel level, the shoulder in the IK I-V relationship is also partially inhibited by apamin,[3] suggesting the presence of small conductance Ca^{2+}-dependent K^+ channels in rabbit cells.

When I_K is recorded after Ca^{2+} currents are washed out or in the presence of Ca^{2+}-channel blockers, only the voltage-dependent component of IK (IK_v) remains. IK_v inactivates during long step depolarizations, but the inactivation is not complete, suggesting that more than one type of channel is contributing to IK_v. In fact, two different components can be isolated using 4-AP[20] (Fig. 4.2B). The inactivating component is fully removed by the application of 1 mM 4-AP (IC_{50} of 0.2 mM) and both the transient and the noninactivating components are sensitive to TEA at concentrations greater than 5 mM. The existence of these two components are confirmed when steady-state inactivation properties are studied. H∞ curves are well fitted with a Boltzman distribution plus a constant component (the noninactivating component) which only represents 10% of the total IK_v.[20] The apparent threshold for activation of IK_v

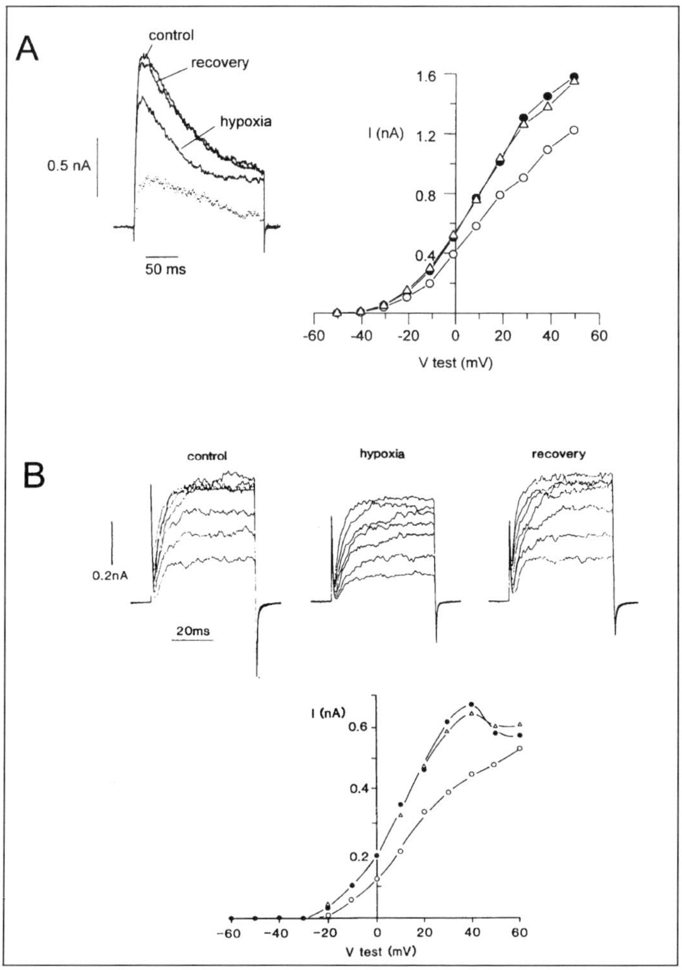

Fig. 4.3. Effects of hypoxia on whole-cell K^+ currents from adult rabbit (A) and neonatal rat (B) cells. I-V relationships of IK recorded in an adult rabbit (A) and in a neonatal rat (B) type I cell before (filled circles), during (open circles) and after (open triangles) exposure of the cell to hypoxia (≈5 mmHg in A, ≈25 mmHg in B). The actual currents obtained at +40 mV as indicated in the rabbit cells, and the difference between control and hypoxia (dotted line) are also shown in A. The whole family of currents obtained in the rat cell are shown in B.

is around -40 mV, and this is also the potential at which the transient current is 50% inactivated in the steady state. The time course of the inactivation is relatively slow, and it can be described by two exponential functions with time constants of 80 and 825 ms.[20] At the single channel level, two different voltage-dependent, Ca^{2+}-insensitive channels have been described from inside-out excised patches.[22] One of them, named SK, has a conductance of 16 pS and exhibits very slow activation and almost no inactivation at all. The other is the most frequently found; it has a conductance of 40 pS and shows activation and inactivation kinetics quite similar to those found in the transient current seen in whole-cell recordings. It has been called Ko_2, because is the only one that is inhibited by hypoxia in excised patches.[22,23]

Cells from rabbit embryos also have Ca^{2+}-dependent and voltage-dependent components, both of which are sensitive to TEA.[5] Whole cell IK has not been studied in detail, but a K^+ channel with a conductance of 137 pS has been recorded in the cell-attached configuration. This channel has an open probability that decreases with depolarization and that depends of the O_2 content of the bathing solution.[24]

IK in neonatal rats have amplitudes of around 0.4 nA at +60 mV (although there is a wide cell-to-cell variability), which is much smaller than the typical values that are obtained in adult rabbit cells (typically in the range 1.5 to 3 nA) (compare Figs. 4.2A and 4.3B). The outward K^+ currents of neonatal rat type I cells have been shown to be sensitive to numerous pharmacological blockers including TEA, 4-AP and Ba^{2+} (see refs. 8 and 25). These currents have been divided into a Ca^{2+}-sensitive component and a voltage-gated, Ca^{2+}-insensitive component (IK_{Ca} and IK_v respectively). Since under the recording conditions most commonly used, $[Ca^{2+}]_i$ is not completely buffered, IK_{Ca} can be selectively inhibited with Ca^{2+} channel blockers,[7,21] because activation of K_{Ca} occurs during cell depolarization by Ca^{2+} influx through voltage-gated Ca^{2+} channels. For this reason, as in rabbit cells (see above), whole-cell I-V relationships also display an outward shoulder,[26] with amplitudes increasing steeply with depolarizations from *ca.* -30 mV to +20 mV, but then declining to varying degrees before once more increasing with membrane potential (Fig. 4.4B). Alternatively, IK_{Ca} can be directly inhibited by the scorpion venom peptide charybdotoxin (ChTx),[26] indicating that the underlying channels are high conductance (Maxi-K or BK) channels. More recently, this has been confirmed using single channel recording techniques which have revealed a channel of approximately 200 pS conductance whose activity is steeply dependent on $[Ca^{2+}]_i$ (ref. 27). Apamin has no effect in type I cells of young rats,[26] a finding which contrasts with its ability to partially inhibit K^+ currents in adult rabbit type I cells.[3] The Ca^{2+}-insensitive IK_v of rat type I cells has been less thoroughly studied than IK_{Ca}, but has been shown to have a linear current-voltage relationship, and to be sensitive to 4-AP.[28]

IK in adult rats have been recently characterized,[9] appearing to be very similar to IK in neonatal rats. Two components of IK, Ca^{2+} and voltage-dependent (IK_{Ca} and IK_v, respectively) are also evident, and as in neonatal rat chemoreceptor cells the ChTx sensitive current is predominant. IK_v is a typical delayed rectifier, exhibiting a slow activation and a very slow inactivation, well described by the sum of two exponentials with $t_1 = 0.68$ and $t_2 = 4.96$ seconds.[9] Interestingly, the component of IK attributable to IK_{Ca} increases with age from 4 day old to 10 day old rats, but is similar in 10 day old and adult rat type I cells.[29] This may be of physiological importance, since IK_{Ca} is O_2 sensitive in rat cells (see below) and the maturation of O_2 sensitivity of the intact carotid body (as determined by carotid sinus nerve activity and catecholamine release)[30] is most evident up to 10 days of age.

EFFECTS OF ACUTE HYPOXIA ON IONIC CURRENTS

A major advancement in our understanding of carotid body chemotransduction came with the observation that hypoxia inhibits IK in type I cells. This was first reported in adult rabbit type I cells,[31] and has subsequently been shown to occur in other type I cell preparations. However, the component of IK sensitive to hypoxia is not the same in adult rabbit as compared with embryonic rabbit or rat cells.[8,9,21,24,32]

There are now numerous pieces of evidence from both whole cell and excised patch experiments, supporting the view that the component of IK modulated by O_2 in rabbit cells is the transient component of IK_v (Fig. 4.3A). Low PO_2 reversibly inhibits IK (IK_v)[31,32] when Ca^{2+} channels are washed out (Fig. 4.3A), and in excised patches decreases the open probability of the inactivating K^+ channel (Ko_2).[22,23] The inhibition of the transient K^+ current increases the firing frequency of action potentials in type I cells,[32,33] which would produce an increase in Ca^{2+} entry to the cell through Ca^{2+} channels and an elevation of intracellular Ca^{2+} (ref. 11 and 34). The mechanisms of modulation of IK by O_2 are still a matter of controversy and there are different hypotheses in the literature. Based on the effect of hypoxia in isolated patches, it has been proposed that O_2 interacts with a membrane sensor directly coupled to Ko_2.[1,34] The nature of that sensor is not known, but López-López and González have shown that CO prevents the hypoxic inhibition of IK, suggesting that the sensor could be a heme-linked protein present in the plasma membrane.[35] Other authors, in spite of the effect of low O_2 in isolated patches, have proposed that the sensor is a NAD(P)H oxidase complex, with some of their components located in the membrane and coupled to the K^+ channel through the generation of a second messenger (H_2O_2)[36] (see chapter 5 by Pérez-García and González).

The membrane model of hypoxic transduction, involving the modulation of cell excitability through the effects of O_2 in a K^+ channel, has been challenged by Biscoe and Duchen.[37] Using the same preparation of adult rabbit carotid bodies and cyanide (histotoxic hypoxia) as a stimulus,[38] they did not find an inhibition of IK, and proposed that the effect of any type of hypoxia on ionic currents would be secondary to an elevation of intracellular Ca^{2+}. However, a lack of effect of hypoxia on IK has been also described occasionally in some preparations, and a good correlation exists between this fact and the total inability of the culture to release dopamine in response to hypoxic stimulation.[39]

The effect on whole cell K^+ currents is quite similar in rabbit embryos than in adult cells.[5,24] However, at the single channel level hypoxia decreases the open probability of a 137 pS channel. This channel has a different voltage dependence than the 40 pS channel inhibited in cells from adult animals (see above).[24] We lack a complete characterization of the single channel properties in these embryonic cells, and in order to compare their properties with those found in adult cells such characterization has to be done.

Hypoxia also inhibits K^+ currents in young.[8,21,28] or adult[9,29] rat type I cells. This effect has been shown to be selective for IK_{Ca} (Fig. 4.3B), although other workers have not determined whether or not hypoxia selectively inhibits a specific subtype of K^+ channel in their preparation. Stea and Nurse reported that hypoxia inhibited K^+ currents regardless of whether recordings were made using conventional whole-cell recordings or using perforated-patch recordings; (i.e., with or without dialysis of the cell interior).[8] This finding would suggest that hypoxic inhibition of K^+ channels did not depend on soluble cytosolic factors. However, no means of gauging the rate or extent of cell dialysis during conventional recordings were reported, so the possible involvement of cytosolic mediators cannot be fully discarded. More recently, single channel studies in young rat type I cells have shown that K_{Ca} channels are unaffected by hypoxia in conventional, excised outside-out patches and inhibition by hypoxia was only seen in perforated vesicle recordings where the channels remain in contact with a small volume of cell cytosol.[27] This finding opened up major discrepancies between findings in adult rabbit and young rat type I cells. In rabbit, hypoxia inhibits a specific Ca^{2+}-insensitive Ko_2 channel via a membrane-delimited mechanism.[22,23] In rat, hypoxic inhibition of K_{Ca} channels was dependent on as yet unidentified cytosolic factors.[27] Such differences are difficult to account for at present, but emerging in the literature is the awareness that O_2-sensitive channels are more widespread than in the carotid body,[40,41] and may not be confined to K^+ channel types, since O_2-sensitive L-type Ca^{2+} channels (both native and recombinant) have recently been documented.[42,43] The O_2 sensitivity of Ca^{2+} channels have been also reported in type I cells from adult rabbits,[33] although Ca^{2+} currents recorded from adult rat type I cells seem to be insensitive to hypoxia.[9] The role of O_2 modulation of Ca^{2+} channels in the chemotransduction process remains to be fully determined, but their voltage-dependent suppression by hypoxia may prevent excessive rises of $[Ca^{2+}]_i$ at inappropriately high PO_2 levels.

The role of IK_{Ca}, as the trigger of hypoxic depolarization required in the membrane model of hypoxic transduction in the rat, has been recently questioned by the observation that pharmacological inhibition of IK_{Ca} fails to stimulate either the intact carotid body[44-46] or isolated type I cells[47] under normoxic conditions. In this regard, Buckler has described a different O_2-sensitive current, carried by a resting (leak) K^+ channel which has little voltage dependence and is insensitive to TEA and 4-AP.[47] Hypoxic inhibition of this current could be the trigger for membrane depolarization, whilst hypoxic inhibition of IK_{Ca} could prevent repolarization during raised $[Ca^{2+}]_i$.

Hypoxic modulation of ionic channels is becoming a very complicated issue. It is conceivable that O_2-sensing mechanisms couple to different channels to varying degrees, and the prevalent effect is determined by species, culture conditions or other undetermined factors. Certainly, the physiological relevance of every reported effect of low O_2 on the different ionic currents of chemoreceptor cells remains to be determined.

EFFECTS OF CHRONIC HYPOXIA ON IONIC CURRENTS

Chronic hypoxia, which is encountered at high altitude or in individuals with hypoxic lung disease, is known to cause an enlargement of the carotid body due to increased size and number of type I cells.[48] This is associated with adaptive ventilatory changes, which have two components with different time-courses. First, and within a time frame of hours to few days there is a sensitization of the chemoreceptor reflex[49] (known also as acclimatization), and second, and within a time frame of several years (in humans) there is a blunting of hypoxic sensitivity.[50] Over the past three years, workers have investigated electrophysiological differences in type I cells which might account for the adaptive changes seen in response to chronic hypoxia. Thus, Stea et al cultured isolated rat type I cells for up to 2 weeks in 6% O_2 and noted that cells increased in size and also dramatically increased expression of Na^+ channels, while Ca^{2+} channel expression was unaffected.[14,51] These workers also noted a small decrease in K^+ channel density.[51] Similar results have been recently reported by Hempleman in neonatal rat carotid body cells following chronic hypoxia in vivo.[10] Such effects would increase excitability of type I cells, which is an attractive explanation for increased chemoreceptor sensitivity during acclimatization to chronic hypoxic conditions. Interestingly, the above-described effects of chronic hypoxia were mimicked by agents which elevate $[cAMP]_i$, which is known to be raised in type I cells under hypoxic conditions.[1] This intracellular messenger may, therefore, mediate adaptive changes of type I cells to long-term hypoxia.

In another study of chronic hypoxic conditions, Wyatt et al[52] isolated type I cells from young rats born and reared in chronic hypoxia (10% O_2). Such animals have a blunted ventilatory response to acutely inspired hypoxic gas mixtures, and may represent a model for long-term adaptive changes seen in experimental animals and in high-altitude residents. Type I cells from such animals were increased in size and number, and whole-cell patch clamp recordings demonstrated that K^+ current density was dramatically reduced (whilst Ca^{2+} current density was unaffected) as compared with age-matched normoxically reared rat pups.[16,52] Reduction in K^+ current density was largely attributed to a loss of K_{Ca} channels, as determined by a greatly reduced sensitivity to ChTx. Nevertheless, the residual K^+ channels could still be reversibly inhibited by acute hypoxia, to the same degree as observed in normoxic cells. This suggested that chronically hypoxic type I cells retained O_2-sensing mechanisms which could couple to K^+ channels other than K_{Ca} channels. Interestingly, despite possessing such O_2-sensitive channels, chronically hypoxic type I cells did not depolarize in acute hypoxia, suggesting that their O_2-sensitive channels were not active at resting membrane potential.[52] Such a lack of depolarizing response might account for the lack of chemoreceptor-mediated ventilatory responses to acute inspired hypoxia seen in animals (and humans) exposed to hypoxic episodes in the early postnatal life (see chapter 12 by Pásaro and Ribas).

RESPONSES TO ACIDIC STIMULI

In addition to hypoxia, type I cells are well known to release transmitters in response to a fall of extracellular pH and/or hypercapnia. In adult rabbit type I cells, this effect has been proposed to occur via Na^+ loading of type I cells (arising from increased activity of Na^+/H^+ exchangers) which leads to a reversal of Na^+/Ca^{2+} exchange, so that Ca^{2+} enters type I cells on this exchanger rather than through voltage-gated Ca^{2+} channels.[53] Indeed, although acidic stimuli inhibit IK in rabbit type I cells, there is a parallel reduction in I_{Na} and I_{Ca}[1], suggesting a nonselective inhibition of currents by hydrogen ions. By contrast, in young rat type I cells acidic transduction mechanisms are comparable with those for hypoxia.[7,26,54] Thus, a lowering of pH_o from 7.4 to 7.0 selectively inhibits K_{Ca} channels[26] and, importantly, this pH shift does not alter Ca^{2+} channel functioning.[7] The effects of pH_o are likely to be mediated via changes in pH_i, since selective intracellular acidosis (caused by application of salts of weak acids) also selectively inhibits K_{Ca} channels.[7] Furthermore, the exquisite sensitivity of the carotid body to acidosis may lie in the observation that, despite possessing numerous pH regulating mechanisms,[55] there is an extremely steep dependence of pH_i on pH_o.[56] In addition, Buckler and Vaughan-Jones have demonstrated that hypercapnic-induced rises of $[Ca^{2+}]_i$ are dependent on membrane depolarization, since voltage-clamping type I cells at their resting membrane potential prevented a 20% CO_2 stimulus from raising $[Ca^{2+}]_i$ (as measured using the Ca^{2+} indicator indo-1), and such rises were also strongly inhibited by organic L-type Ca^{2+} channel blockers.[18] Thus in rat type I cells at least, close parallelisms exist between mechanisms for transduction of hypoxic and hypercapnic stimuli.

CONCLUSIONS

In conclusion, all the carotid body chemoreceptor cells studied so far, from adult or neonatal rabbits or rats possess voltage-dependent currents. However, there are numerous differences in the properties of those currents reported in the literature (see Table 4.1 for a resume). Several possible explanations could account for these differences. First, differences in the stage of development of the cells. The lack of Na^+ currents in rabbit embryos vs. adult rabbit may be an example of that. Secondly, differences occurring between species, as the lack of a transient K^+ current in rat cells, or the different types of K^+ currents modulated by O_2 in rat vs. rabbit. Thirdly, differences in the isolation procedures or the conditions or durations of culturing of the cells may be an important factor. This might explain why Na^+ currents are recorded in neonatal rat cells by some authors that keep cells in culture for longer than 48 h but not by others that use freshly isolated or short-term cultured cells.

Despite these remaining discrepancies and questions, the fundamental scheme for the membrane model for hypoxic transduction, i.e., that hypoxic inhibition of K^+ current leads to depolarization/increased excitability, and thus Ca^{2+} influx through voltage-gated channels leading to transmitter release, appears to be the best framework to keep searching for the actual mechanisms involved in hypoxic chemotransduction.

Acknowledgments

This work has been supported by grant PB92-0267 of the Spanish DGICYT and by

Table 4.1.

	RABBIT		RAT	
	Adult	**Embryo**	**Neonatal**	**Adult**
I_{Na}	TTX sensitive	–	TTX sensitive (from absent to present in 40% of cells)	TTX sensitive <10% of cells
I_{Ca}	Peak ~ 0.4-1 nA (10 Ca^{2+}) L-Type N-Type P-Type	Peak ~ 0.4 nA (10.8 Ca^{2+}) L-Type ?	Peak ~ 0.05 nA (10 Ca^{2+}) L-Type N-Type ?	Peak ~ 0.08 nA (10 Ba^{2+}) L-Type N-Type ?
I_K	1.- Ca^{2+}-dependent -BK (Charybdotoxin ?) -Apamin 2.- Transient 3.- Non Inactivating	1.- Ca^{2+}-dependent 2.- Voltage dependent	1.-Ca^{2+}-dependent (IK_{Ca}) (Charybdotoxin) 2.-Voltage dependent (IK_v)	1.-Ca^{2+}-dependent (IK_{Ca}) (Charybdotoxin) 2.-Voltage dependent (IK_v)
O_2 sensitivity	Transient IK I_{Ca}	Voltage dependent Inward rectifier (?)	IK_{Ca} IK leak	IK_{Ca}

the British Heart Foundation and the Wellcome Trust.

References

1. González C, Almaraz L, Obeso A et al. Carotid body chemoreceptors: from natural stimuli to sensory discharges. Physiol Rev 1994; 74:829-98.
2. Peers C, Buckler KJ. Transduction of chemostimuli by the type I carotid body cell. J Membrane Biol 1995; 144: 1-9.
3. Duchen MR, Caddy KW, Kirby GC et al. Biophysical studies of the cellular elements of the rabbit carotid body. Neuroscience 1988; 26:291-311.
4. Ureña J, López-López J, González C et al. Ionic currents in dispersed chemoreceptor cells of the mammalian carotid body. J Gen Physiol 1989; 93:979-99.
5. Hescheler J, Delpiano MA, Acker H et al. Ionic currents on type-I cells of the rabbit carotid body measured by voltage-clamp experiments and the effect of hypoxia. Brain Research 1989; 486:79-88.
6. Fieber LA, McCleskey EW. L-type calcium channels in type I cells of the rat carotid body. J Neurophysiol 1993; 70: 1378-84.
7. Peers C, Green FK. Intracellular acidosis inhibits Ca^{2+}-activated K^+ currents in isolated type I cells of the neonatal rat carotid body. J Physiol 1995; 437:589-602.
8. Stea A, Nurse CA. Whole-cell and perforated-patch recordings from O_2-sensitive rat carotid body cells grown in short- and long-term culture. Pflugers Archiv—European J Physiol 1991; 418: 93-101.
9. López-López JR, González C, Pérez-García MT. Properties of ionic currents from isolated adult rat carotid body chemoreceptor cells: effect of hypoxia. J Physiol 1997; 499(2):429-41.
10. Hempleman SC. Sodium and potassium current in neonatal rat carotid body cells following chronic in vivo hypoxia. Brain Res 1995; 699:42-50.
11. González C, López López JR, Obeso A et al. Ca^{2+} dynamics in chemoreceptor cells: an overview. Adv Exp Med Biol 1993; 337:149-56.
12. Obeso A, Rocher A, Fidone S et al. The role of dihydropyridine-sensitive Ca^{2+} channels in stimulus-evoked catecholamine release from chemoreceptor cells of the carotid body. Neuroscience 1992; 47:463-72.
13. Montoro R, López-Barneo J. Calcium channels in glomus cells and their regulation by oxygen tension. (Abstract) Biophysical Journal 1995; 68:A209
14. Stea A, Jackson A, Macintyre L et al. Long-term modulation of inward currents in O_2 chemoreceptors by chronic hypoxia and cyclic AMP in vitro. J Neurosci 1995; 15:2192-202.
15. E Silva MJ, Lewis DL. L- and N-type Ca^{2+} channels in adult rat carotid body chemoreceptor type I cells. J Physiol 1995; 489:689-99.
16. Peers C, Carpenter E, Hatton CJ et al. Ca^{2+} channel currents in type I carotid body cells of normoxic and chronically hypoxic neonatal rats. Brain Res 1996; 739:251-7.
17. Lahiri S, Hsiao C, Zhang R et al. Peripheral chemoreceptors in respiratory oscillations. J Appl Physiol 1985; 58:1901-8.
18. Buckler KJ, Vaughan Jones RD. Effects of hypercapnia on membrane potential and intracellular calcium in rat carotid body type I cells. J Physiol 1994; 478(1):157-71.
19. Buckler KJ, Vaughan Jones RD. Effects of hypoxia on membrane potential and intracellular calcium in rat neonatal carotid body type I cells. J Physiol 1994; 476:423-8.
20. López-López JR, De Luis DA, González C. Properties of a transient K^+ current in chemoreceptor cells of rabbit carotid body. J Physiol 1993; 460:15-32.
21. Peers C. Hypoxic suppression of K^+ currents in type I carotid body cells: selective effect on the $Ca^{2(+)}$-activated K^+ current. Neuroscience Lett 1990; 119: 253-6.
22. Ganfornina MD, López Barneo J. Potassium channel types in arterial chemoreceptor cells and their selective modulation by oxygen. J Gen Physiol 1992; 100:401-26.
23. Ganfornina MD, López Barneo J. Gating of O_2-sensitive K^+ channels of arterial chemoreceptor cells and kinetic modifications induced by low pO_2. J Gen Physiol 1992; 100:427-55.

24. Delpiano MA, Hescheler J. Evidence for a PO_2-sensitive K^+ channel in the type-I cell of the rabbit carotid body. FEBS Lett 1989; 249:195-8.
25. Peers C, O'Donnell J. Potassium currents recorded in type I carotid body cells from the neonatal rat and their modulation by chemoexcitatory agents. Brain Res 1990; 522:259-66.
26. Peers C. Selective effect of lowered extracellular pH on Ca^{2+}-dependent K^+ currents in type I cells isolated from the neonatal rat carotid body. J Physiol 1995; 422:381-95.
27. Wyatt CN, Peers C. $Ca^{(2+)}$-activated K^+ channels in isolated type I cells of the neonatal rat carotid body. J Physiol 1995; 483:559-65.
28. Peers C. Effects of D600 on hypoxic suppression of K^+ currents in isolated type I carotid body cells of the neonatal rat. FEBS Lett 1990; 271:37-40.
29. Hatton CJ, Carpenter E, Pepper DR, Kumar P, Peers C. Developmental changes in isolated rat type I carotid body cell K^+ currents and their modulation by hypoxia. J Physiol 1997; 501:49-58.
30. Donnelly DF, Doyle TP. Developmental changes in hypoxia-induced catecholamine release from rat carotid body, in vitro. J Physiol 1994; 475:267-75.
31. López-Barneo J, López-López JR, Ureña J et al. Chemotransduction in the carotid body: K^+ current modulated by PO_2 in type I chemoreceptor cells. Science 1988; 241:580-2.
32. López-López JR, González C, Ureña J et al. Low pO_2 selectively inhibits K channel activity in chemoreceptor cells of the mammalian carotid body. J Gen Physiol 1989; 93:1001-15.
33. Montoro RJ, Ureña J, Fernandez-Chacon R et al. Oxygen sensing by ion channels and chemotransduction in single glomus cells. J Gen Physiol 1996; 107:133-43.
34. López-Barneo J, Benot AR, Ureña J. Oxygen sensing and the electrophysiology of arterial chemoreceptor cells. News in Physiological Sciences 1995; 8:191-5.
35. López-López JR, González C. Time course of K^+ current inhibition by low oxygen in chemoreceptor cells of adult rabbit carotid body. Effects of carbon monoxide. FEBS Lett 1992; 299:251-4.
36. Acker H, Xue D. Mechanisms of O_2 Sensing in the carotid body in comparison with other O_2-sensing cells. NIPS 1995; 10:211-6.
37. Biscoe TJ, Duchen MR. Cellular basis of transduction in carotid chemoreceptors. Am J Physiol 1990; 258:L271-8.
38. Biscoe TJ, Duchen MR. Electrophysiological responses of dissociated type I cells of the rabbit carotid body to cyanide. J Physiol 1989; 413:447-68.
39. Pérez-García MT, Obeso A, López-López JR et al. Characterization of cultured chemoreceptor cells dissociated from adult rabbit carotid body. Am J Physiol 1992; 263:C1152-9.
40. Jiang C, Haddad GG. Oxygen deprivation inhibits a K^+ channel independently of cytosolic factors in rat central neurons. J Physiol 1994; 481(1):15-26.
41. Weir EK, Archer SL. The mechanism of acute hypoxic pulmonary vasoconstriction: the tale of two channels. FASEB J 1995; 9:183-9.
42. Franco-Obregon A, Ureña J, López-Barneo J. Oxygen-sensitive calcium channels in vascular smooth muscle and their possible role in arterial relaxation. Proc Natl Acad Sci USA 1995; 92:4715-9.
43. Fearon IM, Palmer ACV, Balmforth AJ, et al. Hypoxia inhibits the recombinant alpha1C subunit of the human cardiac L-type Ca^{2+} channel. J Physiol 1997: 500:551-556.
44. Donnelly DF. Modulation of glomus cell membrane currents of intact rat carotid body. J Physiol 1995; 489:677-88.
45. Cheng PM, Donnelly DF. Relationship between changes of glomus cell current and neural response of rat carotid body. J Neurophysiol 1995; 74:2077-86.
46. Pepper RD, Landauer RC, Kumar P. Effect of charybdotoxin on hypoxic chemosensitivity in the adult rat carotid body in vitro. J Physiol 1995; (487.P)177P.
47. Buckler KJ. A novel oxygen-sensitive potassium current in rat carotid body type I cells. J Physiol 1997; 498(3):649-62.
48. Dhillon DP, Barer GR, Walsh M. The enlarged carotid body of the chronically hypoxic and chronically hypoxic and hypercapnic rat: a morphometric analysis. Q J Exp Physiol 1984; 69:301-17.

49. Nielsen AM, Bisgard GE, Vidruk EH. Carotid chemoreceptor activity during acute and sustained hypoxia in goats. J Appl Physiol 1988; 65:1796-802.
50. Wach RA, Bee D, Barer GR. Dopamine and ventilatory effects of hypoxia and almitrine in chronically hypoxic rats. J Appl Physiol 1989; 67:186-92.
51. Stea A, Jackson A, Nurse CA. Hypoxia and N6,O2'-dibutyryladenosine 3',5'-cyclic monophosphate, but not nerve growth factor, induce Na^+ channels and hypertrophy in chromaffin-like arterial chemoreceptors. Proc Natl Acad Sci USA 1992; 89:9469-73.
52. Wyatt CN, Wright C, Bee D et al. O_2-sensitive K^+ currents in carotid body chemoreceptor cells from normoxic and chronically hypoxic rats and their roles in hypoxic chemotransduction. Proc Natl Acad Sci USA 1995; 92:295-9.
53. Rocher A, Obeso A, González C et al. Ionic mechanisms for the transduction of acidic stimuli in rabbit carotid body glomus cells. J Physiol 1991; 433: 533-48.
54. Stea A, Alexander SA, Nurse CA. Effects of pHi and pHe on membrane currents recorded with the perforated-patch method from cultured chemoreceptors of the rat carotid body. Brain Res 1991; 567:83-90.
55. Buckler KJ, Vaughan-Jones RD, Peers C et al. Intracellular pH and its regulation in isolated type I carotid body cells of the neonatal rat. J Physiol 1991; 436: 107-29.
56. Buckler KJ, Vaughan-Jones RD, Peers C et al. Effects of extracellular pH, PCO_2 and HCO_3^- on intracellular pH in isolated type-I cells of the neonatal rat carotid body. J Physiol 1991; 444:703-21.

CHAPTER 5

Mechanisms of Sensory Transduction in Chemoreceptor Cells: The Role of Second Messengers

María Teresa Pérez-García and Constancio González

INTRODUCTION

Sensory transduction is concerned with the mechanisms occurring in sensory receptors and by which the stimuli, i.e., changes in the environment or in the interior of the organisms, are transformed into electrical signals intelligible to the nervous system. Implicit in sensory transduction is that the electrical signals carried by the sensory neurons must be a facsimile of the changes detected. The sensory neuron is the element that delivers the detected signals to higher order neurons in the nervous systems, but in different sensory receptors, depending on their structural and functional organization, the sensory neurons may be the primary, secondary or tertiary target for the stimulus. In primary sensory receptors a specialized part of the sensory neuron itself, the sensory nerve ending, is the direct target for the stimulus. The mechanoreceptors of the skin, the arterial baroreceptors and the olfactory receptors are examples of primary sensory receptors. In secondary sensory receptors, the first target for the stimulus is a specialized cell. This specialized cell is linked, usually by a synapse, to the sensory neuron. The specialized cell, or receptor cell, transduces the stimulus into a neurosecretory response, the release of neurotransmitters, which acting on the sensory neuron generate the propagated electrical signals facsimile of the changes detected by the receptor cells. The auditory and vestibular mechanoreceptors and the taste chemoreceptors are well characterized mammalian secondary sensory receptors. In tertiary sensory receptors an additional element is interposed between the sensory receptor and the sensory neuron. The links between the three elements are two synapses. Photoreceptors in the vertebrate retina are linked synaptically to bipolar cells, and these in turn are linked to

The Carotid Body Chemoreceptors,
edited by Constancio González.

the retinal ganglion cells which are the sensory neurons in the visual receptor of vertebrates; there are additional cells linking the photoreceptors to the ganglion cells (horizontal and amacrine cells) which help to fine-tune the transmission of information between photoreceptors and ganglion cells. Quite frequently, in secondary and tertiary sensory receptors the receptor complex (receptor cells, sensory nerve endings or supporting structures) receive a synaptic input from an efferent fiber capable of modulating the sensitivity of the receptor.

The carotid body (CB) was described as a sensory receptor capable of sensing changes in the qualitative composition of the blood by Fernando de Castro.[1] In his original description, the CB was defined as a secondary sensory receptor, in which the glomus, type I or chemoreceptor cells sense the blood and transmit the sensed signals via secretory products to the sensory nerve endings of the carotid sinus nerve (CSN), a branch of the IXth cranial pair. The sensitivity of chemoreceptor cells to the modifications of the PO_2 and PCO_2/pH in their environment is well established.[2] González and Fidone[3] showed for the first time that CBs in vitro, deprived of any nervous input, secreted the neurotransmitter dopamine (DA) when the PO_2 in the bathing solution was reduced. Pérez-García et al[4] showed for the first time that isolated chemoreceptor cells in culture secreted increasingly higher quantities of DA as PO_2 in the bathing solution decreased; there was a close parallelism between the neurosecretory behavior of the isolated cells and that of the intact CBs, and among the neurosecretory responses, the action potential frequency recorded in the CSN[5,6] and ventilation rate in the intact animal (Fig. 5.1). Several groups have confirmed in intact organ or at the single cell level those original findings (see chapter 3 by González et al for references).

On the other hand, it has also been observed that after destruction of the CB, the regenerated CSN fibers-endings lack chemosensory properties;[7] similarly, it has been observed that the presence of synaptic contacts between chemoreceptor cells and the sensory nerve endings of the CSN are necessary for the genesis of propagated hypoxic chemoreceptor activity.[8] Therefore, thesedays it is universally accepted among the workers in the field that the CB is a secondary sensory arterial chemoreceptor.

In modeling the transduction cascade in secondary (or tertiary) sensory receptors, it is useful to divide the entire process into two sequentially related but independent processes: the transduction of the sensory stimuli, concerned with the mechanisms that take place in the sensory cells between the arrival of the stimulus and the release of the neurotransmitters at the synapse, and the neurotransmission, concerned with the genesis of the postsynaptic potentials and the propagated activity in the sensory nerve endings and fibers. However, it also is common in the study of neurotransmission to include many steps taking place in the presynaptic element, such as the synthesis, storage and release of neurotransmitters. As a consequence, the study of the regulation of the transduction can equally be conceived as the study of the regulation of neurotransmission.[2]

In addition to these general considerations, there are some specific difficulties in studying chemosensory transduction in the CB. First, the CB responds to more than one natural stimulus including low PO_2, which is the main natural stimulus, high PCO_2 and low pH. This implies that even when the output of chemoreceptor cells, the release of neurotransmitters, is presumably the same,[9] the mechanisms linking each stimulus to the exocytotic machinery may be completely different. And second, there are well characterized differences in the electrical properties of chemoreceptor cells from different species (see chapter 4 by López-López and Peers), and therefore the existence of differences in the transduction process among species is plausible. A combination of the first and the second point may render difficult or inadequate the generalization of results obtained in one species to the other species.

In the present chapter we will summarize the available information on the mecha-

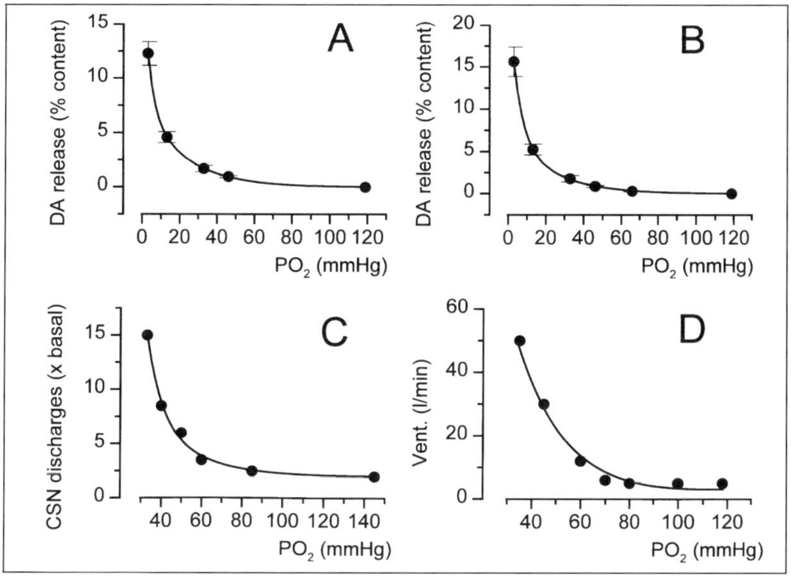

Fig. 5.1. Relationships between bath PO_2 and the release of dopamine (DA) in short-term cultured chemoreceptor cells (A) and intact rabbit carotid bodies (B). Both figures were obtained by incubating the cells or the organs for 10 min in solutions equilibrated at the indicated PO_2. (C) Relationship between arterial PO_2 and carotid sinus nerve (CSN) action potential frequency (discharges). Basal frequency was taken at arterial PO_2 higher than 400 mmHg. (Redrawn with data obtained by several authors in blood perfused in situ preparations of the cat carotid body). (D) Approximate ventilation rate in humans as a function of arterial PO_2.

nisms involved in the transduction of the different stimuli to the CB chemoreceptors. We will underline the differences among species, and emphasize the modulation of the transduction cascades exerted by second messengers and G proteins. The modulation of the sensitivity of the CB chemoreceptors produced by the efferent innervation of the CB receptor complexes is reviewed in chapter 8 by Almaraz et al.

LOW PO_2 TRANSDUCTION

Physiological Hypoxia and Physiological O_2-Sensing

At the outset of this section we would like to devote some discussion to O_2-sensing and transduction in general, and thereafter we will present and discuss the specific case for the CB chemoreceptors. In recent publications,[10,11] we have tried to coin the concept of physiological hypoxia and physiological sensitivity to hypoxia. We have defined physiological hypoxia as a hypoxic hypoxia produced by ambient factors (decrease in barometric pressure), and proceeding without any pathology for the entire lifespan of individuals and from generation to generation. We have set the highest limit of physiological hypoxia at a barometric pressure of around 460 mmHg, corresponding to an inspired PO_2 of ≈87 mmHg, and to an alveolar PO_2 before hyperventilation of ≈40 mmHg (see Fig. 2.1). This barometric pressure corresponds to an altitude of 4,000 m above sea level, where nearly 15 million people live.

The point behind this concept is that humans permanently living at this or lower altitudes, as well as lowlanders ascending temporarily or permanently to these altitudes, develop a triad of adaptative responses, which are directed to reduce the strain produced by the environmental hypoxia. The hyperventilation triggered by the chemoreceptor cells of the carotid body, the polycytemia triggered by the erythropoietin producing cells of the kidney and the moderate pulmonary hypertension generated by the smooth muscle cells of the pulmonary artery are aimed to prevent hypoxia and to maintain metabolic rate and function in body cells.[11] The precise meaning of prevention of hypoxia in body cells is best appreciated when it is considered the relationship between arterial PO_2 and activation of these three cell types. The three cell types have a threshold to hypoxia near an arterial PO_2 of 70 mmHg (corresponding to arterial oxygen content over 95% of that found at sea level), implying that hyperventilation, production of erythropoietin/increase in red cell mass and pulmonary hypoxic vasoconstriction start before there is a significant decrease in the availability of O_2 in the tissues. A consequence of this low threshold for hypoxia is that chemoreceptor cells of the carotid body, erythropoietin producing cells and smooth muscle cells of the pulmonary arteries must possess molecular O_2-sensing mechanisms with low affinity for O_2. On the other hand, the hyperbolic-like shape of the curves relating arterial PO_2 to the function of these three cell types implies that their functional activity increases as arterial PO_2 continues to decrease, and as discussed in chapter 2 by Obeso et al, these cells must possess a metabolic machinery capable of supporting a progressively increasing activity as the intensity of hypoxia increases. Although the experimental data available to support this notion are rather incomplete, it is well documented in a great variety of tissues that sustained increased functional activity requires an increased energetic metabolic rate, and in fact, data obtained in the CB indicate an increase in glucose consumption and maintenance of ATP levels during hypoxia, indicating an increased turnover (synthesis and expenditure) of ATP (see chapter 2 by Obeso et al).

It is the conjunction of these three properties (low threshold, general adaptative/homeostatic purpose of the generated responses, and increased functional and metabolic activity during hypoxia) in chemoreceptor cells of the carotid body, erythropoietin producing cells of the kidney and smooth muscle cells of the pulmonary arteries what defines physiological sensitivity to hypoxia, and distinguishes it from the general sensitivity to hypoxia exhibited by all cells in higher animals. The general sensitivity to hypoxia is characterized by a high threshold, by responses directed to the survival of the hypoxic cells (and not to the entire organism), and by a reduction of functional and metabolic activity of the hypoxic cells.

These considerations call attention to the possibility of a unitary mechanism for O_2-sensing in the three cell types endowed with physiological sensitivity to hypoxia. In fact, in a recent symposium held in Madrid, Spain, attended by workers in the fields of chemoreception, erythropoiesis and pulmonary circulation, one of the general conclusions was that in all likelihood the mechanisms involved in O_2-sensing could be common for the three cell types under consideration, although obviously the transduction cascade would be specific, to adequately couple the O_2-sensor to the effector machinery in each cell type.[12]

Putative O_2-Sensors

Recently developed molecular biology techniques have demonstrated unequivocally that O_2-sensors in prokaryotic cells are hemoproteins located in the cell membrane, and the same appears to be true in yeast.[13] From the point of view of evolution, these findings would lend support to the proposal that O_2-sensors in higher animals also are hemoproteins, but we lack direct experimental data to accept or to reject this proposal. Nonetheless, there are experimental data which are consistent with the notion of the involvement of a hemoprotein or other type of metalloprotein in O_2-sensing.

In the case of the CB, the involvement of a hemoglobin-like pigment in the detection of hypoxia was suggested by Lloyd and coworkers,[14] when they found that a slug of CO while breathing a hypoxic gas mixture reduced hyperventilation like a slug of pure oxygen. Their proposal was that the hemoglobin-like pigment would be desaturated during hypoxia, and that this desaturation would be the signal triggering CB chemoreception; CO would saturate the sensor and cause it to behave as if it were saturated with O_2. Although the mixture of the CO with alveolar gas, and the much higher affinity of hemoglobin for CO than for O_2 would reduce the pressure of CO in arterial blood to very low values, making questionable the interpretation of the observation, the proposal does have the merit of promoting research in this direction using better controlled experimental conditions (see below). Some years later Lahiri's group[15,16] revived the notion that a hemoglobin-like pigment would act as O_2-sensor in the CB based on the resemblance between the CSN response curves for hypoxia at different PCO_2 and the curves for dissociation of hemoglobin; they estimated that the hemoglobin-like chromophore present in the CB would have a P_{50} of ≈40 mmHg and a unique Bohr effect, it being remarkable that Whalen and coworkers[17] measuring CB tissue PO_2 found in some series of experiments a P_{50} of 32 mmHg for the hypoxic CSN action potential frequency. As commented above, an O_2-sensor with a higher P_{50} than hemoglobin would fulfill the requirement for the CB to prevent the hypoxia in the body cells.

The concept that a hemoprotein was involved in O_2-sensing in the CB was reinforced by findings in human hepatoma capable of producing erythropoietin in an O_2-dependent manner. In 1988 Golberg and coworkers[18] reported that the production of erythropoietin mRNA elicited by hypoxia (as well as the production of the hormone itself) were suppressed by CO. The discovery of a K^+ current in chemoreceptor cells that was reversibly inhibited by hypoxia (see below), prompted the exploration of the effects of CO on this current, and it was found that CO prevented the inhibition of the K^+ current produced by hypoxia[19] (Fig. 5.2). Our observation at the K^+ current level was extended by Lahiri and coworkers[20] to the intact CB preparation; using a preparation of the carotid artery bifurcation perfused with cell-free buffered saline it was found that the CSN discharges elicited by hypoxia (perfusion with solutions equilibrated at PO_2 of 43-60 mmHg) were markedly reduced (> 60%) by the introduction of CO at 60-70 mmHg in the equilibrating gas. In that and ulterior articles,[20,21] these authors found that increasing the CO/O_2 ratios produced dual effects, inhibition of the hypoxic response and an excitation, the excitatory effect being light sensitive and associated with a decrease in O_2-consumption by the CB, i.e., the excitatory effect was due to the inhibition of cytochrome oxidase, and thereby comparable to the action of other inhibitors of the respiratory chain such as cyanide. The studies with CO have also been extended to the third system with physiological sensitivity to hypoxia, the pulmonary circulation, and it was found that CO inhibits hypoxic pulmonary vasoconstriction in a reversible manner, and by a mechanism that is independent of the guanylate cyclase system[22] (Fig. 5.2).

These experimental data are the only support to implicate a hemoprotein in O_2-sensing, and therefore caution is needed in proposing that the O_2-sensor in any of the three cell systems possessing physiological sensitivity to hypoxia is in fact a hemoprotein. However, CO is poorly reactive in biological systems; hemoproteins and other O_2-transporting/using iron or copper containing proteins, all of them in their reduced form (Fe^{2+}, Cu^{1+}), beingthe only known ligands for CO.[23,13] Therefore, it would appear that a consideration of the O_2-handling proteins having a P_{50} or a Km for O_2 in the range of 10-40 mmHg and a comparable affinity for O_2 and CO[19] (see above) may be possible candidates for O_2-sensor. In the case of the rabbit CB chemoreceptor cells, a third requisite for the O_2-sensor is that it should be located in the plasma membrane; this is so, because low PO_2 decreases the open probability of K^+-channels in isolated membrane patches recorded in the inside-out configuration,[24] implying that the O_2 sensor is intrinsic to the cell membrane. To our knowledge there is not a metalloprotein fulfilling the three requirements (see Tables 2 and 3 in Coburn and Forman,[23] and Table 2 in Vanderkooi et al).[25]

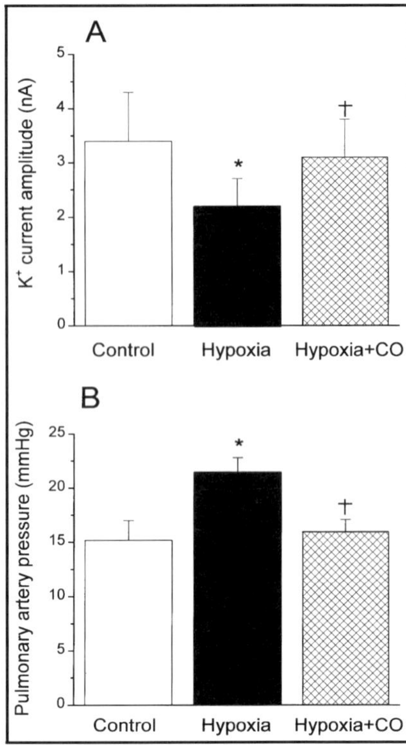

Fig. 5.2. (A) Effects of carbon monoxide (CO) on the amplitude of K^+ currents recorded in rabbit carotid body chemoreceptor cells. The amplitude of control currents was obtained while recording from isolated chemoreceptor cells perfused with solutions equilibrated with air (PO_2 ≈150 mmHg); in the middle column it is shown the amplitude of the currents recorded while perfusing with solutions at a PO_2 of 33 mmHg; and in the left column, hypoxia plus CO, it is shown the amplitude of the currents recorded while perfusing with solutions equilibrated at a PO_2 of 33 mmHg and a PCO of around 66 mmHg. (B) Effects of CO on the pulmonary arterial pressure recorded from an in situ preparation of the rat lung. Control refers to pulmonary arterial pressure recorded with a blood PO_2 of ≈140 mmHg; hypoxia stands for the pulmonary arterial pressure recorded at 23 mmHg; and hypoxia plus CO refers to the pulmonary arterial pressure recorded at a PO_2 of 23 mmHg and a PCO of ≈56 mmHg. *Data are different from controls. †Data are not different from controls. In both preparations CO did not have an effect on normoxic control conditions.

If we limit the restrictions to the two initial requirements, (due to the fact that in rat CB chemoreceptor cells cytoplasmic components are required for low PO_2 to inhibit the O_2-sensitive K^+ channels, which in this species is a charybdotoxin sensitive K^+_{Ca} channel),[26] there are several microsomal and mitochondrial enzymes that could act as O_2-sensors. Many of these enzymes use NAD(P)H as a donor of electrons and are capable of producing oxygen activated species.

One of the enzymes belonging to the latter group and proposed to be the O_2-sensor is the NADPH oxidase,[27,28] which in phagocyte cells is responsible for the oxygen burst and for the production of the hydrogen peroxide. From a kinetic point of view this enzyme is suited to act as an O_2-sensor because reported Km of the enzyme for O_2 oscillate between 5 and 30 mM[29] (3-18 mmHg). There are, however, many facts that do not fit the proposal. First, cytochrome b_{-245} (also known as cytochrome b_{558} because of the absorption maximum of its α-band), which is the last element in the electron transporting mechanism of this enzymatic complex, does not bind CO at all,[30,31] and therefore cannot accommodate the experimental findings described above. And second, Acker's proposal, which included that NADPH oxidase would also be the O_2-sensor in erythropoietin producing cells, is not supported by other data; on the one hand, patients with chronic granulomatosis which lack NADPH oxidase have a normal erythropoiesis,[32] and on the other hand, cells obtained from these patients and transfected with constructs containing O_2-responsive elements exhibit normal responses to low PO_2. In the clinical descriptions of patients with chronic granulomatosis, no mention is made to ventilatory deficits.[33]

Aside from these specific comments on NADPH oxidase, the next point to consider is the coupling of the O_2-sensor to the following elements in the transduction cascade. If the sensor is intrinsic to the plasma membrane, its coupling would not necessarily need a coupling factor, but if the sensor is located in the cell interior there is an absolute requirement for a coupling factor, since the second step in the cascade appear to be the O_2-sensitive K^+ channels (see next paragraph).

The Hypoxic Transduction Cascade

In the case of the chemoreceptor cells of the CB and smooth muscle cells of the pulmonary artery, the involvement of plasma membrane mechanisms in the transduction cascade is accepted by most workers in the field. Thus, the CB being a secondary sensory receptor implies that chemoreceptor cells should release neurotransmitters in parallel to the intensity of the hypoxic stimulus; this extreme has been demonstrated not only for hypoxia and acidosis,[5,6,34] but also for a great variety of pharmacological CB stimulants including cyanide, dinitrophenol and 2-deoxy-glucose.[35,36] It was also found that type I cells were able to release DA in response to high extracellular K^+(ref. 37); high K^+_e induced release was Ca^{2+}-dependent and sensitive to dihydropyridine agonists and antagonists of L-type voltage-dependent Ca^{2+} channels,[38] indicating that neurotransmitter release was triggered by depolarization, and suggesting for the first time that chemoreceptor cells were excitable cells, with a membrane potential dependent on the distribution of K^+ across cell membrane.[37] The secretory response elicited by hypoxia also was dependent on the extracellular Ca^{2+} and sensitive to dihydropyridines, implying that hypoxia depolarizes chemoreceptor cells to activate voltage-dependent Ca^{2+} channels, and thereby, that the mechanisms of O_2 sensory transduction are linked to plasma membrane processes.[38] Additionally, it was observed that tetrodotoxin (a selective blocker of voltage-dependent Na^+ channels) inhibited significantly the release of DA induced by mild to moderate hypoxic stimuli,[39] reinforcing the notion of cell depolarization during hypoxic stimulation. Comparable studies in pulmonary arteries have yielded the same results and allowed identical conclusions, i.e., hypoxia depolarizes pulmonary artery smooth muscle cells.[40] Obviously, the transduction cascade in erythropoietin producing cells must be different since it involves protein synthesis and therefore must have a different time scale (see below).

The study of the electrophysiological properties of the chemoreceptor cells isolated from rabbit and rat CB allowed the direct demonstration of the presence in those cells of voltage-activated Na^+, K^+ and Ca^{2+} channels,[41,42] in addition, it was demonstrated that a transient component of the outward K^+ current in rabbit CB chemoreceptor cells was reversibly inhibited by lowering the PO_2 in the external solution.[41,43] Further studies in excised membrane patches showed that low PO_2 was able to decrease the open probability of the K^+ channels responsible for the low PO_2-sensitive K^+ current, indicating, as mentioned above, that the O_2-sensing mechanism in rabbit CB chemoreceptor cells is a membrane-delimited entity.[24]

The conjunction of the neurochemical, pharmacological and electrophysiological data summarized in this section lead this laboratory to propose a cascade for the transduction of the hypoxic stimulus in the rabbit CB chemoreceptor cells with the following steps.[2,9] A membrane limited O_2-sensor, probably a hemoprotein, would sense the PO_2 in the surroundings of the cells as the degree of saturation/desaturation of the sensor; conformational changes produced upon saturation/desaturation of the sensor (in clear homology to the behavior of hemoglobin) would regulate allosterically the open probability of the O_2-sensitive K^+ channels, in such a way that an O_2-desaturation would lead to a decrease in the opening probability; the resulting decrease in K^+ conductance would lead to cell depolarization, activation of voltage-dependent Ca^{2+} and Na^+ channels, Ca^{2+} entry and release of neurotransmitters. The steps of cell depolarization, activation of Na^+ and Ca^{2+} channels and entry of Ca^{2+} are soundly supported by experimental data[38,39,44] (see above). The mechanism proposed for the coupling between the O_2-sensor and K^+ channels is speculative, and the proposal that the inhibition of the O_2-sensitive K^+ channel is responsible for the cell depolarization is being debated. The O_2-sensitive K^+ channel in the rabbit CB chemoreceptor cells is voltage-dependent with a threshold in the vicinity of -40 mV, and therefore it should be closed at the resting normoxic membrane potential. Only if chemoreceptor cells are firing action potentials spontaneously in normoxia, as it appears to be case,[45] it is conceivable that a decrease in the opening probability of this channel can lead to the observed increase in the firing frequency of the cells during hypoxia.[43,45]

The electrophysiological properties of chemoreceptor cells obtained from neonatal and adult rats are different from those of adult rabbits (see chapter 4 by López-López and Peers), and there are some controversies regarding basic features of the transduction cascade in this species. To start with, the O_2-sensitive K^+ current is Ca^{2+}-dependent, and the channel responsible is a high conductance charybdotoxin-sensitive K^+_{Ca}, both in neonatal[26] and adult rat CB chemoreceptor cells.[46] According to Wyatt and Peers,[26] hypoxic inhibition of the K^+_{Ca} channel in neonatal rat CB chemoreceptor cells leads to the required cell depolarization to activate voltage-dependent Ca^{2+} channels[47] (most of the rat CB chemoreceptor cells lack Na^+ channels) and Ca^{2+} entry; the release of neurotransmitters[48] would follow. These findings, however, have not been confirmed by Buckler,[49] who finds that pharmacological inhibition of the K^+_{Ca} channel does not depolarize the cells (i.e., K^+_{Ca} would not contribute to the resting membrane potential), and describes a new O_2-sensitive K^+ channel which is voltage-independent, and therefore capable upon hypoxic inhibition of generating the required cell depolarization to activate Ca^{2+} channels; findings of Cheng and Donnelly[50] show that charybdotoxin does not alter holding current, membrane resistance or basal CSN discharge but markedly reduced outward currents also speak against a role for K^+_{Ca} in the genesis of resting membrane potential.[51] In the rabbit CB chemoreceptor cells a systematic search for this leaky, voltage-independent and O_2-sensitive K^+ channel is lacking. In conclusion, in spite of the differences among species, it is noteworthy that chemoreceptor cells at any developmental age possess O_2-sensitive K^+ channels, indicating that they constitute key elements in the transduction of the hypoxic stimulus.[52]

We do not want to finish this section on O_2-sensing/transduction without a comment on other proposed O_2-sensors or coupling mechanisms. As discussed in detail in chapter 2 by Obeso et al, there are theoretical bases and experimental data indicating that during hypoxic activation of chemoreceptor cells the NAD(P)H/NAD(P)$^+$ quotient increases and, taking into account the standard potential of this redox pair, it is conceivable that the reduced/oxidized quotients of most redox pairs in the cells would also increase. On the other hand, as discussed above, several O_2-using metalloproteins capable of interaction with CO use NAD(P)H as an electron donor and can generate oxygen active species (H_2O_2, O^-_2,...). Since both the redox state of cell and oxygen active species have been proposed to act as couplers between the stimulus, low PO_2, and the initial effectors in the transduction cascade, the K^+ channels, we should devote some comments to these hypotheses, even though in their formulations it is possible to dissect out several indefinitions.

In the case of the CB the proposal that an increase in NADH could be the signal triggering chemoreception (inhibition of K^+ channels in today's terminology) dates from the early 1970s when Mills and Jöbsis[53] described a low O_2-affinity cytochrome oxidase, that has not been confirmed by other authors.[54] In recent years Weir and Archer[40] have also suggested that an increase in the reduced forms of redox pairs would lead to inhibition of K^+ channels in smooth muscle cells of the pulmonary arteries, the coupling factor would be a cysteine residue presumably present in the β subunit of O_2-sensitive K^+ channels.[55] Although from a biophysical point of view such a proposal is conceivable, it is necessary to demonstrate that the conditions capable of changing the redox state of the cysteine residue take place in the cells.

For example, typical concentrations of glutathione (GSH) in most mammalian cells[56] is around 2 mM with GSH/GSSG ratios greater than 10/1, making observations on K^+ currents obtained with 2 mM GSH or GSSG in the recording pipettes of questionable physiological significance. In addition, the findings obtained with some metabolic blockers do not fit the proposal that an increase in the reduced forms of redox pairs is responsible for the inhibition of K^+ channels; thus, uncouplers, and probably 2-deoxiglucose, *decrease* the NADH/NAD ratio in cells and yet they inhibit K^+ currents in pulmonary artery smooth muscle cells.

Even more difficult to accept are the findings with H_2O_2. H_2O_2 is an oxidant per se, and it can also diminish the concentration of GSH by the action of GSH peroxidase (H_2O_2 + GSH —> GSSG +H_2O). Since there is a direct relation between tissue PO_2 and the production of oxygen active species, the proposal is that during hypoxia there is a cellular decrease in the concentration of these molecular species leading to an increase in GSH and reduced cysteine residues, and to a decrease in the opening probability of K^+ channels.[57,27] First, it is questionable that a decrease in the arterial PO_2 from the normoxic value of ≈93 mmHg to the threshold value of ≈70 mmHg for the detection of physiological hypoxia causes a significant reduction in the production of oxygen active species, especially taking into account that hypoxia increases the metabolic rate of tissues with physiological sensitivity to hypoxia and the parallelism between the electron transport rate in the mitochondria and the production of O_2-active species;[58] for example, uncouplers greatly increase the production of O_2-active species and induce superoxide dismutase to defend cells from them.[57] Second, even accepting the proposed decrease in H_2O_2, the experiments aimed to support the involvement of H_2O_2 in the regulation of K^+ channels activity are of questionable physiological significance; thus, the steady state intracellular concentration of H_2O_2 in many cells is in the range of 10^{-7} to 10^{-9} M,[59] and the concentration of H_2O_2 effective to reduce K^+ currents is 5 x10^{-4} M.[59] Similarly high concentrations (3 x 10^{-4} M or higher) of H_2O_2 were needed to inhibit erythropoietin production in hepatoma cells.[60]

The energy charge of the cell, [ATP]/[ADP][AMP][Pi], has also been considered by many authors as a signal triggering CB chemoreception and hypoxic pulmonary vasoconstriction. It will suffice to state that in both preparations inhibition of K^+ currents is obtained with ATP concentrations in the recording pipettes of 5 mM (see also chapter 2 by Obeso et al). However, it is conceivable that metabolic inhibitors, such as cyanide that reduces ATP levels,[36] or CO at high concentrations that reduces O_2-consumption,[21] can cause ionic disbalances in the cells via reduction of the activity of the Na^+/K^+ pump, leading to cell depolarization and activation of cell responses.

Finally, the hypoxic-triggered long-term responses in the CB involving synthesis of proteins (e.g., induction of tyrosine hydroxylase,[11] induction of Na^+ channels)[61] can, to some extent, be compared with the production of erythropoietin triggered by hypoxia. In the case of the CB, the activation of the tyrosine hydroxylase gene could be mediated at least in part, as it is the case in PC-12 cells, by the products of early responsive oncogenes acting on AP-1 sites present in the gene promoter,[62] because hypoxia greatly increases the expression of c-fos and c-jun proteins in the CB (Obeso and González, unpublished). The actions of hypoxia on voltage-dependent Na^+ channels could be linked to putative CRE-sites in the gene coding for the channel, since cyclic AMP mimicked the effects of hypoxia. In hepatoma cells producing erythropoietin it has been identified as a factor, named hypoxia inducible factor one (HIF-1), that bounds to a specific region of the erythropoietin gene activating its rate of transcription.[63,32]

HIGH PCO_2 /LOW PH TRANSDUCTION

Since isohydric solutions containing weak acids, including isohydric hypercapnic solutions, as well as low pH solutions stimulate the CB chemoreceptors, there is a general agreement that the chemoreceptor signal during natural high PCO_2/low pH stimulation is a decrease in intracellular pH; the speed of the CB response to an increase in PCO_2 being higher than that to a decrease in pH due to the fast diffusion of CO_2 into the cell and the carbonic anhydrase catalyzed hydration to H^+ and bicarbonate.[34,64-67] The available experimental evidence also supports that this increase in $[H^+]_i$ acts as a signal independent of the PO_2, in the sense that acidic/hypercapnic stimulus are effective to increase the activity of the CSN at any level of PO_2. However, the converse is not true, that is, at a PCO_2 low enough or at a pH high enough the CSN nerve is silenced,[68] suggesting that a decrease in $[H^+]$ (pH ≈7.8-8) disrupts the O_2-sensing mechanisms or some step in the hypoxic cascade transduction. At the intermediate ranges of CO_2/pH and PO_2 encountered in physiological or even in most pathological situations, there is a positive interaction between both stimuli with the net result of genesis of CSN responses that are additive, multiplicative or less than additive.[69] The genesis of such interactions can occur at the O_2-sensor (a unique Bohr-like effect)[16] and/or at the level of some steps of the cascade transduction (e.g., at the level of K^+ channels,[70] of intracellular $Ca^{2+}{}_i$ or of the exocytotic machinery).[9]

The transduction cascade for acidic/hypercapnic stimulus has been studied in some detail in the intact rabbit CB[71] and in isolated rat CB chemoreceptor cells.[64,72,65] In the former preparation the experimental approach has been neurochemical, and in the second the transduction cascade has been studied with a combination of electrophysiological and single cell microfluorometric techniques. The results indicate a completely different cascade of transduction in both species.

In the rabbit CB the rationale for the study was the consideration of the transduction cascade as a classical stimulus-secretion coupling process, i.e., the aim of the experiments, involving ionic manipulations and the use of selected pharmacological tools, was to dissect mechanisms coupling the acidic/hypercapnic stimulus to the release of neurotransmitters from chemoreceptor cells. In initial experiments it was demonstrated that the acidic stimulus which induced release of DA from chemoreceptor cells was dependent on the presence of extracellular Ca^{2+} in ≈80%, implying that Ca^{2+} must enter the cells from the external milieu.[34,38] It was also observed that dihydropyridine blockers of Ca^{2+} channels were ineffective to reduce the acidic stimulus-induced release of DA,[38] implying that acidic stimuli do not activate voltage-dependent Ca^{2+} channels, and thereby do not depolarize significantly chemoreceptor cells. Similarly, tetrodotoxin did not reduce the release of DA induced by acidic stimuli, reinforcing the same conclusion.[39] These findings with blockers of voltage-dependent channels were in clear contrast with those described above for the hypoxic stimulus, and yet open the question on the pathway for the Ca^{2+} entry into the cells during acidic stimulation. As a potential pathway for Ca^{2+} entry into chemoreceptor cells the presence of a Na^+/Ca^{2+} exchanger in these cells was explored, and it was found that the inhibition of the Na^+/K^+ pump by ouabain or by the removal of K^+ from the incubating solution and the removal of external Na^+-- maneuvers which decrease or reverse the Na^+ gradient across the cell membrane, induced release of DA that was Ca^{2+} dependent; these findings indicated that in fact chemoreceptor cells have a Na^+/Ca^{2+} exchanger that working in reverse mode is capable of introducing in the cells enough Ca^{2+} as to trigger the release of neurotransmitters.[71] With these data, the critical point was to find a mechanism linking the increase in intracellular hydrogen ion concentration to the functioning of the Na^+/Ca^{2+} exchanger in the reverse mode. Since on intracellular acidification all cells extrude H^+, quite commonly coupled to the influx of Na^+ (Na^+/H^+ and Na^+,$^-HCO_3/H^+$,Cl^- exchangers), we reasoned that this influx of Na^+ could be responsible for the reduction of the Na^+ gradient, and thereby for the working of the

Na^+/Ca^{2+} exchanger in the reverse mode. To test this hypothesis, we blocked in sequential experiments the different H^+ exchangers with ethylisopropylamiloride by eliminating Na^+, $^-HCO_3$ and Cl^- from the bathing solutions, and we found that the release of neurotransmitters induced by acidic stimulation was greatly reduced in every case, leading us to propose the cascade of transduction shown in Figure 5.3.[71]

In contrast, in neonatal and presumably also in adult rats, acidic stimuli inhibit the charybdotoxin-sensitive K^+_{Ca} without affecting the Ca^{2+} currents,[70] and produce an increase in intracellular Ca^{2+} which is dependent on the activation of voltage-dependent Ca^{2+} channels.[65] In other words, the transduction cascades for hypoxic and acidic stimuli would be, for the most part, indistinguishable, although there are no data on the possible actions of acidic stimuli on the O_2-sensitive leaky K^+ current recently described by Buckler[49] (see above and chapter 4).

SECOND MESSENGER SYSTEMS IN THE TRANSDUCTION PROCESS

The modulation of the chemoreceptor cell function by intracellular messengers is an aspect of chemoreception that has only been studied very recently, and, as a consequence, only a few aspects of the overall significance of the second messengers in the CB chemoreceptors are known. There are not data regarding the possible role of second messengers on the regulation of the transduction cascades in the rat CB chemoreceptor cells. Second messengers participate in the regulation of the response of the CB not only to hypoxia, but also hypercapnia as well as other pharmacological stimuli.

ADENYLATE CYCLASE-cAMP SYSTEM

The first intracellular messenger system studied in some detail in the CB chemoreceptor has been the adenylate cyclase-cAMP system. The available literature is consistent in showing that low PO_2 stimulation increases cAMP content in rabbit and cat CB incubated in a variety of different conditions,[73-75] this increase being restricted to chemoreceptor cells.[76] Other stimuli, including high PCO_2/low pH and several pharmacological agents also effectively increased cAMP content in the rabbit CB, but hypoxia was the only stimulus that increased cAMP levels in Ca^{2+}-free media,[73] suggesting a direct, neurotransmitter-independent, activation of an adenylate cyclase by low PO_2 (Fig. 5.4A). Conversely, maneuvers that lead to an increase on cAMP levels (activation

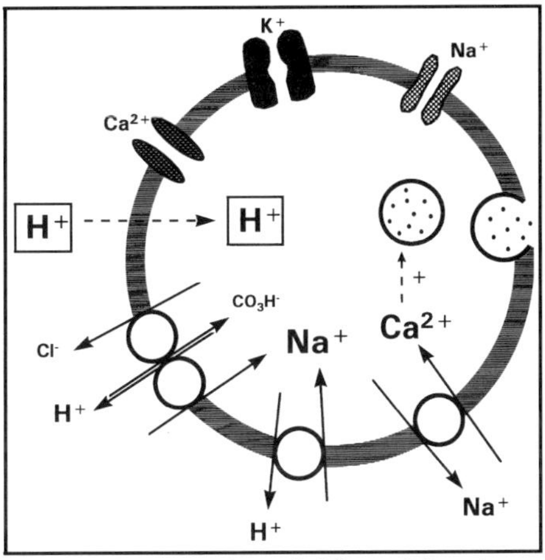

Fig. 5.3. Proposed model for acidic stimulus transduction in rabbit carotid body chemoreceptor cells. The figure shows a scheme of a chemoreceptor cell with voltage-dependent Na^+, K^+ and Ca^{2+} channels, and several countertransport mechanisms in its membrane. Experimental data (see text) support the following cascade of transduction for the acidic stimulus: extracellular H^+ (metabolic and respiratory acidosis, or increased concentrations of weak acids in the extracellular milieu) diffuse to the cell interior and allosterically activate the H+ extruding mechanisms (Na^+/H^+ and $Na^+,HCO^-_3/H^+,Cl^-$ exchangers); this cellular homeostatic response results in a decrease of the original intracellular increase in $[H^+]$, and in an increase in intracellular $[Na^+]$; the increase in intracellular $[Na^+]$ reduces the transmembrane Na^+ gradient and allows the Na^+/Ca^{2+} exchanger to function in reverse mode, extruding Na^+ ions and producing influx of Ca^{2+} ions; the influxing Ca^{2+} activates the exocytotic release of neurotransmitters.

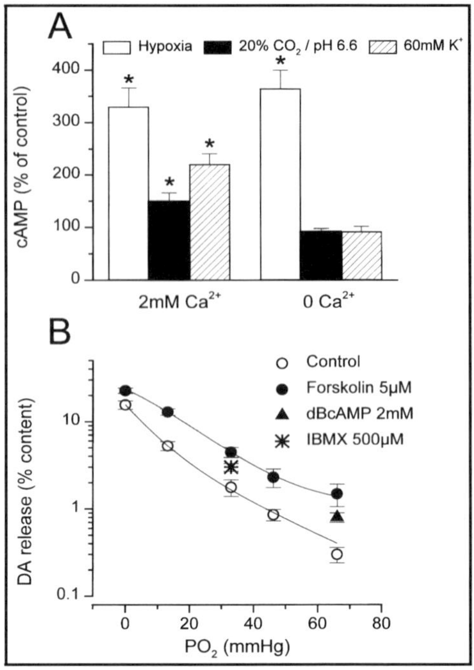

Fig. 5.4. (A) Effect of hypoxic (PO_2 ≈33 mmHg), acidic and high K^+_e stimulation on cAMP levels in rabbit carotid bodies incubated in normal and in 0 Ca^{2+} solutions. In all the cases the stimuli were applied for 10 min, and the levels of the cyclic nucleotide are expressed as percentage of those found in organs incubated in control solutions (PO_2 ≈150 mmHg, 5% CO_2/pH 7.4, and 5 mM K^+e). Hypoxia is the only stimulus producing an increase of cAMP levels in 0 Ca^{2+} solutions. (B) Effect of forskolin (an activator of adenylate cyclase), dibutyryl cAMP and IBMX (isobutylmethylxantine, an inhibitor of the cAMP degrading phosphodiesterase) on the release of dopamine elicited by hypoxic stimuli of different intensities.

of adenylate cyclase with forskolin, inhibition of phosphodiesterase with isobutylmethylxantine or bath application of permeable analogues of cAMP) potentiated the efflux of $^{45}Ca^{2+}$ from previously loaded CB and the release of catecholamines and the CSN response elicited by hypoxia[77] (Fig. 5.4B).

Cyclic AMP seems to activate the hypoxic transduction cascade at least in two different steps. On the one hand, it would inhibit the O_2-sensitive K^+ current, leading to a potentiation of the hypoxic stimulus.[78] In the other hand, it would also modulate the exocytotic machinery of chemoreceptor cells.[77] Bath application of forskolin or dibutyryl cAMP, while recording from isolated rabbit CB chemoreceptor cells in the whole cell configuration, produced an inhibition of the O_2-sensitive transient component of the K^+ current mimicking the action of hypoxia. However, it is important to point out that the nucleotide is not necessary for the low PO_2 inhibition of the K^+ current, because as we have mentioned above, low PO_2 is able to reduce the open probability of the O_2-sensitive K^+ channels in saline perfused inside-out cell membrane patches.[24] It was also observed that neither forskolin nor dibutyryl cAMP were effective in modulating Ca^{2+} currents. The activating effect of cAMP on the exocytotic machinery was inferred from the observation that release of catecholamines induced by ionomycin, the Ca^{2+} ionophore, was potentiated by forskolin. It should be noted, however, that forskolin did not increase, but on the contrary, showed a tendency to decrease the release of neurotransmitters elicited by high external K^+, implying that additional, but not yet defined processes, are targets for the nucleotide or for protein kinase A.[77]

Guanylate Cyclase-cGMP System

This system has been shown to modulate in an inhibitory way the CB response to hypoxic stimulus. Immunohistochemical localization of cGMP demonstrated a moderate level of reactivity in the chemoreceptor cells of the normoxic rat CB, being the reactivity reduced by a short period (10 min) of incubation in a hypoxic solution (5% O_2). On incubations with high external K^+ (100 mM) the reactivity to cGMP increased, and in these conditions the reduction of cGMP produced by the hypoxic incubation was more evident.[76] In another study,[79] atrial natriuretic peptide (ANP) was localized in chemoreceptor cells in coexistence with cGMP, and also demonstrated that ANP greatly increased the levels of this cyclic nucleotide in a dose-dependent manner. Finally, Wang et al[80] demonstrated that ANP and permeable cGMP analogues (but not cGMP itself) were able to inhibit low PO_2 and nicotine induced CSN activity, being ineffective on basal or in high external K^+/O Ca^{2+} induced CSN discharges. It was suggested that the inhibitory actions of ANP and cGMP analogs were produced at the chemoreceptor cell level, although a reduction of the binding or efficiency of neurotransmitters in the postsynaptic membranes (the sensory nerve endings) was not excluded.[81] Consistent with this latter possibility was the observation that ANP and cGMP analogs failed to alter the release of catecholamines induced by hypoxia. Taking into account that common cellular targets for cGMP are K^+_{Ca} (activation) and Ca^{2+} channels (inhibition), it would be interesting to define the actions of cGMP on these channels in chemoreceptor cells to explain the lack of effect of the nucleotide on the release of catecholamines.

Nitric Oxide and Carbon Monoxide

Recent studies have indicated that nitric oxide (NO) and carbon monoxide (CO) may act as chemical messengers in the nervous system, their actions being mediated by the guanylate cyclase-cGMP system. The presence of the enzymatic systems generating NO and CO in the CB, and the possible role of these messengers in chemoreception have been investigated in the last three years. With respect to NO, it has been shown that nitric oxide synthase is present in some petrosal ganglion neurons whose nerve endings terminate in the vicinity of the chemoreceptor/substentacular cell lobules, as well as in neurons located in the microganglia present all along glossopharyngeal and CSN nerves and whose nerve endings terminate in association with the intracarotid body blood vessels.[82] These locations of nitric oxide synthase suggest that NO can modulate the CB reflex activity by vascular and chemoreceptor cell-mediated mechanisms; in chapter 8 by Almaraz et al there is an extensive discussion on the functional significance of this volatile messenger. The role of CO as an inhibitory chemical messenger in the CB chemoreceptors has been proposed by Prabhakar et al.[83] These authors found that the cat CB contains heme oxygenase, the CO synthesizing enzyme, which is selectively located on chemoreceptor cells. Their findings implicate CO as a physiological inhibitor of CB activity. CO formed by glomus cells might inhibit the chemosensory response via the activation of the guanylate cyclase-cGMP system, as it has been described in other systems, and/or by modulating the O_2-sensitive K^+ channel activity acting at the putative oxygen sensor in the cell membrane. The fact that heme oxygenase activity is modulated by changes in PO_2 allows one to propose an attractive hypothesis on the molecular mechanisms for CO modulation of low PO_2 chemoreception: Hypoxia would decrease CO formation by reducing heme oxygenase activity, the decrease in CO would remove the basal inhibition and cause an increase in CSN activity. In spite of the presence of heme oxygenase in the CB tissue and the hypothesis just mentioned, great caution should be used in assigning a physiological role to CO in any given system; first, because the selectivity of heme oxygenase inhibitors commonly used to inhibit the endogenous production of CO is questionable;[84] and second, because the concentrations of CO needed to activate guanylate cyclase are so high that it is dubious that they can ever be reached by endogenous CO production.

Prostaglandins

The role of salicylates as potentiators of the CB responses to hypoxia has been known for many years.[9] Recently, it has been shown that at least part of their effects are mediated by their ability to inhibit prostaglandin synthesis. In an in vitro preparation of rabbit CB, acetylsalicylic acid and indomethacin (inhibitors of cyclooxygenase, the prostaglandin synthesizing enzyme) potentiated low PO_2 and high PCO_2-induced CA release, being these effects reversed by prostaglandin E_2 (PGE_2) application. When PGE_2 was applied alone, it produced a dose-dependent inhibition of the ^{3}H-CA release induced by hypoxia and hypercapnia and high external K^+, and conversely, the natural stimuli augmented the synthesis of endogenous PGE_2 in the intact CB.[85,86] Patch-clamp recordings in isolated cells demonstrated that PGE_2 inhibited Ca^{2+} currents, and thereby probably also the entry of Ca^{2+} in these channels. This action of PGE_2 required GTP and was inhibited by intracellularly applied GDP-β-S, indicating that PGE_2 was acting through a G protein-dependent mechanism.[86] As a whole, these findings indicate that PGE_2, regardless of its origin within the CB, is an important negative modulator of CB chemosensory activity (Fig. 5.5).

The modulation of the sensory transduction in the CB produced by some of the above mentioned second messenger systems implicates the presence of G protein-mediated pathways in the transduction process. In this regard, our laboratory has shown that fluoride (a general activator of G proteins), pertussis toxin (a blocker of the Gi-Go proteins mediated effects) and cholera toxin (and activator of Gs proteins) exert differential effects on the release of ^{3}H-CAs evoked by hypoxic and hypercapnic stimuli in the rabbit CB; these findings are consistent with the notion (see above), that the stimulus-secretion coupling for each stimulus (i.e., their transduction cascade) is different or at least that they are differentially modulated.[87] In spite of the lack of data on the molecular characterization of the G proteins present in chemoreceptor cells, recent studies show that under hypoxic stimulation there is an activation of Gs and Go-Gi proteins.[88] It was also observed that the increase in cAMP levels induced by low PO_2 in the absence of extracellular Ca^{2+} is abolished by pretreatment with PTX, suggesting either the presence of a Go-Gi protein positively coupled to adenylate cyclase or, alternatively, that the O_2-sensing mechanism is coupled to both, a Gs and a Go-Gi protein, so that the α_s subunits of Gs proteins will catalyze the activation of adenylate cyclase with the concurrence of βγ subunits provided by Go-Gi proteins.

CONCLUDING REMARKS AND PERSPECTIVES

The application of patch-clamp techniques to preparations of isolated chemoreceptor cells in primary culture has driven hypoxic and acidic sensory transduction in chemoreceptor cells from the darkness, and brought the CB chemoreceptors to the paths

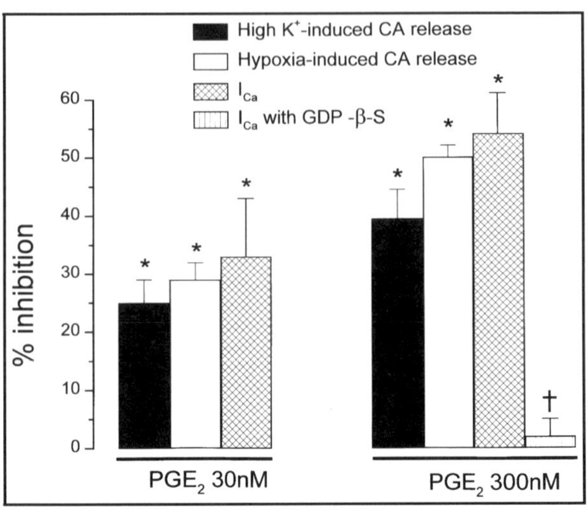

Fig. 5.5. Prostaglandin E2 inhibits the release of catecholamine elicited by hypoxic (PO_2 ≈66 mmHg) and high K^+_e (35 mM) stimulation in the intact rabbit carotid body, and Ca^{2+} currents recorded from short-term cultured rabbit carotid body chemoreceptor cells. Note that prostaglandin E2 inhibition of Ca^{2+} currents was prevented by the inclusion in the recording pipette of GDP-β-S, an analog of GDP that bounds irreversibly to G proteins and blocks their activation.

followed by other sensory receptors. However, the journey has only just started. We must experimentally solve the apparent from the genuine differences among species, and we must enter into the newer pathways of ion channel cloning to test the possibility of the intrinsic O_2-sensitivity of the O_2-sensitive K^+ channels. We should join efforts with researchers in the fields of erythropoietin and pulmonary circulation. If finding references to CB works in articles devoted to O_2-sensing mechanisms in erythropoietin producing and pulmonary artery smooth muscle cells, and the converse, is enlightening, we would define as profitable the joined ventures among researchers of these three fields. The molecular approaches followed in vision and olfaction research have not yet arrived to the arterial chemoreception field, implying that many new pieces must be described and added to the frame delimited by current models of sensory transduction in chemoreceptor cells. However, our minds should not be narrowed by new molecular or biophysical findings; we never should forget that the CB is a small republic made of interrelated individual cells at the service of the entire organism.

Acknowledgments

This work has been supported by Spanish DGICYT grant PB92/0267 and U.S. NIH grants NS 07938 and NS 12636.

References

1. de Castro F. Sur la structure et l'innervation du sinus carotidien de l'homme et des mamifères. Noveaux faits sur l'innervation et la fonction du glomus caroticum. Etudes anatomiques et physiologiques. Trab Lab Invest Biol Univ Madrid 1928; 24:331-380.
2. González C, Almaraz L, Obeso A et al. Oxygen and acid chemoreception in the carotid body chemoreceptors. Trends Neurosci 1992; 15:146-53.
3. González C, Fidone S. Increased release of ^{3}H-dopamine during low O_2 stimulation of rabbit carotid body in vitro. Neurosci Lett 1977; 6: 95-99.
4. Pérez-García MT, Obeso A, López-López, JR et al. Characterization of cultured chemoreceptor cells dissociated from adult rabbit carotid body. Am J Physiol 1992; 263:C1152-9.
5. Fidone S, González C, Yoshizaki K. Effects of low oxygen on the release of dopamine from the rabbit carotid body in vitro. J Physiol Lond 1982; 333:93-110.
6. Rigual R, González E, González C et al. Synthesis and release of catecholamines by the cat carotid body in vitro: effects of hypoxic stimulation. Brain Res 1986; 374:101-109.
7. Verna A. Dense-cored vesicles and cell types in the rabbit carotid body. In: Acker H, Fidone S, Pallot D et al. eds. Chemoreception in the Carotid Body. Berlin: Springer-Verlag, 1977:216-220.
8. Zapata P, Stensaas LJ, Eyzaguirre C. Axon regeneration following a lesion of the carotid nerve: electrophysiological and ultrastructural observations. Brain Res 1976; 113:235-253.
9. González C, Almaraz L, Obeso A et al. Carotid body chemoreceptors: from natural stimuli to sensory discharges. Physiol Rev 1994; 74:829-98.
10. González C, López-López JR, Pérez-García MT et al. Cellular mechanisms of carotid body chemoreception. Respir Physiol 1995; 102:137-147.
11. González C. Sensitivity to physiological hypoxia. In: Weir EK, López-Barneo J, eds. Oxygen Regulation of Ion Channels and Gene Expression. Armonk NY Futura Press, 1997: (in press).
12. López-Barneo J, Weir K. Oxygen Regulation of Ion Channels and Gene Expression. Armonk NY Futura Press, 1997 (in press).
13. Bunn HF, Poyton RO. Oxygen sensing and molecular adaptation to hypoxia. Physiol Rev 1996; 76:839-885.
14. Lloyd BB, Cunningham DJC, Goode RC. Depression of hypoxic hyperventilation in man by sudden inspiration of carbon monoxide. In: Torrance RW, ed. Arterial Chemoreceptors. Oxford, UK: Blackwell, 1968:145-8.
15. Lahiri S, Delaney RG. The nature of response of single chemoreceptor fibers of carotid body to changes in arterial pO_2 and pCO_2-H^+. In: Paintal AS, ed. Morphology and Mechanisms of Chemore-

ceptors. Delhi, India: Vallabhbhai Patel Chest Institute, 1976:18-26.
16. Lahiri S. Introductory remarks: oxygen linked response of carotid chemoreceptors. Adv Exp Med Biol 1977; 78: 185-202.
17. Whalen WJ, Nair P. Tissue PO_2 in the cat carotid body and related functions. Adv Exp Med Biol 1977; 78:225-232.
18. Goldberg M, Dunning SP, Bunn HF. Regulation of the erythropoietin gene: evidence that the oxygen sensor is a heme protein. Science 1988; 242:1412-5.
19. López-López JR, González C. Time course of K^+ current inhibition by low oxygen in chemoreceptor cells of adult rabbit carotid body. Effects of carbon monoxide. FEBS Lett 1992; 299:251-4.
20. Lahiri S, Iturriaga R, Mokashi A et al. CO reveals dual mechanisms of O_2 chemoreception in the cat carotid body. Respir Physiol 1993; 94:227-40.
21. Lahiri S. Carotid body O_2 chemoreception: respiratory and nonrespiratory aspects. Biol Signals 1995; 4:257-262.
22. Tamayo L, López-López JR, Castañeda J et al. Carbon monoxide inhibits hypoxic pulmonary vasoconstriction in rats by a cGMP-independent mechanism.Pflügers Arch 1997 (in press).
23. Coburn RF, Forman HJ. Carbon monoxide toxicity. In: Fishman AP, ed. The Respiratory System. Bethesda: Amer Physiol Soc 1987:439-456.
24. Ganfornina MD, López-Barneo J. Single K^+ channels in membrane patches of arterial chemoreceptor cells are modulated by O_2 tension. Proc Natl Acad Sci USA 1991; 88:2927-30.
25. Vanderkooi JM, Erecinska M, Silver IA. Oxygen in mammalian tissue: methods of measurement and affinities of various reactions. Am J Physiol 1991; 260: C1131-C1150.
26. Wyatt CN, Peers C. Ca^{2+}-activated K^+ channels in isolated type I cells of the neonatal rat carotid body. J Physiol Lond 1995; 483:559-565.
27. Acker H. Cellular oxygen sensors. Ann NY Acad Sci 1994; 718:3-10.
28. Acker H, Xue D. Mechanisms of O_2 sensing in the carotid body in comparison with other O_2-sensing cells. NIPS 1995; 10:211-6.
29. Cross AR, Jones OTG. Enzymatic mechanisms of superoxide production. Biochim Biophys Acta 1991; 1057:281-298.
30. Lizuka T, Kanegasaki S, Makino R et al. Studies on neutrophil b-type cytochrome in situ by low temperature absorption spectroscopy. J Biol Chem 1985; 260: 12049-12053.
31. Parkos CA, Dinauer MC, Walker LE et al. Primary structure and unique expression of the 22-kilodalton light chain of human neutrophil cytochrome b. Proc Natl Acad Sci USA 1988; 85:3319-3323.
32. Ratcliffe PJ, Ebert BL, Ferguson DJP et al. Regulation of the erythropoietin gene. Nephrol Dial Transplant 1995; 10:18-27.
33. Wintrobe MM, Lee GR, Boggs DR et al. Clinical Hematology. New York: Lea & Febiger, 1977:1327-1355.
34. Rigual R, López-López JR, González C. Release of dopamine and chemoreceptor discharge induced by low pH and high PCO_2 stimulation of the cat carotid body. J Physiol Lond 1991; 433:519-531.
35. Obeso A, Almaraz L, González C. Effects of 2-deoxy-D-glucose on in vitro cat carotid body. Brain Res 1986; 371:25-36.
36. Obeso A, Almaraz L, González C. Effects of cyanide and uncouplers on chemoreceptor activity and ATP content of the cat carotid body. Brain Res 1989; 481: 250-7.
37. Almaraz L, González C, Obeso A. Effects of high potassium on the release of [^{3}H]dopamine from the cat carotid body in vitro. J Physiol Lond 1986; 379: 293-307.
38. Obeso A, Rocher A, Fidone S et al. The role of dihydropyridine-sensitive Ca^{2+} channels in stimulus-evoked catecholamine release from chemoreceptor cells of the carotid body. Neuroscience 1992; 47:463-472.
39. Rocher A, Obeso A, Cachero MT et al. Participation of Na^+ channels in the response of carotid body chemoreceptor cells to hypoxia. Am J Physiol 1994; 267:C738-44.
40. Weir EK, Archer SL. The mechanism of acute hypoxic pulmonary vasoconstriction: the tale of two channels. FASEB J 1995; 9:183-189.
41. López-Barneo J, López-López JR, Ureña J et al. Chemotransduction in the carotid

body: K^+ current modulated by PO_2 in type I chemoreceptor cells. Science 1988; 241:580-2.
42. Duchen MR, Caddy KW, Kirby GC et al. Biophysical studies of the cellular elements of the rabbit carotid body. Neuroscience 1988; 26:291-311.
43. López-López JR, González C, Ureña J et al. Low pO_2 selectively inhibits K channel activity in chemoreceptor cells of the mammalian carotid body. J Gen Physiol 1989; 93:1001-1015.
44. González C, López López JR, Obeso A et al. Ca^{2+} dynamics in chemoreceptor cells: an overview. Adv Exp Med Biol 1993; 337:149-156.
45. Montoro RJ, Ureña J, Fernández-Chacón R et al. Oxygen sensing by ion channels and chemotransduction in single glomus cells. J Gen Physiol 1996; 107:133-143.
46. López-López JR, González C, Pérez-García MT. Properties of ionic currents from isolated adult rat carotid body chemoreceptor cells: Effect of hypoxia. J Physiol Lond 1997; 499:429-441.
47. Peers C. O_2 sensing in the carotid body. Prim Sensory Neuron 1996; 1:197-208.
48. Donnelly DF. Electrochemical detection of catecholamine release from rat carotid body in vitro. J Appl Physiol 1993; 74:2330-2337.
49. Buckler KJ. A novel oxygen-sensitive potassium current in rat carotid body type I cells. J Physiol Lond 1997; 498:649-662.
50. Cheng PM, Donnelly DF. Relationship between changes of glomus cell current and neural response of rat carotid body. J Neurophysiol 1995; 74:2077-2086.
51. Donnelly DF. Modulation of glomus cell membrane currents of intact rat carotid body. J Physiol Lond 1995; 489:677-688.
52. Peers C, Buckler KJ. Transduction of chemostimuli by the type I carotid body cell. J Membrane Biol 1995; 144: 1-9.
53. Mills E, Jöbsis FF. Simultaneous measurement of cytochrome a_3 reduction and chemoreceptor afferent activity in the carotid body. Nature 1970; 225:1147-1149.
54. Acker H, Eyzaguirre C. Light absorbance changes in the mouse carotid body during hypoxia and cyanide poisoning. Brain Res 1987; 409:380-385.
55. Rettig J, Heinemann S, Wunder F et al. Inactivation properties of voltage-gated K^+ channels altered by presence of b-subunit. Nature 1994; 369:289-294.
56. Halliwell B, Gutteridge JMC. Free radicals in biology and medicine. New York: Oxford University Press, 1987.
57. Archer SL, Huang J, Henry T et al. A redox-based O_2 sensor in rat pulmonary vasculature. Circ Res 1993; 73:1100-1112.
58. Chance B, Sies H, Boveris A. Hydroperoxide metabolism in mammalian organs. Physiol Rev 1979; 59:527-605.
59. Vega Saez de Miera E, Rudy B. Modulation of K^+ channels by hydrogen peroxide. Biochem Biophys Res Commun 1992; 186:1681-1687.
60. Fandrey J, Frede S, Jelkmann W. Role of hydrogen-peroxide in hypoxia-induced erythropoietin production. Biochem J 1994; 303:507-510.
61. Stea A, Jackson A, Nurse CA. Hypoxia and N6,O2'-dibutyryladenosine 3',5'-cyclic monophosphate, but not nerve growth factor, induce Na^+ channels and hypertrophy in chromaffin-like arterial chemoreceptors. Proc Natl Acad Sci USA 1992; 89:9469-9473.
62. Czyzyk-Krzeska MF, Furnari BA, Lawson EE et al. Hypoxia increases rate of transcription and stability of tyrosine hydroxylase mRNA in pheochromocytoma (PC12) cells. J Biol Chem 1994; 269: 760-764.
63. Wang GL, Semenza GL. General involvement of hypoxia-inducible factor 1 in transcriptional response to hypoxia. Proc Natl Acad Sci USA 1993; 90:4304-4308.
64. Buckler KJ, Vaughan-Jones RD, Peers C et al. Effects of extracellular pH, PCO_2 and HCO_3^- on intracellular pH in isolated type-I cells of the neonatal rat carotid body. J Physiol 1991a; 444:703-721.
65. Buckler KJ, Vaughan Jones RD. Effects of acidic stimuli on intracellular calcium in isolated type I cells of the neonatal rat carotid body. Pflugers Arch 1993; 425: 22-27.
66. Iturriaga R, Mokashi A, Lahiri S. Dynamics of carotid body responses in vitro in the presence of CO_2-HCO_3^-: role of carbonic anhydrase. J Appl Physiol 1993; 75:1587-1594.
67. Lahiri S, Iturriaga R, Mokashi A et al. Adaptation to hypercapnia vs. intracellular pH in cat carotid body: responses

in vitro. J Appl Physiol 1996; 80:1090-1099.
68. Hayes MW, Balwant KM, Torrance RW. Reduction of the responses of carotid chemoreceptors by acetazolamide. In: Paintal AS, ed. Morphology and Mechanisms of Chemoreceptors. Delhi, India: Vallabhbhai Patel Chest Institute, 1976: 36-47.
69. Torrance RW. Prolegomena. In: Torrance RW, ed. Arterial Chemoreceptors. Oxford: Blackwell Scientific Publication, 1968:1-40.
70. Peers C, Green FK. Inhibition of Ca^{2+}-activated K^+ currents by intracellular acidosis in isolated type I cells of the neonatal rat carotid body. J Physiol Lond 1991; 437:589-602.
71. Rocher A, Obeso A, González C et al. Ionic mechanisms for the transduction of acidic stimuli in rabbit carotid body glomus cells. J Physiol Lond 1991; 433: 533-48.
72. Buckler KJ, Vaughan-Jones RD, Peers C et al. Intracellular pH and its regulation in isolated type I carotid body cells of the neonatal rat. J Physiol Lond 1991b; 436:107-129.
73. Pérez-García MT, Almaraz L, González C. Effects of different types of stimulation on cyclic AMP content in the rabbit carotid body: functional significance. J Neurochem 1990; 55:1287-93.
74. Delpiano MA, Acker H. Hypoxia increases the cyclic AMP content of the cat carotid body in vitro. J Neurochem 1991; 57:291-7.
75. Wang WJ, Cheng GF, Yoshizaki K et al. The role of cyclic AMP in chemoreception in the rabbit carotid body. Brain Res 1991; 540:96-104.
76. Wang ZZ, Stensaas LJ, de Vente J et al. Immunocytochemical localization of cAMP and cGMP in cells of the rat carotid body following natural and pharmacological stimulation. Histochemistry 1991; 96:523-30.
77. Pérez-García MT, Almaraz L, González C. Cyclic AMP modulates differentially the release of dopamine induced by hypoxia and other stimuli and increases dopamine synthesis in the rabbit carotid body. J Neurochem 1991; 57:1992-2000.
78. López-López JR, De Luis DA, González C. Properties of a transient K^+ current in chemoreceptor cells of rabbit carotid body. J Physiol Lond 1993; 460:15-32.
79. Wang ZZ, He L, Stensaas LJ et al. Localization and in vitro actions of atrial natriuretic peptide in the cat carotid body. J Appl Physiol 1991; 70:942-6.
80. Wang WJ, He L, Chen J et al. Mechanisms underlying chemoreceptor inhibition induced by atrial natriuretic peptide in rabbit carotid body. J Physiol Lond 1993; 460:427-441.
81. Kupfermann I. Functional studies of cotransmission. Physiol Rev 1991; 71: 683-732.
82. Wang ZZ, Stensaas LJ, Bredt DS et al. Localization and actions of nitric oxide in the cat carotid body. Neuroscience 1994; 60:275-86.
83. Prabhakar NR, Dinerman JL, Agani FH et al. Carbon monoxide: a role in carotid body chemoreception. Proc Natl Acad Sci USA 1995; 92:1994-7.
84. Meffert MK, Harley JE, Schuman EM et al. Inhibition of hippocampal heme oxygenase, nitric oxide synthase and long-term potentiation by metalloporphyrins. Neuron 1994; 13:1225-1233.
85. Gómez-Niño A, Almaraz L, González C. In vitro activation of cyclo-oxygenase in the rabbit carotid body: effect of its blockade on [^{3}H]catecholamine release. J Physiol Lond 1994a; 476:257-67.
86. Gómez-Niño A, López-López JR, Almaraz L et al. Inhibition of [^{3}H] catecholamine release and Ca^{2+} currents by prostaglandin E2 in rabbit carotid body chemoreceptor cells. J Physiol Lond 1994b; 476:269-77.
87. Cachero TG, Rocher A, Rigual R et al. Effects of fluoride and cholera and pertussis toxins on sensory transduction in the carotid body. Am J Physiol 1995; 269 (Cell Physiol. 38):C1271-9.
88. Cachero TG, Rigual R, Rocher A et al. Cholera and pertussis toxins reveal multiple regulation of cAMP levels in the rabbit carotid body. Eur J Neurosci 1996; 8:2320-2327.

CHAPTER 6

Chemosensory Activity in the Carotid Nerve: Effects of Physiological Variables

Patricio Zapata

INTRODUCTION

What is known today as the *carotid (sinus) nerve* was initially called "*Sinusnerv*" by Hering[1] in 1924 (although the same name had been used as early as 1885 by Ph. Knoll—see Heymans and Neil[2]), "*nerf intercarotidien*" by de Castro[3] and "*nerf carotidien*" by Hovelacque et al.[4] It is a branch of the glossopharyngeal (IXth cranial) nerve.

FIBER COMPONENTS OF CAROTID NERVE

The carotid nerve mainly contains: 1) barosensory fibers from the carotid sinus; 2) chemosensory fibers from the carotid body. Thus, the name "carotid nerve" will be used here because it recognizes both neural components, while the name "sinus nerve" appears appropriate for only one component, the one not concerned with the present book. The carotid nerve also contains: 3) a variable but small number of preganglionic parasympathetic fibers directed to the carotid bifurcation,[5,6] 4) postganglionic sympathetic fibers originated from the superior cervical ganglion, coursing through the ganglio-glomerular nerves (internal carotid nerve), bypassing carotid body tissues and ascending through the carotid nerves to an unknown destination;[7] and 5) a few postganglionic sympathetic fibers from the superior cervical ganglion, which ascend to the glossopharyngeal nerve trunk and then descend through the carotid nerve towards the carotid bifurcation.[8] (See Fig. 6.1; see also chapters 1 and 8 by Verna and Almaraz et al, respectively).

Because of the above, recordings from the intact carotid nerve will reveal centripetal impulses from afferent fibers and centrifugal impulses from efferent autonomic fibers. After cutting the carotid nerve at its emergence from the glossopharyngeal nerve, recordings from

The Carotid Body Chemoreceptors,
edited by Constancio González.

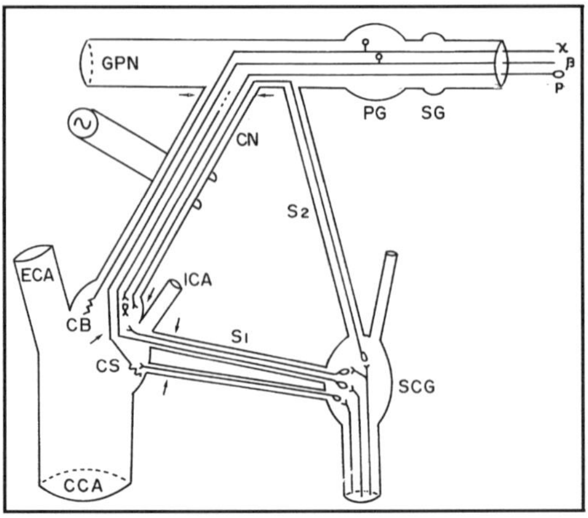

Fig. 6.1. Schematic diagram of the innervation of the carotid bifurcation, signaling the origin and destination of fibers contained within the carotid (sinus) nerve (CN). CB, carotid body; CCA, common carotid artery; CS, carotid sinus; ECA, external carotid artery; GPN, glosso-pharyngeal nerve; ICA, internal carotid artery; P, preganglionic parasympathetic neuron synapsing on postganglionic neuron in the capsule of the carotid body; PG, petrosal ganglion; SCG, superior cervical ganglion; SG, superior (Ehrenritter's) ganglion; S1, postganglionic sympathetic fibers contained within ganglio-glomerular nerves; S2, postganglionic sympathetic fibers directed to the glossopharyngeal nerve and entering the carotid body through the carotid nerve; β, barosensory neuron; χ, chemosensory neuron. Between arrows, sections required for recording pure chemosensory activity from the carotid nerve.

its peripheral end consist mostly of sensory discharges, but dominated by pulse-related bursts of the usually larger action potentials of carotid sinus barosensory fibers.[9] Further section of the ganglio-glomerular nerves eliminates the few ascending sympathetic fibers and leaves only the afferent discharges. (See Fig. 6.1). Uncontaminated recordings of the chemosensory fibers from the carotid bodies may be obtained by: 1) isolation of single or few chemosensory fibers by dissection of filaments from the nerve (single or pauci-fiber recordings);[10] 2) microelectrode recordings from petrosal ganglion cells,[11,12] where most of the perikarya of carotid chemosensory fibers are concentrated; 3) dissection of perivascular connections between the carotid body and sinus,[13-15] to eliminate barosensory fibers (multifiber recordings); 4) reducing intrasinusal or systemic arterial blood pressure below the firing threshold of carotid sinus baroreceptors,[13,16] procedures which, however, increase the resting rate of chemosensory discharges (see later).

The carotid nerve of the cat contains myelinated (A) and unmyelinated (C) fibers, with diameters of from 1 to 9 mm and from 0.1 to 0.3 mm, respectively,[7] and they comprise chemosensory, barosensory and autonomic fibers. Electrophysiologically identified chemosensory fibers occur in both groups: the conduction velocities of A fibers range from 3 to 53 m/s, whereas those of C fibers range from 0.5 to 2.0 m/s.[12,17]

Recordings of Carotid Chemosensory Activity

It was Fernando de Castro's idea,[3] prompted from anatomical studies, that the carotid body "tastes" the blood for chemical substances. However, the first reported recordings of well defined chemosensory activity in the carotid nerve were those of Zotterman.[13] Recording of afferent nerve impulses provides a simple, precise and powerful method for the analysis of the neural output of receptor organs. Thus, it has mostly replaced the indirect method of assessing the responsiveness of arterial chemoreceptors through the elicitation of ventilatory and cardiovascular reflex reactions (see chapter 10). Single unit recordings are amenable to analyses of frequencies of nerve impulses (minimal, mean and peak frequencies), the time course of such discharges (continuous measurements of mean frequencies or instantaneous frequencies--the last ones representing the reciprocals of intervals between contiguous impulses) or more detailed analyses of pulse intervals (histograms of distribution, probability densities and autocorrelations between nonsuccessive spikes). All of them have been used for the analysis of the afferent discharges recorded from chemosensory units. On the other hand, the advantages of multifiber recordings from the entire nerve have been summarized by Fitzgerald and Osborne[18] as follows: 1) they present better stability than single fiber preparations, especially during prolonged recordings; 2) they minimize the problem of individual fiber variability, necessitating larger numbers of experiments to obtain statistically significant data; 3) the whole nerve responses are virtually identical to the mean responses of individual fibers.

Recordings of chemosensory activity from the carotid nerves have been obtained from different preparations: 1) carotid bodies in situ with their intact circulation (e.g., Eyzaguirre and Lewin[10]); 2) carotid bodies in situ which are vascularly isolated and perfused with blood or saline solutions (see O'Regan[19,20]); 3) carotid bodies in vitro superfused with saline solutions;[21] 4) carotid bodies in vitro perfused and superfused with saline solutions.[22,23] Preparations 1 and 3 may be recorded with slow decay for prolonged periods of time (up to 12 hours, by personal experience of this author).

Concerning their responses to chemical stimuli, the chemosensory fibers of the carotid nerve form a very homogeneous population, as shown by the fact that stimulus-response curves for single fibers are very similar to those of the whole nerve.[24] Each fiber responds to changes in the concentrations of oxygen, carbon dioxide and hydrogen ions. Furthermore, temporal correlations of the rates of discharges of pairs of fibers recorded at different levels of chemical stimulation result in straight lines with intercepts near zero, suggesting similar thresholds and patterns of responses, although differing in the ranges of the frequencies they sustain.[25] However, chemosensory C fibers have higher thresholds and latencies, but lower maximal discharge rates in response to injections of NaCN and acids than their A fiber counterparts.[17]

SPONTANEOUS CHEMOSENSORY DISCHARGES UNDER BASAL CONDITIONS

Some early observations on the electrical activity recorded from carotid nerves and on reflex effects evoked from the carotid bifurcation suggested that the chemosensory fibers of the carotid nerves were active only when oxygen in the blood fell below normal range and carbon dioxide exceeded certain levels. These ideas were abandoned after Eyzaguirre and Lewin[10] showed the presence of nerve impulses in these fibers (either isolated or recorded from the entire carotid nerve) under eupneic conditions (normocapnic normoxia) in artificially ventilated, paralyzed and anesthetized cats. Furthermore, the existence and importance of a resting rate of chemosensory inflow through the carotid nerves upon eupneic breathing is revealed by the immediate reflex reduction in ventilation after the animals breathe pure oxygen for a few seconds[26] or after receiving i.v. injections of dopamine,[27] a substance that may briefly silence arterial chemoreceptor discharges (see chapter 7). These reflex effects are mostly due to the withdrawal of carotid chemosensory discharges since they are still observed after severance of the aortic nerves.[27] Thus, ongoing activity through the carotid nerves drives ventilation in steady-state normoxia.[28,29]

Superfusing carotid bodies in vitro under conditions mimicking those of in situ preparations[21,30] shows the presence of spontaneous chemosensory discharges. Based on the hypothesis that this is due to some transmitter(s) released from glomus cells, probably requiring the entry of extracellular calcium (Ca^{2+}_e), the effects of changes in

$[Ca^{2+}]_e$ on spontaneous chemosensory activity had been studied.[31,32] Bathing the carotid body in a Ca^{2+}-free solution increased temporarily the basal frequency of discharge, an effect probably due to decreased nerve ending threshold, after which the basal fell below control levels and the chemosensory responses to hypoxia, acidity and flow interruption were reduced. Otherwise, adding Mg^{2+} to the superfusate markedly depressed basal chemosensory activity and the responses to acidity and flow interruption.

Stochastic Distribution of Carotid Chemosensory Discharges

Single fiber recordings from carotid nerves from cat carotid bodies in situ revealed that their spontaneous discharges under basal conditions were aperiodic,[10] a characteristic that is valuable to differentiate them from carotid barosensory fibers, exhibiting prominent pulse related bursting discharges. Statistical analyses of the intervals between chemosensory impulses from single-fiber recordings obtained from normally circulated or artificially perfused carotid bodies in cats showed that interval histograms had exponential distributions and that the standard deviation of intervals equaled the mean intervals, thus satisfying two criteria for a random pattern of discharges.[33] Recordings from preparations superfused in vitro, in which stimulant levels are kept constant, also showed that the histograms of their interval distributions were very close to those expected for random events.[30] A later study confirmed that 70% of spike trains did not differ significantly from the exponential distribution characteristic of Poisson's type random processes, whereas the remaining 30% presented some degree of sequential ordering (i.e., intervals of similar duration tend to occur together).[34] A similar analysis applied to the interspike intervals recorded from chemosensory fibers of carotid bodies in situ under hypoxic-hypercapnic conditions revealed mild degrees of serial correlations,[35] suggesting the presence of a modulatory process limiting variation about mean frequency. Such modulation was eliminated by treating the preparations with haloperidol, a dopaminergic blocker.[36]

Recordings of isolated chemosensory units in cats anesthetized, paralyzed and artificially ventilated revealed that the mean discharge frequencies of carotid fibers were nearly twice those of aortic fibers (2-4 Hz vs. 1-2 Hz) under normoxic normocapnia.[37] Otherwise, carotid fibers always discharged at higher frequencies than aortic fibers when subjected to hypoxic or hypercapnic challenges.

Rhythmic Fluctuations in Carotid Chemosensory Discharges

Carotid chemosensory discharges recorded in situ in spontaneously breathing or artificially ventilated paralyzed cats show prominent fluctuations of their instantaneous frequencies when ventilatory rates are low. These "respiratory oscillations" in chemosensory rate[38] follow the respiratory fluctuations of arterial PCO_2,[39,40] pH[41] and PO_2.[42] Carotid chemosensory fibers in the cat may follow these oscillations up to imposed ventilatory rates of 70 cycles/min,[43] as increases in respiratory rate proportionally decrease the amplitudes of variations of blood gases.[44] Contrarily, as the heart is operating as a mixing chamber, a decrease in heart rate will attenuate the oscillations in arterial blood gases[45] and thus the respiratory fluctuations in chemosensory discharges.

Cross correlations between single fiber discharges of carotid nerve and cardiac cycles revealed respiratory fluctuations in more than half of the experiments and cardiac rhythmicity in one-third of the chemosensory fibers recorded in cats artificially ventilated.[46] However, the ganglio-glomerular nerves of those preparations were intact, opening the possibility that the fluctuations of chemosensory discharges were dependent on sympathetic bursts with respiratory and cardiac timings. Superimposed cardiac and respiratory rhythmicities are a prominent feature of nerve impulses recorded from the ganglio-glomerular nerves.[47] However, respiratory fluctuations in carotid chemosensory rate persist after eliminating the sympathetic nerve supply to the carotid body,[48] reinforcing the idea that they are due to oscillations in arterial blood gases (see ref. 29).

The ventilatory oscillations in carotid chemosensory discharges opened a discussion on the possibility that arterial chemoreceptors would operate as detectors not of the levels but of the rates of changes of chemical stimuli in the blood. However, recent observations indicate that when 1 to 3 inspirations are omitted in artificially ventilated cats, the fluctuations in carotid chemosensory discharges reach progressively higher frequencies for those prolonged cycles, as it would be expected from a proportional receptor, instead of maintaining the same frequency, as it would be expected from a differential receptor.[49]

Carotid Chemosensory Activity in Fetal and Neonatal Ages

The problem of the initiation and resetting of chemosensory activity in the carotid nerves has been studied in lambs by Blanco et al.[50] Such activity was detected in all exteriorized fetuses of 90 to 143 days of gestational age, showing mean chemosensory frequencies of about 5 Hz at an oxygen pressure in the arterial blood (P_aO_2) of 25 Torr. Recordings in near-term fetuses whilst the umbilical cord was ligated and ventilation in air had started revealed that the chemosensory frequency (f_x) increased by 200-500% as P_aO_2 fell, but then decreased below control values as P_aO_2 increased. No spontaneous chemosensory impulses were detected on the day of birth in lambs delivered vaginally or by Caesarean section at 135-146 days, but it could be evoked by hypercapnia. Spontaneous chemosensory activity was again recorded in lambs more than 2 days old. Thus, carotid chemoreceptors are active and responsive in fetuses, quiescent at birth when P_aO_2 has risen and reset to the adult range over next few days (see chapter 11 by D. Donnelly).

The above results explain why silencing of arterial chemoreceptors by breathing 100% oxygen for 15-20 s produces no changes in ventilation on the day of birth in vaginally born rats or in near-term pups delivered by Caesarean section, but produced a significant decrease in ventilation after 1 day, which became more pronounced after 7 days of age.[51] Similarly, oxygen tests of 30 s do not change ventilation in healthy humans studied 2 to 6 h after birth, but a 10% decrease in ventilation is observed in 2-6 day old infants.[52]

The influence of carotid chemoreceptors on ventilatory drive shortly after birth is illustrated by the hypoventilation in

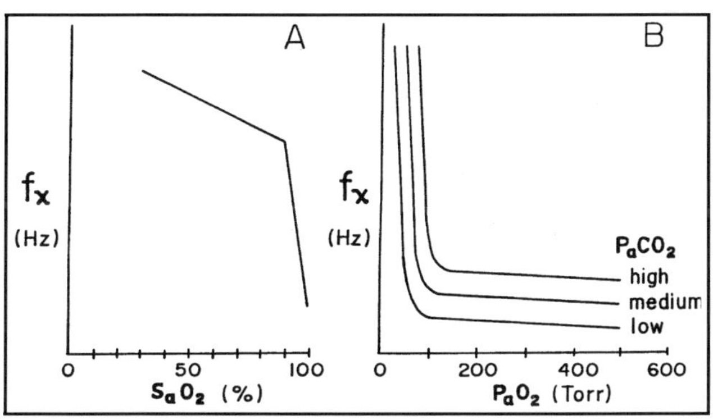

Fig. 6.2. Schematic diagram of relationships between steady levels of oxygen (abscissae) and frequency of chemosensory impulses (fx; ordinates). Ordinates given without numerical scale because similar trends are observed for single chemosensory units as for the entire nerve chemosensory discharge. A. Effects of changes in oxygen saturation of the arterial blood (SaO_2). B. Effects of changes in partial pressure of oxygen in arterial blood (PaO_2), studied at different levels of partial pressure of carbon dioxide in arterial blood ($PaCO_2$).

normoxia, increased frequency and duration of apneas and high mortality in young piglets (less than 9 days old) subjected to bilateral section of the carotid nerves[53] (see chapter 11).

CHEMOSENSORY RESPONSES TO OXYGEN CHANGES

The carotid chemosensory discharges recorded in response to varying pressures of oxygen largely depend on the conditions set by the simultaneous influences of other physiological variables, such as PCO_2, pH and temperature. But, for an orderly discussion, the effects of changing PO_2 on chemosensory discharges will be analyzed first, assuming that other relevant stimuli are kept constant at the center of their physiological ranges; then these effects will be reanalyzed, taking into consideration different levels of other concomitant physiological stimuli.

Chemosensory Activity at Different Steady Levels of Oxygen

Von Euler et al[54] ventilated cats with different mixtures of O_2 (3-30%) in N_2, thus modifying the saturation of oxygen in the arterial blood (S_aO_2) between 50 and 100%, and observed that the frequency of impulses recorded from the entire carotid nerve was linearly and inversely related to S_aO_2. If the observations of Lahiri et al[55] on the frequency of chemosensory discharges in single carotid nerve fibers recorded at different steady-state levels of P_aO_2 are replotted to relate them to calculated levels of S_aO_2, the lineal inverse relationship is confirmed for the range between 50 and 90%, but further increases in S_aO_2 toward 100% produce a sharper drop in chemosensory frequency (see Fig. 6.2A).

A hyperbolic function is the best description of the relationship observed between the impulse frequency in single carotid chemosensory fibers and P_aO_2[56] as P_aO_2 is raised from *ca.* 40 to 90 Torr, f_x decreases rapidly, but further raises of P_aO_2 up to 600 Torr result in small decreases in f_x. Nevertheless, chemosensory units are not maintained completely silenced even at extremely high values of P_aO_2, an indication that the carotid chemoreceptors do not possess a real threshold for oxygen sensitivity. Thus the carotid bodies are not only excited during hypoxia, but also during normoxia and even during prolonged periods of hyperoxia.

The hyperbolic relationship between f_x and P_aO_2 has been confirmed in many recordings obtained from single fibers[57] and entire carotid nerves, but the curve may be displaced to the right and upward by increasing steady levels of carbon dioxide (Fig. 6.2B). In carotid bodies superfused in vitro with saline solutions saturated with different concentrations of O_2 in N_2, a similar relationship has been observed between f_x and the oxygenation of the medium.[30]

Chemosensory Responses to Abrupt Changes in Oxygenation

In anesthetized and moderately hypoxic cats, inhalation of 100% O_2 along two ventilatory cycles led within 3 s to a deep reduction in the f_c recorded from one carotid nerve, immediately followed by a 10-15% decrease in tidal volume after 10 s of beginning O_2 administration; both reductions disappeared within 1 min.[58] These observations account for the transient reductions in ventilation on rapidly shifting from a normoxic environment to a hyperoxic one, observed in unanesthetized humans and dogs, and revealing the presence of a previous ventilatory drive from carotid chemoreceptors in normoxia.[26,59] The ventilatory depressions induced by hyperoxic tests are transient because the ventilatory responses themselves lead to increased P_ACO_2 and then P_aCO_2 which excite both central and arterial chemoreceptors, which in turn reflexly increase ventilation to a level close to that observed in the initial normoxic condition.

In adult cats, a sudden transition from normoxia to hypoxia led to a rapid increase in f_c from the carotid nerve, not followed by adaptation to intermediate levels of chemosensory discharges,[60] even when hypoxia was sustained for 30 min.[61] However, prolonged exposures of rabbit carotid bodies in situ to isocapnic hypoxia produce a maximal increase in f_x to *ca.* 650% within 2-5 min, followed by a progressive decline (adaptation), reaching *ca.* 560% of the baseline at the end of 60 min.[62] Nevertheless, upon exposure of goats to eucapnic hypoxia for up to 4 h, recordings from single carotid chemosensory fibers reveal a slow progressive increase in the frequency of discharges between the 1st and 4th hour,[63] a phenomenon which may contribute to the time-dependent progressive increase in ventilation on ascent to altitude, known as ventilatory acclimatization to hypoxia.[64]

When recording chemosensory discharges from carotid bodies superfused in vitro, sudden shifts to solutions equilibrated with higher concentrations of O_2 produce reductions of f_x, while shifting to superfusates equilibrated with lower concentrations of O_2 produce increases of f_x[21]. Superfusing with solutions equilibrated with 100% N_2 induces a vigorous increase of f_x followed by a progressive reduction of chemosensory discharges.[30]

Studies on carotid bodies perfused and superfused in vitro show that hypoxic perfusates produced faster and larger chemosensory responses when perfused with saline solutions equilibrated with CO_2-HCO_3^- than when perfused with solutions devoid of these substances, the responses to NaCN being also potentiated in the presence of CO_2-HCO_3^-.[65] Similarly, the chemosensory responses of cat carotid bodies in vitro to 100% N_2-equilibrated saline, NaCN and flow interruption are faster and more intense after adding acetate to the perfusate and superfusate[66] (see also González et al[29]). This suggests that, even when the extracellular pH is maintained normal, the intracellular acidosis induced by acetate enhances the chemosensory responses to hypoxic, cytotoxic and stagnant hypoxia.

Based on the hypothesis that hypoxic chemoreception involves an enhanced release of transmitter(s) from glomus cells to make sensory nerve fibers to discharge at higher frequencies, the effects of changes in $[Ca^{2+}]_e$ on chemosensory discharges have been extensively studied. Recordings from cat carotid bodies in vitro[32] reveal that low Ca^{2+} superfusates reduce the chemosensory responses to hypoxic stimulation. Furthermore, recordings from cat carotid bodies in situ[67] show that Ca^{2+}-free perfusates decrease chemosensory responses to hypoxia, a similar effect being obtained by perfusates containing the calcium channel blockers verapamil, diltiazem or nifedipine. In cat carotid bodies superfused in vitro, the chemosensory responses to NaCN are similarly attenuated by these blockers of voltage-gated calcium channels (Sanhueza and Zapata, unpublished results). For a characterization of calcium currents in glomus cells, see González et al[29] (see also chapter 4 by López-López and Peers).

The Nature of the Oxygen Stimulus

What is really important for stimulation of carotid body chemoreceptors is the level of tissue O_2 utilization. Robin[68] proposed the term *dysoxia* for the result of any process leading to reduced O_2 utilization within the cell.

Dysoxia may be *secondary* to: 1) environmental hypoxia, such as the reduced PO_2 observed in poorly oxygenated environments or at high altitude; 2) pulmonary disturbances reducing P_AO_2 or O_2 diffusion from the alveoli to the lung capillaries (reduced P_aO_2); 3) hypoxemia due to reduced transport capacity of the blood, such in anemia or reduced affinity of hemoglobin for O_2 (reduced S_aO_2); 4) stagnant hypoxia, due to systemic (decreased cardiac output, systemic hypotension, increased affinity of hemoglobin for O_2) or local (vasoconstriction, ischemia, arterio-venous anastomoses) causes; 5) decreased capillary, interstitial or intracellular transport of O_2. All of the above reduce O_2 inflow to the mitochondria and, therefore, are more or less capable of exciting carotid and aortic chemoreceptors (see Fidone and González[69]). Thus, breathing carbon monoxide (CO), to produce varying degrees of carboxyhemoglobinemia and thus reducing the O_2 transport capacity, increases the frequency of discharge of carotid chemosensory fibers, although less intensely than that of aortic chemosensory fibers.[55] It must be noted, however, that very brief exposures to CO (along a single ventilatory cycle) in blood perfused preparations produce a sharp rise in P_aO_2 and a very transient inhibition of carotid chemosensory discharges.[70]

Furthermore, dysoxia may be the *primary* disturbance that occurs in spite of normoxia or even hyperoxia, during circumstances formerly referred to as histotoxic or cytotoxic hypoxia, and attributable to abnormally enhanced or depressed mitochondrial O_2 consumption.[68] The intense chemosensory discharges elicited by 2,4-dinitrophenol or cyanide administration (see Anichkov and Belen'kii[71]) are illustrative of the stimulant effects of primary dysoxia. Increases in chemosensory discharges recorded from the carotid nerve of anesthetized normoxic cats have been reported in response to intravenous or intra-arterial injections of: 1) inhibitors of the electron transport chain, such as cyanide, azide and antimycin A; 2) uncouplers of oxidative phosphorylation, such as 2,4-dinitrophenol and carbonyl cyanide *p*-trifluoromethoxyphenylhydrazone (FCCP) and; 3) inhibitors of ADP phosphorylation, such as oligomycin.[72,73] Blocking this last phase of ATP formation by oligomycin made carotid chemosensory fibers unresponsive to the effects of the inhibitors of the earlier phases of mitochondrial metabolism.

Prolonged hyperoxia may lead to the accumulation of free radicals within tissues and thus become toxic (hyperoxic dysoxia). Lahiri et al[74] observed in cats that 3 days exposure to isocapnic hyperoxia attenuated the carotid chemosensory responses to hypoxia and cyanide, while those to hypercapnia were accentuated.

CHEMOSENSORY RESPONSES TO CARBON DIOXIDE CHANGES

As early as 1935, increases in the frequency of impulses were recorded from the carotid nerve in cats after either occluding the trachea for 30 s, breathing 10% CO_2 or increasing P_aCO_2 above 35 Torr.[13,75] The first response (asphyxia) should be ascribed to either hypoxia, hypercapnia or both, but, since spontaneously breathing animals hyperventilate when exposed to increased concentrations of CO_2, the chemosensory responses to the second and third conditions indicate that hypercapnia alone is a suitable stimulus for carotid chemoreceptors. For a full discussion of interactions between PO_2, PCO_2 and pH in chemoreceptor transduction, see González et al.[29]

Chemosensory Activity at Different Steady Levels of Carbon Dioxide

Recordings from carotid nerves in cats revealed direct sigmoid functions between resting levels of f_x and alveolar pressures of carbon dioxide (P_ACO_2), in the range between 10 and 60 Torr, even when O_2 was the remaining inspiratory gas; the entire sigmoid curve was progressively displaced upward when the inspiratory fraction of oxygen (F_IO_2) was reduced to 50, 20 and 10%.[10] Later recordings from single chemosensory fibers[56,76] showed sigmoidal increases in f_x in response to augmented levels of P_aCO_2, even when pH_a was kept constant (*ca.* 7.45) by i.v. administration of $NaHCO_3$; the curves were displaced upward when pH_a was kept at more acidic levels (*ca.* 7.25), downward when P_aO_2 was kept high (*ca.* 270 Torr) and exhibited increased initial slopes and saturation under hypoxic conditions (see Fig. 6.3A). The lines fitting steady f_x's recorded from single carotid nerve fibers at 3 levels of P_aCO_2 became progressively steeper as P_aO_2 levels were decreased from 400 to 25 Torr.[77]

Studies on carotid bodies in vitro have confirmed that carotid nerve discharges were directly dependent on the levels of CO_2 at which the superfusing solutions had been equilibrated.[30]

Chemosensory Responses to Abrupt Changes in Carbon Dioxide

A sudden transition from normocapnia to hypercapnia leads to a rapid and pronounced increase in f_x (overshoot), followed by a slow decline to an intermediate level of chemosensory discharges. Withdrawal of the hypercapnic stimulus results in an undershoot in f_x before regaining basal chemosensory activity. These adaptive reactions are typical of chemosensory responses to CO_2 changes.[60,78] The overshoots in chemosensory responses to hypercapnic stimuli are blocked by acetazolamide (Diamox®), an inhibitor of carbonic anhydrase.

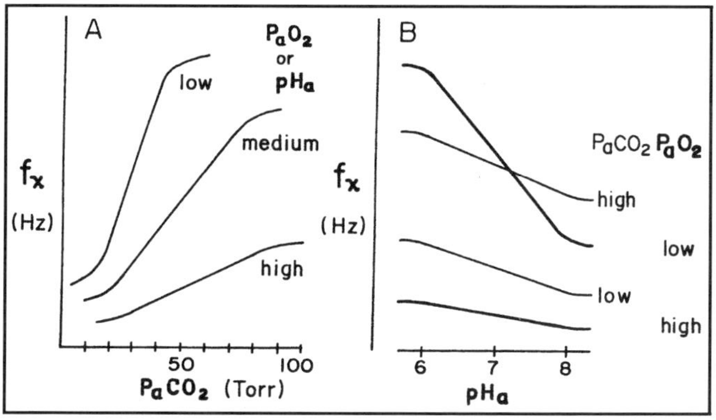

Fig. 6.3. Schematic diagram of relationships between steady levels of carbon dioxide and acidity (abscissae) and frequency of chemosensory impulses (f_x; ordinates). Ordinates are given without numerical scale because similar trends are observed for single chemosensory units as for the entire nerve chemosensory discharge. (A) Effects of changes in partial pressure of carbon dioxide in arterial blood ($PaCO_2$), studied at different levels of partial pressure of oxygen (PaO_2) or pH (pH_a) in arterial blood. (B) Effects of changes in pH of arterial blood (pH_a), studied at different levels of partial pressures of oxygen (PaO_2; thin lines) or carbon dioxide ($PaCO_2$; thick lines) in arterial blood.

When the cat carotid body was perfused with Ringer's solution, decreasing the pH from 7.4 to 7.1 through either a decrease in HCO_3^- or an increase in PCO_2 gave chemosensory responses of the same magnitude, but the response to CO_2 occurred approximately twice as rapidly as it did in response to reduction of HCO_3^-. However, when an increase in PCO_2 of 30 Torr was accompanied by a proportional increase in HCO_3^-so that pH was held constant, the chemosensory response was only transient, the discharge returning to control level within 30 s.[79]

Simultaneous recordings of ventilation and carotid chemosensory discharges in pentobarbitone-anesthetized cats have revealed that brief inhalations (along 2 or 3 ventilatory cycles) of 8% CO_2 caused brisk parallel increases in ventilation and chemosensory discharges.[80] Since the ventilatory reaction was delayed, slowed and weakened in chemodenervated awake dogs,[81] it was concluded that the initial ventilatory response to a moderate and brief increase in CO_2 was of chemoreflex origin.

A study of the time course of carotid chemosensory responses to step changes in blood gases in cats revealed that those to CO_2 had a latency of 0.2-0.3 s and a time to peak of 1.2-2.2 s, whereas those to O_2 and pH were slightly slower.[82] The sensitivity of carotid chemoreceptors to small rapid changes in P_aCO_2 explains their contribution to the ventilatory oscillations induced by within-breath changes in P_aCO_2[40] (see also previous section on rhythmic fluctuations in carotid chemosensory discharges).

Studies on carotid bodies perfused and superfused in vitro show higher basal levels of chemosensory discharges when perfused with saline solutions equilibrated with CO_2-HCO_3^- than when perfused with solutions devoid of these substances, but hypercapnic perfusates produced similar increases in chemosensory frequency above baselines under both conditions, with prominent overshoots followed by adaptation to intermediate levels of chemosensory discharges. However, in the presence of CO_2-HCO_3^-, a prominent undershoot was observed after switching from hypercapnic to normocapnic perfusates.[65]

CHEMOSENSORY RESPONSES TO PH CHANGES

An increase in the frequency of impulses recorded from the carotid nerve in cats after injections of diluted acids in the femoral vein was reported by Zotterman[13] in 1935. Several authors later showed that while chemosensory activity and ventilation are increased by metabolic acidosis, they are decreased by metabolic alkalosis.

The specificity of pH effects on the activity of chemosensory fibers of the carotid nerve was checked by comparing these effects with those induced on the discharges of the barosensory fibers of the same nerve, in in vitro preparations superfused with Locke's solution equilibrated with O_2 50% + N_2 50%, in the absence of CO_2. Reducing pH (by changing HCl concentration) from 7.45 to 7.35 resulted in a significant and maintained increase in the frequency of chemosensory discharges, while it was necessary to reduce pH below 4.0 to obtain a change in barosensory discharges (originated from the carotid sinus), consisting of a decrease in frequency to the same stretch applied longitudinally.[31]

When studying the chemosensory discharges from cat carotid bodies perfused and superfused in vitro with CO_2-HCO_3^--free Tyrode's solution, adding 30 mM acetate to the perfusate and superfusate—even when maintaining the extracellular pH at 7.4—increases the frequency of chemosensory discharge up to about 570% of control.[66] This suggests that the intracellular acidosis of glomus cells induced by acetate[83] increases chemosensory discharges, even when the extracellular pH is kept unmodified (see chapter 5).

Chemosensory Activity at Different Steady Levels of pH

Recordings of the integrated chemosensory activity of carotid nerves in cats allowed researchers to separate the effects of steady H^+ concentrations in the blood from those of P_aCO_2, by comparing and combining the effects of respiratory and metabolic acidosis and alkalosis.[84] These studies showed that the relationship between f_x and $[H^+]$ was direct but nonlinear.

Recordings from single chemosensory fibers from cat carotid nerves in situ showed sigmoidal increases in f_x in response to augmented concentrations of hydrogen ions (decreased pH_a from 7.6 to 6.9), produced either by increasing the P_aCO_2 or by i.v. infusions of alkaline or acid solutions; in the latter case, the curves were displaced downward when P_aCO_2 was kept low (*ca.* 17 Torr)[56] (See Fig. 6.3B).

Studies on carotid bodies in vitro have confirmed that the frequency of carotid nerve discharges had an inverse relationship to the pH of the superfusing solution. The curve was almost linear and horizontal when the superfusing solution was equilibrated with 100% O_2, but became steep and sigmoidal when saline was equilibrated with 10% O_2.[30]

Chemosensory Responses to Changes in pH

Slow i.v. injections of lactic acid, to reduce pH_a from 7.45 to 7.22 in cats, produced larger increases in f_x in single or paucifiber recordings from carotid nerves than those of aortic nerves.[85] The increases in carotid chemosensory discharge induced by the rapid isocapnic changes in pH_a provoked by i.v. infusions of lactic acid in pentobarbitone anesthetized cats occurred during ventilation with either air or 100% O_2.[86] On the other hand, slow i.v. injections of $NaHCO_3$, increasing pH_a from 7.32 to 7.55, produced sustained decreases in f_c recorded from carotid nerves and reduced ventilation at all levels of P_aO_2 and P_aCO_2 (ref. 87).

A study of the time course of carotid chemosensory responses in cats revealed that those produced by sudden increases and decreases in pH_a (by switching to cross circulation from another cat) had longer latencies than those responses to changes in P_aO_2 and P_aCO_2.[82] Simultaneous recordings of carotid chemosensory activity, respiration and carotid pH_a in cats showed that the instantaneous f_x followed the oscillation in pH_a, the maximal rates in neural discharges attained at the most acid points of pH oscillations.[40]

CHEMOSENSORY RESPONSES TO CHANGES IN KALEMIA

In classical experiments on crossed-circulation,[88] the hind limbs muscles of one dog ("neural dog") were stimulated to exercise levels, while blood from its inferior cava vein was diverted to another dog ("humoral dog"), whose abdominal aorta pumped arterial blood into the hind limbs of the neural dog. Exercise enhanced ventilation in both neural and humoral dogs, providing evidence for the participation of both neural and humoral factors in the initiation of reflex adjustments in ventilation in response to exercise. However, when the carotids of the humoral dog were perfused with blood from a third ("supporting") dog, ventilation of the humoral dog was unchanged by exercising the neural dog. These experiments suggested that exercising muscles produced a humoral stimulus for the carotid chemoreceptors that induced a reflex ventilatory enhancement. However, the nature of this humoral agent is unknown.

Jarish et al[89] observed dose-dependent increases in carotid nerve discharges in response to intracarotid injections of KCl, and hyperpnea if the nerve was intact. Linton and Band[90] observed that i.v. injections of KCl that transiently increased K^+ concentration in arterial blood from 3 mmol/l (basal) to 6 mmol/l also induced transient increases in carotid nerve chemosensory discharges and ventilation in the cat, with similar temporal profiles (increases lasted from 2 to 6 s). Burger et al[91] studied the effects of prolonged (> 6 min) hyperkalemia (*ca.* 6 mmol/l), produced by i.v. infusions of KCl, on chemosensory discharges obtained at different end tidal levels of PO_2 and PCO_2, observing that hyperkalemia significantly increased the frequency of discharges at low and normal PCO_2 levels (more effectively at low PO_2), but not at the high PCO_2 level (at any PO_2). Otherwise, when KCl and lactic acid were simultaneously infused i.v. to pentobarbitone anesthetized cats, the increase in the mean frequency of carotid chemosensory impulses was larger than when lactic acid was infused alone.[92]

From the above observations, Linton and Band[90] suggested that K^+ released from muscle during exercise may excite carotid chemoreceptors and contribute to the reflexly increased ventilation observed in such condition. In fact, the ventilatory stimulation induced by hyperkalemia was abolished by peripheral chemoreceptor denervation.[93] This suggestion received support from the observation by Sneyd et al[94] that muscle exercise induced in pentobarbitone anesthetized cats doubled normal levels of kalemia, and that i.v. infusions of KCl increasing kalemia to such levels augmented pulmonary ventilation (from 300 to 500 ml/min) within 15 s and induced alveolar hyperventilation (decreased $P_{ET}CO_2$). Similarly, in ketamine sedated monkeys, Paterson et al[95] observed that hyperkalemia during both normoxia (P_aO_2 ~ 100 Torr) and hypoxia (P_aO_2 ~ 40 Torr) augmented ventilation (by 40% and 250%, respectively), but that the enhanced chemosensory drive of ventilation evoked by hyperkalemia was virtually abolished by abrupt switches to 100% O_2 in inspired gas. It has been recently[96] confirmed that the decerebrate hypoxic cat and the hypoxic and normoxic rhesus monkey increase their ventilation in response to hyperkalemia, and that this effect is dependent on PO_2, being abolished by abrupt switches of inspiratory gas to 100% O_2. Finally, in humans subjected to progressive exercise until exhaustion, a linear relationship was observed between kalemia and breath-to-breath minute ventilatory volume, from which it was concluded that changes in plasmatic levels of K^+ can stimulate exercise hyperpnea, through excitation of arterial chemoreceptors.[97]

More recent experiments on rat carotid bodies superfused in vitro[98] showed the effect of raising the extracellular K^+ concentration ($[K^+]_o$) from 3 to 17 mM upon chemoreceptor responses. Increasing $[K^+]_o$ augmented chemoreceptor discharges at any level of PO_2 and PCO_2, but in a PO_2- and PCO_2-independent manner.

CHEMOSENSORY RESPONSES TO CHANGES IN GLYCEMIA

The possibility that carotid chemoreceptors would operate as glucoreceptors has received recent attention. Alvarez-Buylla and Alvarez-Buylla[99] observed that intracarotid infusions of 0.5 ml of 20% glucose solutions caused a decrease in carotid chemosensory discharges, while infusions of mannitol (in same volumes and concentrations) did not modify such discharges, thus ruling out the possibility that the response could be ascribed to osmolality changes. They further observed that cyanide-induced stimulation of carotid chemoreceptors increased the output of hepatic glucose, a reflex effect abolished by carotid nerve section. The same authors[100] have more recently reported that perfusion of the rat carotid bifurcation with hyperglycemic blood from a donor animal decreased brain glucose retention, while perfusion of the same area with hypoglycemic blood had the opposite effect and induced a noticeable hyperglycemia in the arterial and venous blood. Thus, the carotid body chemoreceptors may participate in the homeostatic regulation of glycemia.

It is known that the presence of glucose in the superfusion media contributes to the maintenance of chemosensory activity from carotid bodies in vitro. After *ca.* 1 h of superfusion of the carotid body with glucose-free Tyrode solution, a spontaneous increase in carotid chemosensory activity is observed, followed by decreased basal activity and unresponsiveness to hypoxic stimulation.[101] However, the responsiveness to hypoxia, acidity and acetylcholine was maintained if pyruvate replaced glucose.[102] In carotid bodies superfused with zero glucose Locke's solution, chemosensory responses to hypoxia were progressively reduced to one-third within 180 min, but they were maintained within control limits when pyruvate replaced glucose.[103] In carotid bodies perfused and superfused in vitro, the chemosensory responses to flow interruption and nicotine were also rapidly depressed in the absence of metabolic substrates, while they persisted in the presence of adequate concentrations of either glucose, glutamate or a mixture of amino acids.[104] Chemosensory responses were increased by exposure to 2-deoxy-d-glucose, a glucose analogue entering the cell by the same carrier as glucose, but more effectively when previously superfused with pyruvate-containing than glucose-containing Tyrode solution.[102]

CHEMOSENSORY RESPONSES TO THERMAL CHANGES

It has been known since the early work of Bernthal and Weeks[105] that increasing the temperature of blood perfusing the vascularly isolated carotid bodies of dogs leads to reflex increases in breathing. Studies on cat carotid bodies in situ[106] have shown that the discharge frequency of chemosensory fibers recorded from the carotid nerve increases when warming the blood circulating through the carotid bifurcation and decreases when cooling such blood. The barosensory fibers of the same nerve, innervating the adjacent carotid sinus, were less sensitive to thermal changes.

Studies on carotid bodies in vitro have shown that brisk increases in temperature of the superfusate produce fast increases in f_x (dynamic component) followed by declines to intermediate rates of discharge (static component). When recording from the entire nerve, the discharge at low temperatures (*ca.* 32°C) is contributed by a few fibers firing infrequent impulses, but their rate increases as temperature is augmented and previously silent fibers are recruited.[107] For carotid bodies superfused with saline equilibrated with 100% O_2, thermal increases by 0.5°C steps between 36.0 and 38.5°C resulted in sustained increases in f_x[108] (see Fig. 6.4A).

Recordings from single chemosensory fibers of carotid bodies in vitro[109] superfused at different temperatures have allowed determinations of the temperature coefficient (Q_{10}) and apparent activation energy (μ) of chemosensory frequencies, giving values which are extremely high and characteristic of *thermoreceptor* organs. However, temperature had no uniform effects on the re-

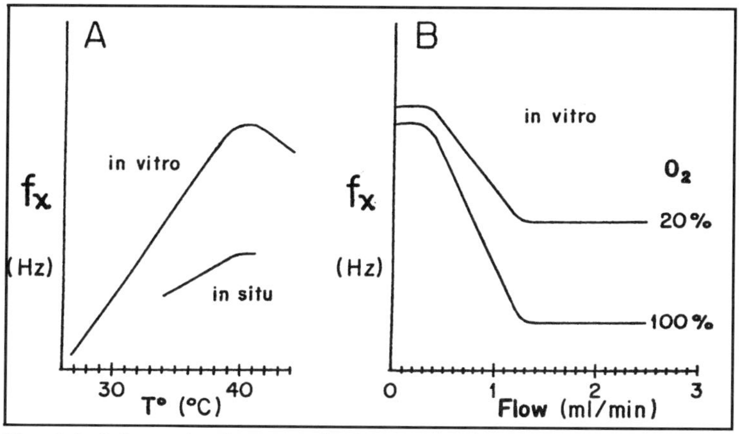

Fig. 6.4. Schematic diagram of relationships between steady levels of temperature and flow (abscissae) and frequency of chemosensory impulses (f_x; ordinates). Ordinates are given without numerical scale because similar trends are observed for single chemosensory units as for the entire nerve chemosensory discharge. (A) Effects of changes in temperature (T°), studied in cat carotid body preparations in situ and in vitro. (B) Effects of changes in flow of cat carotid body preparations superfused in vitro with Tyrode's solution equilibrated with different concentrations of oxygen (20% and 100%) in nitrogen.

sponses of chemosensory fibers to chemical agents introduced into the superfusate.[110]

The above observations led to a study on the effects of changes in body core temperature on the f_x recorded from one carotid nerve in situ, while recording the simultaneous changes in pulmonary and alveolar ventilation in cats.[111] Raising body temperature from 35° to 40°C progressively increased f_x in some cats (see Fig. 6.4A), most commonly after section of the contralateral carotid nerve, but the effect was blunted in other cats by the simultaneously increased alveolar ventilation. Similarly, raising body temperature from 37° to 40°C by external heat in pentobarbitone-anesthetized cats with intact carotid nerves increased respiratory frequency, tidal volume and frequency of spontaneous gasps; the last two changes were not observed after bilateral section of the carotid nerves.[112]

Thus, the carotid nerves may convey thermally-dependent signals to the solitary tract nuclei,[113] which in turn project to thermosensitive regions of the hypothalamus.[114,115] However, the possibility that the carotid nerves would mediate homeothermic adjustments is not sustained by reports of unchanged rectal temperature in awake cats after bilateral section of these nerves.[116] Furthermore, when cats are artificially ventilated to maintain $P_{ET}CO_2$ within normal range and the ventilatory output is measured by the phrenic integrated electroneurogram, raising body temperature from 35.5 to 37.5°C and then to 40.2°C did not modify the mean f_x recorded from one carotid nerve, while the frequency of phrenic bursts increased.[117]

CHEMOSENSORY RESPONSES TO OSMOTIC CHANGES

Verney,[118] in 1947, demonstrated that intracarotid injections of hyperosmotic solutions reduced urinary flow in dogs, an effect attributed to stimulation of hypothalamic "osmoreceptors" and subsequent release of antidiuretic hormone (ADH). However, it was later found that hypoxic perfusion of the carotid bodies led to reflex increases in ADH in vagotomized, thoracotomized and constantly ventilated dogs.[119] Furthermore, increased ADH release was reported during electrical stimulation of the carotid nerves.[120] Similarly, only in cats in which the carotid nerves were intact, slow intracarotid injections of CO_2 saturated Ringer solution increased the frequency of discharges of supraoptic nuclei neurons in the hypothalamus, an effect similar to that evoked by intravenous injections of NaCN.[121] Also, the exaggerated drinking of rats, induced by subcutaneous administration of hypertonic, polyethylene glycol, angiotensin II or 18 h water deprivation was significantly attenuated by bilateral section of the aortic and carotid nerves.[122] In this context, a role for the carotid bodies in controlling the osmolarity of body fluids has been discussed (see Honig[123]).

When the carotid bifurcation area of cats is isolated and perfused in situ with solutions of various concentrations of NaCl, mannitol and glucose, an increase in the osmolality of the perfusing fluid causes an augmented frequency of discharges of single chemosensory fibers of the carotid nerve.[124]

The idea that the carotid bodies may serve as *osmoreceptors* prompted studies on preparations superfused in vitro, in which vascular effects are avoided. It was found that hyperosmotic solutions (+15 to +31%) increased the frequency of single chemosensory fibers of the carotid nerve, whereas hyposmotic solutions (-8 to -23%) reduced the frequency of those discharges.[109] However, opposite effects were observed in cat carotid bodies perfused in situ with isosmotic solutions of NaCl (9 g/l), and made hyperosmotic by adding sucrose or NaCl and hyposmotic by reducing the NaCl content; these effects were attributed to osmolality effects upon the vascular smooth muscle of the glomera.[125]

CHEMOSENSORY RESPONSES TO FLOW CHANGES

As early as 1836, Sir Astley Paston Cooper[126] reported increases in ventilation and heart frequency upon ligation of the common carotid arteries in dogs. The effect was then ascribed to cerebral anemia. However, the increased ventilation evoked by clamping the carotid below its bifurcation was later shown to be due to an augmented discharge of chemosensory fibers of the carotid nerve.[54] It was also shown that the increased discharge from these chemosensory fibers also contributed to the rise of systemic blood pressure, mainly derived from the withdrawal of barosensory impulses evoked by clamping both carotids.[127] More recent observations indicate that while barosensory withdrawal during carotid occlusion is mostly responsible for reflex hypertension and tachycardia, chemosensory excitation induced by this maneuver is the major cause of reflex hyperventilation.[128]

The effect of common carotid artery occlusion on the afferent activity recorded from carotid nerves has been studied in pentobarbitone anesthetized cats.[129] Ipsilateral occlusions lowered intrasinus pressure down to 15-100 Torr, depending on previous pressures, and resulted in silencing of barosensory impulses. For cats breathing room air and with mean systemic arterial pressures below 125 Torr, chemosensory excitation was induced whenever these occlusions lasted 5 s or longer and persisted during 10 min occlusions. The chemosensory excitation had a delay of *ca.* 4 s and the maximal f_x was attained at nearly 30 s. For ipsilateral occlusions performed under 100% O_2 breathing, the delay of excitation was increased to *ca.* 20 s and the maximal f_x attained only 30-40% of that attained for the same animal breathing room air. Bilateral occlusions caused deeper falls in intrasinus pressure and stronger chemosensory excitation. Also, i.v. injections of NaCN further increased f_x during occlusions, indicating that blood flow through the carotid bodies was not arrested.

The problem of whether carotid body chemoreceptors are sensitive to minor changes in systemic blood pressure is hard to analyze, since blood circulation through the organ presents some autoregulation[130] and it is under sympathetic control.[22,131] Nevertheless, it has been reported that moderate falls in systemic arterial pressure, while keeping constant the levels of $P_{ET}O_2$ and $P_{ET}CO_2$, produce minor and delayed increases in f_x recorded from carotid nerve fibers, in comparison with the pronounced and fast increases recorded simultaneously from aortic nerve fibers.[132] In fact, hypotensions to 80 Torr in cats vigorously excite all aortic chemosensory fibers, but only slightly some carotid chemosensory fibers, further hypotensions down to 50 Torr being required to excite all carotid chemosensory fibers.[133]

Studies on carotid bodies superfused in vitro demonstrated that interruption of saline flow induces a rapid and pronounced increase in f_x that can be maintained for a prolonged period of time, whereas increases in superfusing flow produce the opposite effect.[21] Interestingly, flow arrests in preparations superfused with saline equilibrated with 100% N_2 produce further increases in f_x, which are transiently reduced by stirring the saline around the carotid body. When flow had been arrested in preparations superfused with saline equilibrated with 100% O_2, stirring produces further increases in f_x[32]. These experiments posed the question that the carotid body may behave as a *rheoreceptor* (flow receptor).

Further studies on cat carotid bodies in vitro superfused with Tyrode's solutions flowing at various steady rates (range 0.15-2.95 ml/min), but kept at constant temperature (37.7°C), revealed that the mean frequency of chemosensory discharges was higher at low rates of superfusing flow with saline equilibrated with 20% O_2 than with that equilibrated with 100% O_2, the best fitting between basal f_x and superfusing flow being provided by inverse sigmoid curves ($r = -0.84$ and -0.90, at 20% and 100% O_2, respectively), and with maximal gains at about 0.86 and 0.78 ml/min, respectively[134] (see Fig. 6.4B). It was concluded that the chemosensory discharge frequency recorded from carotid bodies in vitro was determined by the superfusion flow, when all other chemoreceptor stimuli were held constant.

Experiments on carotid bodies perfused and superfused in vitro[65] (Iturriaga and Lahiri, 1991) have shown shorter delays and faster increases in f_x when interruption of perfusate flow was performed in Tyrode's solutions containing CO_2-HCO_3^- than in their absence, even when their pH's and PO_2's were the same and the superfusion was maintained.

CONCLUDING REMARKS: IS THE CAROTID BODY A MULTIMODAL RECEPTOR?

The evidence presented above indicates that the carotid body signals not only different submodalities of chemical stimuli (hypoxia, hypercapnia, acidosis, hyperkalemia, glycemia?), but also different modalities of stimuli (chemical, thermal, osmotic, flow). This is not a consequence of an heterogeneous group of sensory units, since a single chemosensory unit may respond to various kinds of stimuli. This implies that the "discharges carried by each sensory fiber or by the entire group of chemosensory fibers innervating the carotid body do not apparently provide information with regard to the exact nature of the actual stimulus originating those discharges."[135]

The operation of each carotid chemosensory unit or the entire population of carotid body chemosensory fibers as the output of a "multimodal receptor" poses a problem for the specificity and therefore adequacy of reflex responses originated from this organ. Fortunately, that is beyond the scope of the present chapter!

Acknowledgments

Thanks are due to Mrs. Carolina Larrain for her continuous help in the laboratory as well as in the preparation of manuscripts.

I express my sincere appreciation to Prof. Carlos Eyzaguirre, Department of Physiology, University of Utah School of Medicine, USA, for his critical reading of an earlier version of this paper.

The work of the author has been supported by grants from FONDECYT (National Fund for Scientific and Technological Development) and DIPUC (Research and Postgraduate Division, Catholic University of Chile).

References

1. Hering HE. Die Sinusreflexe vom Sinus caroticus werden durch einen Nerven (Sinusnerv) vermittelt, der ein Ast des Nervus glossopharyngeus ist. Münch Med Wochenschr 1924; 71:1265-1266.

2. Heymans C, Neil E. Reflexogenic Areas of the Cardiovascular System. London: Churchill. 1958:271.
3. de Castro F. Sur la structure et l'innervation du sinus carotidien de l'homme et des mammifères: nouveaux faits sur l'innervation et la fonction du glomus caroticum. Trav Lab Rech Biol Univ Madrid 1928; 25:330-380.
4. Hovelacque A, Maes J, Binet L, Gayet R. Le nerf carotidien. Étude anatomique et physiologique. Pr Méd 1930; 38:449-453.
5. Berger AJ. The distribution of the cat's carotid nerve afferent and efferent cell bodies using the horseradish peroxidase technique. Brain Res 1980;190:309-320.
6. De Groat WC, Nadalhaft I, Morgan C, Schauble T. The central origin of efferent pathways in the carotid sinus nerve of the cat. Science 1979; 205:1017-1018.
7. Eyzaguirre C, Uchizono K. Observations on the fibre content of nerves reaching the carotid body of the cat. J Physiol, London 1961; 159:268-281.
8. Biscoe TJ, Sampson SR. Rhythmical and nonrhythmical spontaneous activity recorded from the central cut end of the sinus nerve. J Physiol, London 1968; 196:327-338.
9. Bronk DW, Stella G. Afferent impulses in the carotid sinus nerve. I. The relation of the discharge from single end organs to arterial blood pressure. J Cell Comp Physiol 1932; 1:113-130.
10. Eyzaguirre C, Lewin J. Chemoreceptor activity of the carotid body of the cat. J Physiol, London 1961; 159:222-237.
11. Vidruk EH, Dempsey JA. Carotid body chemoreceptor activity as recorded from the petrosal ganglion in cats. Brain Res 1980; 181:455-459.
12. Belmonte C, Gallego R. Membrane properties of cat sensory neurones with chemoreceptor and baroreceptor endings. J Physiol, London 1983; 342: 603-614.
13. Zotterman Y. Action potentials in the glossopharyngeal nerve and in the chorda tympani. Skand Arch Physiol 1935; 72: 73-77.
14. Alvarez-Buylla R. Disociación de las actividades quimiorreceptoras y barorreceptoras en el gato. Arch Inst Cardiol Méx 1954; 24:26-37.
15. Zapata P, Hess A, Eyzaguirre C. Reinnervation of carotid body and sinus with superior laryngeal nerve fibers. J Neurophysiol 1969; 32:215-228.
16. Zapata P, Hess A, Bliss El, Eyzaguirre C. Chemical, electron microscopic and physiological observations on the role of catecholamines in the carotid body. Brain Res 1969; 14:473-496.
17. Fidone SJ, Sato A. A study of chemoreceptor and baroreceptor A and C-fibres in the cat carotid nerve. J Physiol, London 1969; 205:527-548.
18. Fitzgerald RS, Osborne JL. The chemoreception of hypoxia and hypercapnia: further evidence for a dual sensing mechanism. In: Ribeiro JA, Pallot DJ, eds. Chemoreceptors in Respiratory Control. London: Croom Helm 1987:228-236.
19. O'Regan RG. Oxygen usage of the cat carotid body perfused with cell-free solutions. Irish J Med Sci 1979a; 148:69-77.
20. O'Regan RG. Responses of the chemoreceptors of the cat carotid body perfused with cell-free solutions. Irish J Med Sci 1979; 148: 78-85.
21. Eyzaguirre C, Lewin J. Effect of different oxygen tensions on the carotid body in vitro. J Physiol, London 1961b; 159: 238-250.
22. Belmonte C, Eyzaguirre C. Efferent influences on carotid body chemoreceptors. J Neurophysiol 1974; 37:1131-1143.
23. Iturriaga R, Rumsey WL, Mokashi A, Spergel D, Wilson DF, Lahiri S. In vitro perfused-superfused cat carotid body for physiological and pharmacological studies. J Appl Physiol 1991; 70:1393-1400.
24. Fitzgerald RS. Single fiber chemoreceptor responses of carotid and aortic bodies. In: Paintal AS, ed. Morphology and Mechanisms of Chemoreceptors. Delhi: Patel Chest Institute. 1976:27-35.
25. Lahiri S, DeLaney RG. The nature of response of single chemoreceptor fibers of carotid body to changes in arterial PO_2 and PCO_2-H^+. In: Paintal AS, ed Morphology and Mechanisms of Chemoreceptors. Delhi: Patel Chest Institute. 1976:18-26.
26. Dejours P. Intérêt méthodologique de l'étude d'un organisme vivant à la phase de rupture d'un équilibre physiologique. Compt Rend Acad Sci Paris 1957; 245: 1946-1948.

27. Zapata P, Zuazo A. Respiratory effects of dopamine-induced inhibition of chemosensory inflow. Respir Physiol 1980; 40:79-92.
28. Eugenin J, Larrain C, Zapata P. Correlative contribution of carotid and aortic afferences to the ventilatory chemosensory drive in steady-state normoxia and to the ventilatory chemoreflexes induced by transient hypoxia. Arch Biol Med Exp 1989; 22:395-408.
29. González C, Almaraz L, Obeso A, Rigual R. Carotid body chemoreceptors: from natural stimuli to sensory discharges. Physiol Rev 1994; 74:829-898.
30. Eyzaguirre C, Koyano H. Effects of hypoxia, hypercapnia, and pH on the chemoreceptor activity of the carotid body in vitro. J Physiol, London 1965; 178:385-409.
31. Eyzaguirre C, Zapata P. Pharmacology of pH effects on carotid body chemoreceptors in vitro. J Physiol, London 1968; 195:557-588.
32. Eyzaguirre C, Zapata P. A discussion of possible transmitter or generator substances in carotid body chemoreceptors. In: Torrance RW, ed. Arterial Chemoreceptors. Oxford: Blackwell, 1968:213-251.
33. Biscoe TJ, Taylor A. The discharge pattern recorded in chemoreceptor afferent fibres from the cat carotid body with normal circulation and during perfusion. J Physiol, London 1963; 168:332-344.
34. Nolan WF, Donnelly DF, Smith EJ, Dutton RE. Nonrandom chemoreceptor activity during superfusion in vitro. Brain Res 1984; 292:194-197.
35. Donnelly DF, Nolan WF, Smith EJ, Dutton RE. Interspike interval dependency from arterial chemoreceptors. J Appl Physiol 1985; 59:1566-1570.
36. Donnelly DF, Nolan WF, Smith EJ, Dutton RE. Effect of dopamine antagonism on carotid chemoreceptor interspike intervals. Brain Res 1987; 407: 195-198.
37. Lahiri S, Mokashi A, Mulligan E, Nishino T. Comparison of aortic and carotid chemoreceptor responses to hypercapnia and hypoxia. J Appl Physiol 1981; 51:55-61.
38. Black AMS, Torrance RW. Respiratory oscillations in chemoreceptor discharge in the control of breathing. Respir Physiol 1971; 13:221-237.
39. Goodman NW, Nail BS, Torrance RW. Oscillations in the discharge of single carotid chemoreceptor fibres of the cat. Respir Physiol 1974; 20:251-269.
40. Band DM, McClelland M, Phillips DL, Saunders KB, Wolff CB. Sensitivity of the carotid body to within-breath changes in arterial PCO_2. J Appl Physiol 1978; 45:768-777.
41. Linton Raf, Band DM. The relationship between arterial pH and chemoreceptor firing in anaesthetized cats. Respir Physiol 1988; 74:49-54.
42. Kumar P, Nye PCG, Torrance RW. Do oxygen tension variations contribute to the respiratory oscillations of chemoreceptor discharge in the cat? J Physiol, London 1988; 395:531-552.
43. Fitzgerald RS, Leitner L-M, Liaubet MJ. Carotid chemoreceptor response to intermittent or sustained stimulation in the cat. Respir Physiol 1969; 6:395-402.
44. Purves MJ. Fluctuations of arterial oxygen tension which have the same period as respiration. Respir Physiol 1966; 1:281-296.
45. Yokota H, Kreuzer F. Alveolar to arterial transmission of oxygen fluctuations due to respiration in dogs. Pflügers Arch 1973; 340:291-306.
46. Gehrich JL, Moore GP. Statistical analysis of cyclic variations in carotid body chemoreceptor activity. J Appl Physiol 1973; 35:642-648.
47. Biscoe TJ, Purves MJ. Observations on carotid body chemoreceptor activity and cervical sympathetic discharge in the cat. J Physiol, London 1967; 190:413-424.
48. Biscoe TJ, Purves MJ. Observations on the rhythmic variation in the cat carotid body chemoreceptor activity which has the same period as respiration. J Physiol, London 1967; 190:389-412.
49. Torrance RW, Iturriaga R, Zapata P. Effects of expiratory duration on chemoreceptor oscillations. Adv Exp Med Biol 1994; 360:241-243.
50. Blanco CE, Dawes GS, Hanson MA, McCooke HB. The response to hypoxia of arterial chemoreceptors in fetal sheep and new-born lambs. J Physiol, London 1984; 351:25-37.

51. Hertzberg T, Hellström S, Lagercrantz H, Pequignot JM. Development of the arterial chemoreflex and turnover of carotid body catecholamines in the newborn rat. J Physiol, London 1990; 425:211-225.
52. Hertzberg T, Lagercrantz H. Postnatal sensitivity of the peripheral chemoreceptors in newborn infants. Arch Dis Childhood 1987; 62:1238-1241.
53. Donnelly DF, Haddad GG. Prolonged apnea and impaired survival in piglets after sinus and aortic nerve section. J Appl Physiol 1990; 68:1048-1052.
54. Euler US von, Liljestrand G, Zotterman Y. The excitation mechanism of the chemoreceptors of the carotid body. Skand Arch Physiol 1939; 83:132-152.
55. Lahiri S, Mulligan E, Nishino T, Mokashi A, Davies RO. Relative responses of aortic body and carotid body chemoreceptors to carboxyhemoglobinemia. J Appl Physiol 1981; 50:580-586.
56. Biscoe TJ, Purves MJ, Sampson SR. The frequency of nerve impulses in single carotid body chemoreceptor afferent fibres recorded in vivo with intact circulation. J Physiol, London 1970; 208:121-131.
57. Lahiri S, DeLaney RG. Relationship between carotid chemoreceptor activity and ventilation in the cat. Respir Physiol 1975; 24:267-286.
58. Leitner L-M, Pagès B, Puccinelli R, Dejours P. Étude simultanée de la ventilation et des décharges des chémorécepteurs du glomus carotidien chez le chat. I. Au cours d'inhalations brèves d'oxygène pur. Arch Intl Pharmacodyn Thér 1965; 154:421-426.
59. Dejours P. Control of respiration by arterial chemoreceptors. Ann N Y Acad Sci 1963; 109:682-695.
60. Black AMS, McCloskey DI, Torrance RW. The responses of carotid body chemoreceptors in the cat to sudden changes of hypercapnic and hypoxic stimuli. Respir Physiol 1971; 13:36-49.
61. Andronikou S, Shirahata M, Mokashi A, Lahiri S. Carotid chemoreceptor and ventilatory responses to sustained hypoxia and hypercapnia in the cat. Respir Physiol 1988; 72:361-374.
62. Li K, Ponte J, Sadler CL. Carotid body chemoreceptor response to prolonged hypoxia in the rabbit: effects of domperidone and propranolol. J Physiol, London 1990; 430:1-11.
63. Nielsen AM, Bisgard GE, Vidruk EH. Carotid chemoreceptor activity during acute and sustained hypoxia in goats. J Appl Physiol 1988; 65:1796-1802.
64. Bisgard GE. The role of arterial chemoreceptors in ventilatory acclimatization to hypoxia. Adv Exp Med Biol 1994; 360: 109-122.
65. Iturriaga R, Lahiri S. Carotid chemoreception in the absence and presence of CO_2—HCO_3^-. Brain Res 1991; 568: 253-260.
66. Iturriaga R. Acetate enhances the chemosensory response to hypoxia in the cat carotid body in vitro in the absence of CO_2-HCO_3^-. Biol Res 1996; 29:237-243.
67. Shirahata M, Fitzgerald RS. Dependency of hypoxic chemotransduction in cat carotid body on voltage-gated calcium channels. J Appl Physiol 1991; 71:1062-1069.
68. Robin DE. Dysoxia. Abnormal tissue oxygen utilization. Arch Int Med 1977; 137:905-910.
69. Fidone SJ, González C. Initiation and control of chemoreceptor activity in the carotid body. In: American Physiological Society, eds. Handbook of Physiology. 1986; 2:247-312.
70. Nye PCG, Torrance RW, Folgerin H. Arterial chemoreceptor inhibition by a single inspirate containing carbon monoxide is accounted for by raised arterial PO_2. Pflügers Arch 1982; 393:313-317.
71. Anichkov SV, Belen'kii ML. Pharmacology of the Carotid Body Chemoreceptors. NY: Macmillan 1963:225.
72. Mullingan E, Lahiri S, Storey BT. Carotid body O_2 chemoreception and mitochondrial oxidative phosphorylation. J Appl Physiol 1981; 51:438-446.
73. Mullingan E, Lahiri S. Dependence of carotid chemoreceptor stimulation by metabolic agents on P_aO_2 and P_aCO_2. J Appl Physiol 1981; 50:884-891.
74. Lahiri S, Mulligan E, Andronikou S, Shirahata M, Mokashi A. Carotid body chemosensory function in prolonged normobaric hyperoxia in the cat. J Appl Physiol 1987; 62:1924-1931.

75. Samaan A, Stella G. The response of the chemical receptors of the carotid sinus to the tension of CO_2 in the arterial blood of the cat. J Physiol, London 1935; 85:309-319.
76. Fitzgerald RS, Dehghani GA. Neural responses of the cat carotid and aortic bodies to hypercapnia and hypoxia. J Appl Physiol 1982; 52:596-601.
77. Lahiri S, DeLaney RG. Stimulus interaction in the responses of carotid body chemoreceptor single afferent fibers. Respir Physiol 1975; 24:249-266.
78. Lahiri S, Mulligan E, Mokashi A. Adaptive response of carotid body chemoreceptors to CO_2. Brain Res 1982; 234: 137-147.
79. Gray BA. Response of the perfused carotid body to changes in pH and PCO_2. In: Torrance RW, ed Arterial Chemoreceptors. Oxford: Blackwell. 1968:297-299.
80. Leitner L-M, Pagès B, Puccinelli R, Dejours P. Étude simultanée de la ventilation et des décharges des chémorécepteurs du glomus carotidien chez le chat. II. Au cours d'inhalations brèves d'anhydride carbonique. Arch Intl Pharmacodyn Thér 1965; 154:427-433.
81. Bouverot P, Flandrois R, Puccinelli R, Dejours P. Étude du rôle des chémorécepteurs artériels dans la régulation de la respiration pulmonaire chez le chien éveillé. Arch Intl Pharmacodyn Thér 1965;157:253-271.
82. Ponte J, Purves MJ. Frequency response of carotid body chemoreceptors in the cat to changes of P_aCO_2, P_aO_2, and pH_a. J Appl Physiol 1974; 37:635-647.
83. Sato M. Effects of CO_2, acetate and lowering extracellular pH on Ca^{2+} and pH on cultured glomus cells of the newborn rabbit carotid body. Neurosci Lett 1994; 173:159-162.
84. Hornbein TF, Roos A. Specificity of H ion concentration as a carotid chemoreceptor stimulus. J Appl Physiol 1963; 18:580-584.
85. Pokorski M, Lahiri S. Aortic and carotid chemoreceptor responses to metabolic acidosis in the cat. Am J Physiol 1983; 244:R652-R658.
86. McLoughlin P, Linton RAF, Band DM. Effects of intravenous infusion of lactic acid on chemoreceptor discharge in anaesthetized cats ventilated with room air or 100% O_2. Adv Exp Med Biol 1994; 360:249-252.
87. Pokorski M, Lahiri S. Relative peripheral and central chemosensory responses to metabolic alkalosis. Am J Physiol 1983; 245:R873-R880.
88. Kao FF. An experimental study of the pathways involved in exercise hyperpnoea employing cross-circulation techniques. In: Cunningham DJC, Lloyd BB, eds. The Regulation of Human Respiration. Oxford: Blackwell; Philadelphia: Davis. 1963:461-502.
89. Jarish A, Landgren S, Neil E, Zotterman Y. Impulse activity in the carotid sinus nerve following intracarotid injection of potassium chloride, veratrine. sodium citrate, adenosinetriphosphate and α-dinitrophenol. Acta Physiol Scand 1952; 25:195-211.
90. Linton Raf, Band DM. The effect of potassium on carotid chemoreceptor activity and ventilation in the cat. Respir Physiol 1985; 59:65-70.
91. Burger RE, Estavillo JA, Kumar P, Nye PCG. The excitation of cat carotid body chemoreceptors by hyperkalaemia depends on PO_2 and PCO_2. J Physiol, London 1986; 374:25P.
92. McLoughlin P, Linton RAF, Band DM. Effects of intravenous infusions of KCl and lactic acid on chemoreceptor discharge in anaesthetized cats. Adv Exp Med Biol 1994; 360:245-247.
93. Band DM, Linton RAF, Kent R, Kurer FL. The effect of peripheral chemoreceptor denervation on the ventilatory response to potassium. Respir Physiol 1985; 60:217-225.
94. Sneyd JR, Linton RAF, Band DM. Ventilatory effects of potassium during hyperoxia, normoxia and hypoxia in anaesthetized cats. Respir Physiol 1988; 72:59-64.
95. Paterson DJ, Dorrington KL, Bergel DH, Kerr G, Miall RC, Stein JF, Nye PCG. Effect of potassium on ventilation in rhesus monkey. Exp Physiol 1992; 77: 217-220.
96. Paterson DJ, Nye PCG. Effects of oxygen tests on the ventilatory responses of the cat and rhesus monkey to changes in

arterial potassium. Adv Exp Med Biol 1993; 337:365-369.
97. Yoshida T, Chida M, Ichioka M, Makiguchi K, Eguchi J-I, Udo M. Relationship between ventilation and arterial potassium concentration during incremental exercise and recovery. Eur J Appl Physiol 1990; 61:193-196.
98. Pepper DR, Landauer RC, Kumar P. Extracellular potassium and chemosensitivity in the rat carotid body, in vitro. J Physiol, London 1996; 493:833-843.
99. Alvarez-Buylla R, Alvarez-Buylla ER. Carotid sinus receptors participate in glucose homeostasis. Respir Physiol 1988; 72:347-360.
100. Alvarez-Buylla R, Alvarez-Buylla ER. Changes in blood glucose concentration in the carotid body-sinus modify brain glucose retention. Brain Res 1994; 654: 167-170.
101. Almaraz L, Obeso A, González C. Metabolic dissociation of carotid body chemoreceptors responses to different types of stimulation: Preliminary findings. In: Pallot DJ, ed. The Peripheral Arterial Chemoreceptors. London: Croom Helm 1984:141-151.
102. Obeso A, Almaraz L, González C. Effects of 2-deoxy-D-glucose on in vitro cat carotid body. Brain Res 1986; 371:25-36.
103. Delpiano MA. Evidence for glucose uptake in the rabbit carotid body. Adv Exp Med Biol 1993; 337:111-116.
104. Spergel D, Lahiri S, Wilson DF. Dependence of carotid chemosensory responses on metabolic substrates. Brain Res 1992; 596:80-88.
105. Bernthal T, Weeks WF. Respiratory and vasomotor effects of variations in carotid body temperature. Am J Physiol 1939; 127:94-105.
106. McQueen DS, Eyzaguirre C. Effects of temperature on carotid chemoreceptor and baroreceptor activity, J Neurophysiol 1974; 37:1287-1296.
107. Eyzaguirre C, Zapata P. Perspectives in carotid body research. J Appl Physiol 1984; 57:931-957
108. Alcayaga J, Sanhueza Y, Zapata P. Thermal dependence of chemosensory activity in the carotid body superfused in vitro. Brain Res 1993; 600:103-111.
109. Gallego R, Eyzaguirre C, Monti-Bloch L. Thermal and osmotic responses of arterial receptors. J Neurophysiol 1979; 42:665-680.
110. Ito H, Eyzaguirre C. Effects of temperature on the response of chemoreceptor fibers to chemical agents. Brain Res 1983; 279:286-290.
111. Loyola H, Fadic R, Cardenas H, Larrain C, Zapata P. Effects of body temperature on chemosensory activity of the cat carotid body in situ. Neurosci Lett 1991; 132:251-254.
112. Fadic R, Larrain C, Zapata P. Thermal effects on ventilation in cats. Participation of carotid body chemoreceptors. Respir Physiol 1991; 86:51-63.
113. Zapata P, Larrain C, Fadic R, Ramirez B, Loyola H. Thermal effects upon the chemosensory drive of ventilation. Adv Exp Med Biol 1993; 337:371-378.
114. Banks D, Harris MC. Activation of hypothalamic arcuate but not paraventricular neurons following carotid body chemoreceptor stimulation in the rat. Neuroscience 1988; 24:967-976.
115. Calaresu FR, Ciriello J. Projections to the hypothalamus from buffer nerves and nucleus tractus solitarius in the cat. Am J Physiol 1980; 239:R130-R136.
116. Jennings DB, Szlyk PC. Carotid chemoreceptors and the regulation of body temperature. In: Cooper KE, Lomax P, Schonbaum E, Veale WL, eds. Homeostasis and Thermal Stress. Basel: Karger. 1986:30-33.
117. Iturriaga R, Larrain C, Zapata P. Phrenic nerve activity during artificial ventilation at different body temperatures and its relationships with carotid chemosensory activity. Biol Res 1994; 27:145-157.
118. Verney EB. The antidiuretic hormone and the factors which determine its release. Proc Roy Soc London (ser B) 1947; 135:25-105.
119. Share L, Levy MN. Effect of carotid chemoreceptor stimulation on plasma hormone titer. Am J Physiol 1966; 210: 157-161.
120. Michaelis LL, Gilmore JP. Renal effects of electrical stimulation of the carotid sinus nerve. Surgery 1969; 65:797-801.
121. Yamashita H. Effect of baro- and chemoreceptor activation on supraoptic nuclei

neurons in the hypothalamus. Brain Res 1977; 126:551-556.
122. Rettig R, Johnson AK. Aortic baroreceptor deafferentation diminishes saline-induced drinking in rats. Brain Res 1986; 370:29-37.
123. Honig A. Role of the arterial chemoreceptors in the reflex control of renal function and body fluid volumes in acute arterial hypoxia. In: Acker H, O'Regan RG, eds. Physiology of the Peripheral Arterial Chemoreceptors. Amsterdam: Elsevier. 1983:395-429.
124. Trzebski A, Chruscielewski L, Majcherczyk S. Effect of hyperosmic solutions on the carotid baroreceptor and chemoreceptor discharges in cats. Eur J Clin Invest 1977; 7:236 (Abstract).
125. Gallego R, Belmonte C. The effects of blood osmolality changes on cat carotid body chemoreceptors in vivo. Pflügers Arch 1979; 380:53-58.
126. Cooper A. Some experiments and observations on tying the carotid and vertebral arteries, and the pneumogastric, phrenic and sympathetic nerves. Guy's Hosp Rep 1836; 1:457-475.
127. Euler US von, Liljestrand G. The rôle of the chemoreceptors of the sinus region for the occlusion test in the cat. Acta Physiol Scand 1943; 6:319-323.
128. Iturriaga R, Alcayaga J, Zapata P. Contribution of carotid body chemoreceptors and carotid sinus baroreceptors to the ventilatory and circulatory reflexes produced by common carotid occlusion. Acta Physiol Pharmacol Latinoam 1988; 38:27-48.
129. Alcayaga J, Iturriaga R, Zapata P. Carotid body chemoreceptor excitation produced by carotid occlusion. Acta Physiol Pharmacol Latinoam 1986; 36:199-215.
130. McCloskey DI, Torrance RW. Autoregulation of blood flow in the carotid body. Respir Physiol 1971; 13:23-35.
131. O'Regan RG. Responses of carotid body chemosensory activity and blood flow to stimulation of sympathetic nerves in the cat. J Physiol, London 1981; 315:81-98.
132. Lahiri S, Nishino T, Mulligan E, Mokashi A. Relative latency of responses of chemoreceptor afferents from aortic and carotid bodies. J Appl Physiol 1980; 48:362-369.
133. Lahiri S, Nishino T, Mokashi A, Mulligan E. Relative responses of aortic body and carotid body chemoreceptors to hypotension. J Appl Physiol 1980; 48: 781-788.
134. Alcayaga J, Iturriaga R, Zapata P. Flow dependent chemosensory activity in the carotid body superfused in vitro. Brain Res 1988; 455:31-37.
135. Zapata P. Transduction, signal transference, and encoding in composite chemoreceptors: A comparison between gustatory and arterial chemoreceptors. In: Hidalgo C, Bacigalupo J, Jaimovich E, Vergara J, eds. Transduction in Biological Systems. NY: Plenum. 1990:87-98.

CHAPTER 7

Chemosensory Activity in the Carotid Nerve: Effects of Pharmacological Agents

Patricio Zapata

INTRODUCTION: SITES OF ACTIONS

The initial studies on the pharmacology of carotid body chemoreceptors rested on the *reflex changes in ventilation* evoked by certain drugs, which effects were abolished by surgical interruption of the carotid (sinus) nerves. However, very soon, the effects of most drugs were *directly assayed on chemosensory activity*, recorded from the carotid nerves of several mammalian species, most commonly cats, rabbits, dogs and rats, in that order. Recordings of pure chemosensory discharges may be obtained from the carotid nerve, after eliminating the discharges of barosensory and autonomic fibers contained within this nerve, as analyzed in the previous chapter (see chapter 6).

Observing a change in carotid nerve chemosensory activity in response to a drug does not necessarily imply that such drug acts upon the *chemoreceptive sites* ordinarily activated by physiological stimuli. These chemoreceptive sites are assumed to be located in the glomus (type I) cells of the carotid body parenchyma (see discussion in Eyzaguirre and Zapata[1]). Several sites for inducing changes in chemosensory activity may be considered (Fig. 7.1).

Considering *glomus cells* themselves, drugs may act (Fig. 7.1) not only upon their chemoreceptive sites, but they may: 1) modify chemoreceptor stimulants in their passage to chemoreceptive sites; 2) interfere with the transfer of chemoreceptor stimuli from the blood to the chemoreceptive sites; 3) promote or impede the release of transmitters or modulators from glomus cells. Drugs may also: 4) interfere with such transmitters or modulators at the level of recepto-neural junctions, particularly mimicking (analogues or agonists) or blocking (antagonists) their actions; 5) facilitate or impede the generation of nerve impulses (action potentials) at the level of *chemosensory nerve endings* (see Zapata and Eyzaguirre[2]).

The Carotid Body Chemoreceptors,
edited by Constancio González.

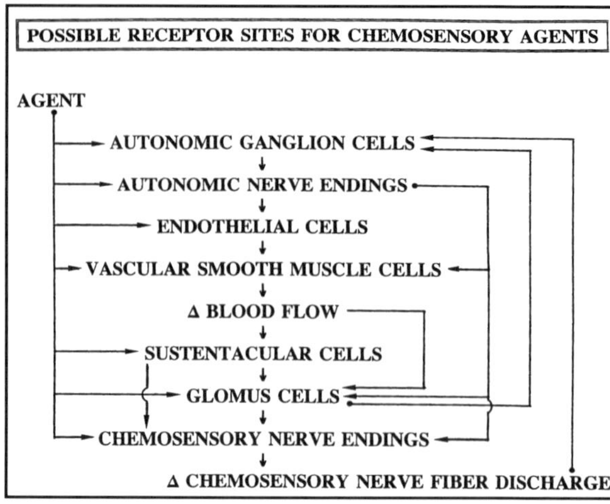

Fig. 7.1. Diagram of possible sites where physiological or pharmacological agents may initiate changes within carotid body chemoreceptor complex leading to changes in the frequency of chemosensory discharges. See text for explanation of interactions between different elements.

Apart from glomus cells and nerve endings, drugs may act upon other elements of carotid body tissue, which in turn may modify chemosensory nerve activity (Fig. 7.1). Even locally applied drugs may act upon the few *autonomic ganglion cells* located within the carotid body, and whose dendrites receive synapses from glomus cells processes,[3,4] or upon the sympathetic ganglion cells of the superior cervical ganglion, situated very close to the carotid body, receiving circulation from branches of the glomic artery[5] and projecting to the carotid body through the ganglioglomerular nerves[6] (see also Fig. 6.1). A few drugs may also act upon the nerve endings (varicosities) of autonomic nerve fibers.[7] By whichever mechanism, postganglionic nerve fibers control the local tonic activity of *vascular smooth muscle cells*, or such cells may be stimulated or inhibited by drugs themselves, resulting in *changes in blood flow* through the carotid body. Changes in local blood flow are known to modify chemosensory nerve activity (see chapter 6). Furthermore, norepinephrine released from sympathetic nerve varicosities may reach glomus cells and chemosensory nerve endings.[7] It must be noted that preparations of carotid bodies superfused in vitro (see chapter 6) have the advantage that effects of drugs there observed cannot be attributed to changes in flow.

Another site to be theoretically considered as target for drugs within the carotid body is the *sustentacular cell*. This element extensively encloses several glomus cells and their attached sensory nerve endings,[8] probably creating a barrier around recepto-neural junctions, but the same element appears interposed in many places between capillaries and glomus cells, thus creating a barrier for the easy access of blood borne substances to chemoreceptive glomus cells. Little is known about the role of sustentacular cells in chemoreceptive function, but it is conceivable that these glial-like cells may provide signals for glomus cells and chemosensory nerve endings (Fig. 7.1), and serve as sinks for substances released from glomus cells.

It must be noted that *endothelial cells* do not apparently constitute a barrier for intravascularly injected drugs to reach the carotid body parenchyma. Glomoids (islands of glomus cells) are organized around capillaries provided with a thin fenestrated endothelium and a thin basal lamina[5] (see also chapter 1). This endothelium allows the access of high molecular weight substances, such as horseradish peroxidase[9] and colloidal Trypan blue,[10] to the intercellular spaces and histiocytes of the carotid body, respectively. Furthermore, endothelial cells may release substances capable of making the vascular smooth muscle cells of the carotid body contract or relax (Fig. 7.1).

CHOLINERGIC ANALOGUES AND ANTAGONISTS

ACETYL-CHOLINE (ACH)

At the 15th International Congress of Physiological Sciences (Leningrad, 1935), two communications (by Anichkov et al and Heymans et al) reported that intracarotid injections of ACh produced intense but brief reflex respiratory excitation in cats and dogs, respectively (see refs. 11 and 12). The first evidence of increased discharge of carotid chemosensory fibers in response to ACh was provided by von Euler et al.[13]

The reflex hyperventilation induced by ACh led Schweitzer and Wright[14] to propose ACh as the physiological transmitter for carotid chemoreceptors, an idea enthusiastically supported by Heymans.[15] Further support was provided by the demonstration of endogenous ACh within the carotid body, persisting after denervation of the organ,[16,17] suggesting that ACh was probably stored within glomus cells and thus could play the role of a junctional transmitter between those cells and chemosensory nerve endings. Indeed, using a bioassay, Metz[18] demonstrated ACh release from the dog carotid body in situ during hypoxic-hypercapnic stimulation. Very recently, Fitzgerald and Shirahata,[19] using high performance liquid chromatography followed by electrochemical detection, confirmed the release of ACh from the cat carotid body in vitro during perfusion with an hypoxic-hypercapnic solution.

The excitatory effect of ACh observed on cat carotid bodies superfused in vitro[20] discarded the possibility that the ACh effect was vascularly mediated. Studies in situ and in vitro demonstrated that ACh activates both A- and C-carotid chemosensory fibers.[21]

The rabbit carotid body poses a particular problem. In this species, intracarotid injections of ACh cause an immediate depression of ventilation, which is greatly reduced after section of the ipsilateral carotid nerve,[22] and a dose-dependent inhibition of chemosensory discharges, which is blocked by atropine.[23] In confirmation, a reduction of the frequency of single chemosensory fibers in response to ACh applied to the carotid body surface or intracarotidally injected has also been reported.[24] Furthermore, ACh decreased the frequency of discharge of single chemosensory units recorded from rabbit carotid bodies superfused in vitro.[25]

Intracellular recordings from cat carotid body chemosensory endings in vitro[26] revealed that ACh induced increased frequencies of spontaneous depolarizing potentials and action potentials, and slow prolonged depolarizations. Mass recordings from cat carotid bodies in vitro[27] and in situ[2] revealed that ACh evoked focal slow potentials of negative polarity, correlated to the ensuing increases in frequency of carotid nerve chemosensory discharges. These observations suggest that ACh induces post-junctional depolarizations of chemosensory nerve endings, responsible for generating the increases in frequency of the discharges recorded along carotid nerves chemosensory fibers.

It has recently been reported that choline-acetyl-transferase (ChAT)-marker for cells capable of synthesizing ACh- is colocalized with dopamine-β-hydroxylase (DβH)—marker for cells capable of synthesizing norepinephrine—in 85% of glomus cells of cat carotid bodies.[28] This means that a large number of glomus cells would be capable of releasing ACh as a transmitter.

ANTICHOLINESTERASES

Working with cat carotid bodies superfused in vitro, Eyzaguirre and Zapata[29] studied the dose-dependent excitatory effects of ACh and observed that the threshold dose (5.5×10^{-8} M) was 1,000-fold displaced to the left (5.5×10^{-11} M) and that the maximal responsiveness was much enhanced in the presence of *eserine* (Fig. 7.2). This pronounced supersensitivity allowed them to superfuse two carotid bodies in series, using one of them as "detector" for the ACh released from the other one ("donor") when electrically stimulated, even after its chronic denervation.

Addition of eserine to the superfusing solution of cat carotid bodies in vitro evokes an initial intense stimulation of chemosensory fibers, which slowly disappears; at this time, responses to ACh are enhanced

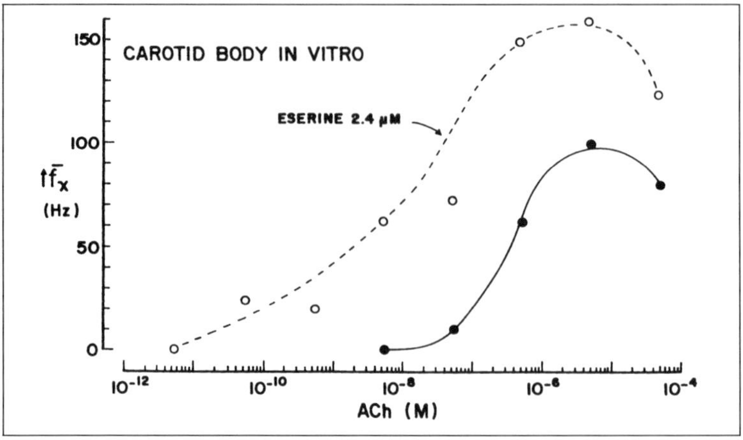

Fig. 7.2. Dose-response curves for increases in the frequency of chemosensory impulses (–f_x; ordinate) elicited by increasing concentrations of acetylcholine (ACh; abscissa), in control conditions (filled circles and continuous line) and after adding eserine 2.4 μM (open circles and interrupted line). Each point, mean obtained from 4 different experiments. Cats carotid bodies superfused in vitro with Locke's solution, pH 7.44 at 35°C, equilibrated with 50% O_2 in N_2, flowing at 0.8 ml/min. (Data replotted from Eyzaguirre and Zapata[29]).

and prolonged, while those to acid stimulation are not consistently modified.[30] However, chemosensory responses to CO_2 stimulation had been found clearly increased in the presence of eserine.[20]

Intracarotid injections of eserine in cats have been found to increase chemosensory activity during hypoxic, normoxic and hyperoxic conditions.[31] However, chemosensory responses to NaCN injections remained unchanged, in spite of the potentiation of chemosensory responses to ACh injections.[32]

Intracarotid injections of *prostigmine*, *diisopropylfluorophosphate* (DFP) and *tetraethyl-pyrophosphate* (TEPP) in cats have also been reported to produce transient increases in chemosensory activity.[31]

Drugs Affecting ACh Uptake and Release

Studies on cat carotid bodies superfused in vitro showed that low concentrations of *hemicholinium-3*—which prevents high affinity choline uptake and thus ACh synthesis, storage and release in the presynaptic side—produced progressive depression of chemosensory responses to hypoxia and acidity, without affecting those to ACh.[30] Studies on preparations in situ confirmed that this drug provoked progressive and marked depression of responses to NaCN, while ACh responses remained unchanged,[33] or failed to show changes in NaCN responses.[32]

Intracarotid or i.v. injections of *4-aminopyridine*—releaser of ACh from motor nerve terminals—did not modify the frequency of carotid chemosensory discharges, in spite of increasing ventilation in cats.[34]

Intracarotid administration of *β-bungarotoxin*—which prevents presynaptic release of ACh--produces little or no change of chemosensory responses to either ACh or NaCN.[32]

Nicotinic Analogues

The intense hyperpnea reflexly evoked by intracarotid injections of *nicotine* and *lobeline*[35] was part of the first observations on the pharmacology of carotid chemoreceptors. Both drugs were later found to increase chemosensory discharges in the carotid nerves of cats[25,36] and rabbits,[25] even in carotid body preparations superfused in vitro (Fig. 7.3). Increased frequency of carotid

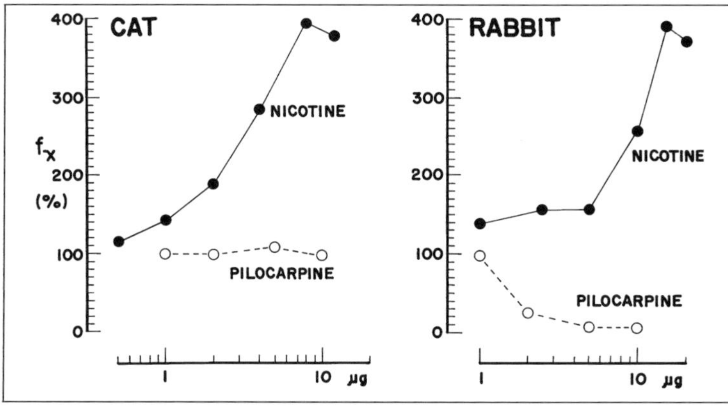

Fig. 7.3. Dose-response curves for changes in the frequency of chemosensory impulses (f_x; ordinates) elicited by increasing doses of cholinergic analogues (abscissae). Responses to nicotine tartrate (filled circles and continuous lines) and pilocarpine hydrochloride (open circles and interrupted lines), injected into the superfusate of carotid bodies in vitro, obtained from cats (left) and rabbits (right). Maximal responses to each dose expressed in percentages of basal chemosensory activity. (Data replotted from Monti-Bloch and Eyzaguirre[25]).

chemosensory discharges and reflex hyperpnea in cats are evoked by i.v. injections of nicotine in doses as low as 1 µg/kg.[37] This explains why the hyperpnea and hypertension caused by inhalation of tobacco smoke in cats[38] and by smoking a regular cigarette in humans,[39] as well as their increased ventilatory responses to hypoxia during cigarette smoking[40] are attributable to the presence of nicotine and mediated through excitation of carotid chemoreceptors.

Carotid chemoreceptors are also excited by *suberyldicholine*[41] (also known as corconium; Anichkov and Belen'kii[11]), *carbachol* (carbamycholine)[25] and *1,1-dimethyl-4-phenyl-piperazinium*.[42] The allegedly nicotinic agonist *piperidil* also increases carotid chemosensory discharges,[43] but this effect is not blocked by the nicotinic antagonist hexamethonium.[42]

Philippot[44] studied the reflex respiratory effects of a long list of *choline derivatives* injected into the carotid of chloralose anesthetized dogs, observing a strong correlation between the intensity of carotid chemoreceptor excitation and the strength of nicotinic actions of these compounds on other organs (see also Anichkov and Belen'kii[11]).

Muscarinic Analogues

Studies searching reflex ventilatory stimulation indicated that cholinomimetics characterized by muscarinic activity but devoid of nicotinic activity were unable to stimulate carotid chemoreceptors (see Anichkov and Belen'kii[11]). The moderate excitatory action of *methacholine* (acetyl-b-methylcholine) on carotid chemosensory discharges, at least 10 times less potent than that of ACh in cats, was explained by its nicotinic action,[45] since it was blocked by mecamylamine but not by atropine (see later). Similarly, the excitatory actions of *McN A-343* were consistently abolished by tetraethylammonium,[46] suggesting the mediation of nicotinic cholinoceptors. However, the purely muscarinic agonists *pilocarpine* and *bethanechol* (carbamyl-b-methylcholine) were without effect upon spontaneous chemosensory activity recorded from the cat carotid body in situ[25,46] (Fig. 7.3).

A particular condition refers to carotid chemosensory activity in the rabbit, since this is inhibited by *pilocarpine*[25] (Fig. 7.3) and *bethanechol*.[23] Thus, the predominantly inhibitory effect of ACh on rabbit chemosensory discharges both in situ[23] and in vitro[25] may be explained by a predominance of muscarinic cholinoceptors in this species (see chapter 3).

NICOTINIC ANTAGONISTS

The excitatory effects of ACh on carotid chemosensory discharges recorded from carotid body preparations superfused in vitro are blocked by *mecamylamine*, *hexamethonium* (C_6) and *d-tubocurarine*, in that order of potency[29] (see Fig. 7.4). However, spontaneous chemosensory discharges persisted in the presence of such blockers, as well as the increases in those discharges in response to acidity, hypoxia and flow interruption, but becoming of reduced strength in the presence of hexamethonium, *d*-tubocurarine[20] and especially mecamylamine.[30,47] Furthermore, mecamylamine reduced the chemosensory excitation induced by electric current applied to the carotid body[48] and that recorded from the "detector" carotid body in response to electrical and asphyxic stimulation of the "donor" carotid body, in serially superfused preparations.[29]

There is conflicting reports on *mecamylamine* effects in situ. Sampson[49] observed that mecamylamine 0.24-6.00 mg/kg i.v. abolished the chemosensory response to ACh, but not those to hypoxia, acidity and NaCN. Nishi and Eyzaguirre[33] observed that mecamylamine 2-10 mg given intracarotidally blocked chemosensory responses to both ACh and NaCN. McQueen[32] observed that intracarotid administration of mecamylamine 1-5 mg/kg, producing transient inhibition of spontaneous chemosensory activity and substantial block of ACh responses, was without effect on NaCN responses.

Transient reductions in spontaneous chemosensory carotid nerve activity had been reported as result of intracarotid injections of *d-tubocurarine* and *decamethonium* (C_{10}).[31] Significant reductions in normoxic levels of chemosensory activity and hypoxic responses have been observed in dogs receiving i.v. injections of *d*-tubocurarine.[50]

Reports that doses of *tetraethylammonium* (TEA)[51] and *hexamethonium*,[52] capable of blocking chemoreflex responses to injected ACh and nicotine, did not depress those to NaCN and asphyxia, served as serious objections to the hypothesis that release of endogenous ACh from glomus cells was involved in the natural excitation of chemosensory nerve fibers. Later, Nishi and Eyzaguirre[33] observed that hexamethonium depressed the responses to both ACh and NaCN in one-fourth of carotid chemosensory units examined, was without effect in another one-fourth of such units, and blocked ACh-induced responses without affecting those to NaCN in the remaining half of chemosensory units studied.

Intracarotid injections of *α-bungarotoxin* are reported to reduce chemosensory responses to ACh and slightly depress those to NaCN,[53] and slightly enhance those to hypoxia, without affecting those to nicotine.[54] It has also been found that intracarotid administration of large doses of the highly penetrating blocker *dihydro-b-erythroidine*, which reduced chemosensory responses to ACh, was without effect on those to NaCN and CO_2.[53] When tested in vitro, dihydro-b-erythroidine was found to provoke an initial marked increase of spontaneous chemosensory discharge.[30]

It must be noted that many recordings from carotid nerve chemosensory fibers have been obtained in situ from animals paralyzed with *gallamine* (Flaxedil) (e.g., refs 32, 49, 55 and 56). Since gallamine is a nicotinic cholinergic blocker, this means that spontaneous chemosensory activity and its changes in response to physiological stimuli are resistant to block by this cholinergic antagonist at the dose used to obtain muscle paralysis.

Landgren et al[31] reported that *succinylcholine* increases the discharges from carotid body chemoreceptors recorded in situ. Apart from being an effective blocker of neuromuscular junctions and autonomic ganglia, succinylcholine also increases mechanosensory discharges from muscle spindles.[57] Furthermore, it must be noted that the depressant chemosensory actions of hexamethonium, *d*-tubocurarine and mecamylamine on carotid body preparations

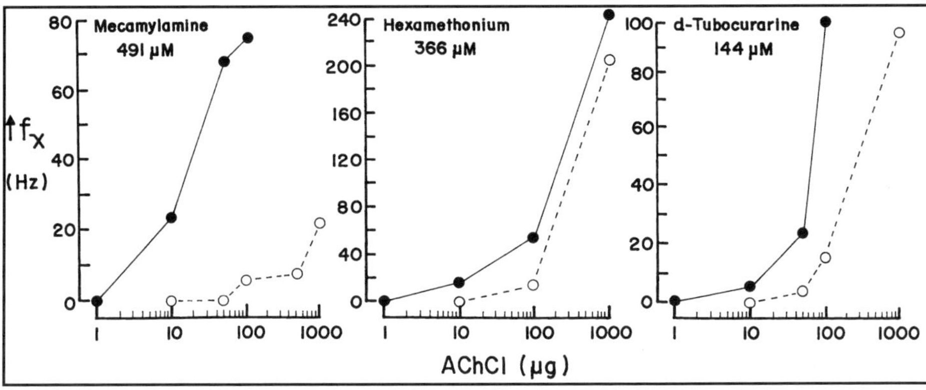

Fig. 7.4. Dose-response curves for increases in the frequency of chemosensory impulses (↑ f_x; ordinates) elicited by increasing doses of acetylcholine chloride (AChCl; abscissae), in control conditions (filled circles and continuous line) and after (open circles and interrupted line) adding mecamylamine 491 µM (left), hexamethonium 366 µM (middle) and d-tubocurarine 144 µM (right). Cat carotid bodies superfused in vitro with Locke's solution, pH 7.42-7.49 at 35°C, equilibrated with 50% O_2 in N_2, flowing at 1.1-1.2 ml/min. (Data replotted from Eyzaguirre and Zapata[29]).

superfused in vitro may be preceded by periods of enhanced spontaneous chemosensory activity (see Figs. 11 and 13 in reference 20, and Fig. 11 in reference 30).

Muscarinic Antagonists

Compared to nicotinic antagonists, *atropine* is a poor blocker of ACh actions on carotid chemosensory activity recorded from cat carotid bodies superfused in vitro,[29] and may initially increase the basal level of chemosensory discharges, before producing a moderate depression of chemosensory responses to flow interruption and acidity.[30] In situ, low doses of atropine--capable of reducing chemosensory responses to ACh--were usually without effect on the spontaneous level of discharge and the responses to NaCN, while large doses of atropine—markedly blocking ACh responses—also depressed NaCN responses.[33] Combined i.v. and intracarotid administration of atropine slightly depressed ACh-induced chemosensory responses, without changing or minimally depressing NaCN-evoked responses.[32]

It must be noted that the chemosensory inhibition induced by electrical stimulation of the carotid nerve itself was consistently blocked by atropine,[46] pointing to the possibilities of centrifugal modulation of chemoreceptor activity or vascular effect mediated by muscarinic cholinoceptors.

The inhibitory effects exerted by ACh and bethanechol on rabbits' carotid chemosensory activity are blocked by atropine.[23]

Based on the hypothesis that both nicotinic and muscarinic receptors may participate in a process of cholinergic transmission between glomus cells and chemosensory nerve endings, Fitzgerald and Shirahata[58] studied the effect of a cocktail of cholinergic antagonists (α-bungarotoxin, mecamylamine and atropine) selectively perfusing the carotid bifurcation of the cat on the chemosensory response to hypoxia, observing a dose-dependent reduction of such response, while barosensory activity was not affected. These data support the participation (probably not exclusive) of ACh in hypoxic chemoreception.

ADRENERGIC AGONISTS AND ANTAGONISTS

Adrenaline (Epinephrine)

Suppression of circulating adrenaline, by bilateral adrenal medullectomy in dogs, decreases ventilation.[59] On the contrary, i.v. infusions of adrenaline induce hyperventilation in humans,[60] dogs[61] and cats.[62,63] That this is a reflex effect originated from the arterial chemoreceptors was demonstrated by its absence while breathing 100% O_2 or after sectioning the buffer nerves.[62]

Recordings from the carotid nerves in situ confirmed that adrenaline increased chemosensory discharges in cats.[62] However, adrenaline-induced chemosensory excitation was assumed to be mediated by vascularly changes, since it was not observed in carotid bodies superfused in vitro.[64]

Intracarotid injections of adrenaline in rabbits[65] provoked brief discrete ventilatory depression followed by more pronounced and prolonged ventilatory excitation, the last response being prevented by phenoxybenzamine and thus ascribed to α-adrenoceptor mediation.

Noradrenaline (NA; Norepinephrine)

It has been found that dopamine-β-hydroxylase (DβH)—a marker of NA synthesizing cells—is colocalized with TH in 91% of glomus cells of the cat carotid bodies.[66] This means that a large number of catecholamine-synthesizing glomus cells are capable of producing NA in the carotid body of cats. Otherwise, the sympathetic outflow to carotid body vasculature is mediated by noradrenergic postganglionic fibers (see chapter 6) and the electrical stimulation or physiological activation of these fibers modifies the carotid chemosensory responses to other agents.[67,68] Thus NA effects on chemosensory responses may reproduce those of sympathetic stimulation.

It is known that i.v. infusions of NA provoke hyperventilation in humans,[60,69,70] the respiratory minute volume being doubled when plasmatic NA attained values similar to those observed during submaximal exercise.[71] The observation that this respiratory effect was reversed by breathing 100% O_2 pointed to the possibility that it was originated by excitation of arterial chemoreceptors. The hyperventilation observed in cats during i.v. infusions of NA proved to be of chemoreflex origin, since it was abolished by section of the carotid nerves.[62] Intracarotid injections of NA in rabbits provoked slight transient depression of ventilation, followed by prolonged intense hyperventilation, the last one being blocked by the α-adrenergic blocker phenoxybenzamine.[65]

Intravenous infusions of NA do indeed increase the frequency of carotid chemosensory discharges in cats[62,72] and rabbits.[73] Bolus intracarotid or i.v. injections of NA in cats may provoke biphasic chemosensory responses: brief slight inhibition followed by prolonged intense excitation, the last effect being eliminated by the α-adrenergic blocker dibenamine.[74] Another report[68] indicates that intracarotid infusions of NA in doses between 0.1 and 5 μg/min inhibit carotid chemosensory activity, while doses of 10 and 20 μg/ml augment such activity; the chemoreceptor inhibition was blocked by the α_2-adrenergic antagonist SKF-86466.

In spite of the above, experiments with carotid bodies superfused in vitro failed to show chemosensory excitation.[64] From this, it was concluded that the increased chemosensory discharge observed in situ in response to NA boluses or infusions should be mediated by vascular changes, probably by stagnant asphyxia caused by vasoconstriction within the carotid body.[75]

Noradrenaline occasionally produces a brief reduction of chemosensory discharges in vitro[76] and in situ,[74,77] but this inhibition is less intense and of shorter duration than that caused by dopamine (see later). This inhibitory effect of NA is not mediated by α-adrenoceptors (it is enhanced after dibenamine), but probably by low-affinity to dopamine receptors (it is blocked after haloperidol) (see later).

Bisgard et al[78] have found that intracarotid infusions of NA depress ventilation in awake goats, an effect not observed when the infusion is made on the side of a previously denervated carotid body. Dopaminergic blockade with domperidone (see later) effectively prevented the NA-induced depression of ventilation. Furthermore, recording of carotid nerve discharges in one anesthetized goat confirmed an abrupt and maintained inhibition of chemosensory dis-

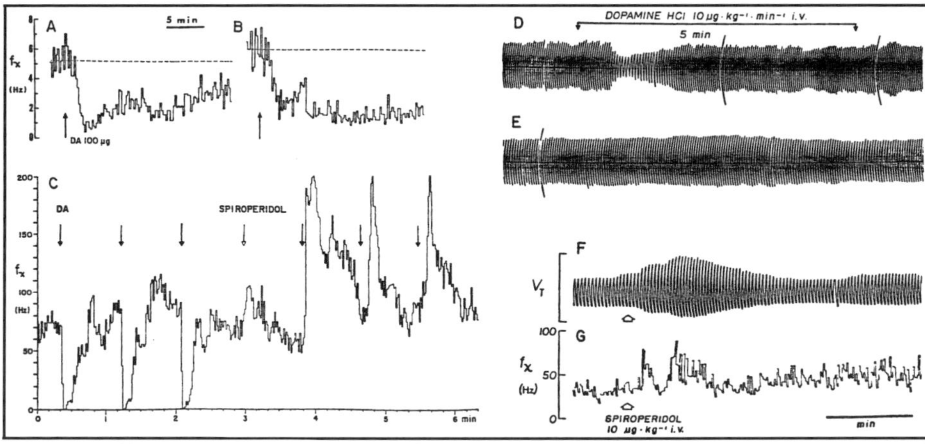

Fig. 7.5. Effects of dopamine (DA) and spiroperidol (SP) on chemosensory activity and ventilation in cats. (A-B) Recording from a single chemosensory fiber in preparation in vitro superfused with Locke's solution 2 ml/min at 37°C. Interrupted horizontal lines, mean basal chemosensory frequencies for the 2-min preceding each injection. Dopamine hydrochloride 100 mg injected into superfusate at arrows, before (A) and after (B) 70 min of application of dibenamine hydrochloride 250 mg (Modified from Zapata[76]). (C) Recording of chemosensory discharges from entire carotid nerve in preparation in situ. Repeated ipsilateral intracarotid injections of dopamine hydrochloride 5 mg (filled headed arrows) before and after i.v. injection of spiroperidol 5 mg/kg (open headed arrow). (Modified from Llados and Zapata[105]). (D-E) Pneumographic recording of ventilation. Intravenous infusions of dopamine hydrochloride 10 mg/kg/min along 5 min (between arrows) before (D) and after (E) bilateral section of the carotid nerves. (Modified from Zapata and Zuazo[72]). (F-G) Simultaneous recording of tidal volume (VT) by pneumotachograph (F) and frequency of chemosensory impulses (f_x) of one cut carotid nerve (G). Contralateral carotid nerve still intact, to mediate reflex ventilatory effects. Spiroperidol 10 mg/kg injected i.v. at arrows. (Reproduced from Zapata and Zuazo[132]).

charges during a 2-min intracarotid infusion of NA, an effect mimicked by the α_2-adrenoceptor agonist guanabenz.

Clonidine

Intravenous injections of this agonist for central α-adrenoceptors reduced for several minutes the frequency of spontaneous chemosensory discharges recorded from one carotid nerve in cats.[74] These injections also provoked brief hypertension followed by prolonged hypotension, and a moderate decrease in respiratory tidal volume if the contralateral carotid nerve was intact.

Isoprenaline (isoproterenol) has been tested as a model of β-adrenoceptor agonist. Isoprenaline infusions induce hyperventilation in man.[70,79,80] Its i.v. injection produced an early and intense hyperpnea, which was reduced to a small and late hyperpnea during thermal blockade of the carotid nerves[81] or after their sectioning[82] in cats, as well as after carotid bodies resection in rabbits.[83] Isoprenaline injected i.v. increased the frequency of carotid chemosensory discharges,[74,81,84] an effect temporally correlated with systemic hypotensive reactions.[74] Intracarotid injections of isoprenaline also induced transient increases in the frequency of chemosensory discharges.[74,77]

The excitatory chemosensory effects of isoprenaline were partially or completely blocked by β-adrenergic antagonists propranolol,[74,85] metoprolol,[77] atenolol[85] and dichloro-isoproterenol (DCI),[74] without affecting the chemosensory responses to hypoxic stimulation.

Adrenergic Antagonists

In previous paragraphs, it has been mentioned that the excitatory effects of NA and adrenaline on carotid chemosensory discharges are blocked by α-adrenergic antagonists (dibenamine [dibenzyline], phenoxybenzamine), while the excitatory effects of isoprenaline are blocked by β-adrenergic antagonists (propranolol, metoprolol, DCI).

Intravenous injections of phenoxybenzamine and dibenamine in cats provoked increases in chemosensory activity, but they were correlated in time and intensity with the falls in systemic arterial pressure.[74]

Intravenous injections of propranolol and metoprolol in cats and rabbits have been found to decrease resting chemosensory activity and almost to abolish chemosensory responses to hypoxia,[77] which may explain the ventilatory depression induced by i.v. infusions of propranolol in man.[70] However, blockade of β-adrenoceptors with propranolol in dogs did not affect reflex respiratory stimulation induced by hypoxia and NaCN.[86]

The chemosensory responses evoked in vitro by hypoxia and ACh were reportedly blocked by DCI,[87] but this effect was later accounted for by nerve fiber block.[64]

DOPAMINERGIC AGONISTS AND ANTAGONISTS

Dopamine

The detection of high levels of dopamine within the carotid bodies of all mammalian species studied[1] prompted a systematic search for its effects upon chemoreflexes and chemosensory activity.

In spite of initial reports of reflex hyperpnea caused by intracarotid injections of DA in dogs,[88,89] later publications indicate that intravenous or intracarotid injections or infusions of DA mostly depress ventilation in cats[72,88,90] (Fig. 7.5D), dogs,[50,61,91] rabbits,[92] rats,[93] goats[94] and newborn lambs.[95] Such effect disappears after section of the carotid nerves (Fig. 7.5E). Thus, ventilatory depression is ascribed to reflex effects of the DA-induced withdrawal of chemosensory impulses. Intravenous infusions of DA in humans also depress ventilation in normoxia[96-99] and hypoxia[100] as well as the slopes of the ventilatory responses to hypoxia[101] and hypercapnia,[102] effects abolished after administration of haloperidol[97] or droperidol,[101] respectively.

Dopamine inhibits the chemosensory discharges from cat carotid bodies in situ[103-107] (Fig. 7.5C). The inhibitory effect of dopamine is observed in both adult and neonatal (4-7 days) cats.[108] That this effect is not mediated by vascular changes is shown by the chemosensory inhibition of cat carotid bodies superfused in vitro in response to low doses of DA[76,109] (Fig. 7.5A), but this response fades (desensitization) after several applications of this substance, giving way to biphasic responses (chemosensory inhibition followed by excitation), and then to delayed and prolonged excitatory responses to larger doses of DA.

Mass recordings from cat carotid bodies in situ[2] and in vitro[25,110] revealed that DA evoked focal slow potentials of positive polarity, i.e., of inverse polarity to those induced by chemosensory stimulants (hypoxia, NaCN, ACh, nicotine). These observations suggest that DA induces postjunctional hyperpolarization of chemosensory nerve endings, responsible for decreasing or silencing the discharges recorded along carotid nerves chemosensory fibers. However, DA also produces membrane depolarization of 76% of glomus cells of rabbit carotid bodies and hyperpolarization of the remaining 24%, with increases in input resistance in all of them.[111]

Dopamine-induced inhibition seems characteristic of arterial chemoreceptors, since the small doses provoking this reaction are without effect on mechanoreceptors and larger doses are required to produce potentiation of barosensory discharges from the carotid sinus in vitro.[76]

In dogs, intracarotid and i.v. injections of low doses of DA caused chemosensory inhibition, while larger doses induced inhibition preceded by excitation.[50] In rabbits, intracarotid injections of DA produced chemosensory inhibition,[22,24,77,112] although preparations in vitro exhibited chemosensory excitation in response to DA.[25,113]

When simultaneously applied to cat carotid bodies superfused in vitro, the excitatory chemosensory responses to ACh may be canceled by the inhibitory effects of DA, but—on sequential applications—the excitatory responses to ACh were enhanced after repeated exposures to DA.[76] Cancellation of opposite effects between concurrent injections of DA and NaCN has been observed in vitro[76] and in situ.[106] However, interactions may be more complex, since intracarotid infusions of DA that reduced the basal level of chemosensory discharges did not change the increase above basal discharges caused by i.v. injections of NaCN.[109] Later, it was found that slow i.v. infusions of DA decrease chemosensory sensitivity to injections of low doses of NaCN, but increase the reactivity to high doses of such chemoreceptor stimulating agent.[114]

Dopaminergic Agonists and Depletors

Apomorphine and *amantadine* have been shown to mimic the inhibitory effects of DA on cat carotid chemosensory activity.[105,106] Similarly, the selective D_2 agonist LY-141865 was equipotent with DA in decreasing chemosensory discharges in rabbit carotid bodies, while the selective D_1 agonist SK&F-38393 was much less effective.[112] However, agents that should release endogenous DA from glomus cells—such as *amphetamine* and *tyramine*—were without noticeable effects on spontaneous chemosensory activity in the cat.[105]

The initial i.v. injections of several *ergoloids* and *ergolines* also induced a transient depression of carotid chemosensory activity, but this effect was followed by blockade of the inhibitory effects of consecutive injections of DA.[115] This dopaminergic agonistic-antagonistic activity of ergot alkaloids is also exhibited on other tissues.[116]

The dopaminergic toxin *6-hydroxydopamine*, when injected intracarotidally in cats, acted initially as a dopaminergic agonist, since it produced transient inhibition of chemosensory discharges, but the drug did not impair chemosensory activity or responses to DA and stimulants for the following 48 hours.[117] It has been reported, however, that depletion of catecholamine stores by treating rabbits with *reserpine* or *α-methyl-p-tyrosine* results in reduced spontaneous chemosensory activity and reduced chemosensory responses to hypoxia and hypercapnia of their carotid bodies superfused in vitro.[118,119]

Dopaminergic Antagonists

The inhibitory effects of DA on carotid chemosensory activity have been found to be blocked by several groups of compounds: 1) *butyrophenones*, such as droperidol,[120] haloperidol,[25,50,90,105] spiroperidol[76,105] and trifluperidol[106] (Fig. 7.5C); 2) *phenothiazines*, such as chlorpromazine,[105,120] fluphenazine[121] and perphenazine;[105] 3) *thioxanthenes*, such as α-flupenthixol;[23,103] 4) *ergoloids*, such as dihydroergotamine,[46,50,109,115,122] dihydroergotoxine, ergometrine, methylergometrine, ergotamine and 2-Br-α-ergocryptine;[115] 5) *benzamides*, such as metoclopramide and sulpiride;[112,123] 6) *aralkylpiperidines*, such as pimozide[120] and domperidone.[112,124-126] However, it must be noted that chronic domperidone treatment (8 weeks and then withdrawn for 4-9 days) in rabbits results in an increased sensitivity to the chemodepressant effects of DA.[127]

Calculation of the inhibition constants (K_i) of some of these compounds on carotid chemosensory activity result in the following order of DA-antagonistic efficiency: spiroperidol > haloperidol > fluphenazine > perphenazine > chlorpromazine.[121]

With regard to the excitatory chemosensory effects of DA observed in rabbit carotid bodies in vitro, they were resistant to the dopaminergic blockers haloperidol and (+)-butaclamol.[113]

To complete the pharmacological characterization of DA effects on carotid chemosensory discharges, mention must be made to possible interference by adrenergic blockers. Although the α-adrenergic blocker phenoxybenzamine was initially reported as an antagonist of DA effects on carotid body,[46] later observations indicated that this drug did not directly antagonize DA actions.[74,106,121] Furthermore, DA inhibitory chemosensory effects were unchanged after treatment with dibenamine[74] (Fig. 7.5B) or phentolamine.[46,106] Dopamine inhibition was also resistant to β-adrenergic blockers, such as propranolol and dichloroisoproterenol (DCI).[74]

Particular attention must be given to the effects of perphenazine, haloperidol and spiroperidol, since these antagonists not only block DA-induced inhibitory effects on carotid chemosensory activity, but reverse them into excitatory ones[105,121,128] (Fig. 7.C). The same occurred after i.v. injections of 2-Br-α-ergocryptine (bromocryptine).[115] Reversal of DA-inhibitory effects into excitatory ones also occurred in preparations in vitro after repeated exposures to DA.[76]

The above observations led to the proposal that inhibitory and excitatory dopaminoceptors (DA_i and DA_e) occur in carotid body tissues,[105] in accordance with Cools and van Rossum's[129] classification of dopaminoceptors in other tissues. Inhibitory dopaminoceptors of cat carotid bodies are presumably not linked to adenylate cyclase, since chemosensory excitation is induced by the second messenger cAMP[130] and by drugs that increase its levels, such as caffeine and theophylline.[131] The different chemosensory effects exhibited by DA in diverse species and the biphasic responses observed in some preparations may be explained by the relative preponderance and affinities of $D\alpha_i$ and DA_e receptors. Furthermore, the presence of two different dopaminoceptors in arterial chemoreceptors provides adequate mechanisms for a complex modulation of chemosensory activity by DA[109] (see chapter 3).

Increases in the resting levels of cat carotid chemosensory discharges were observed after applying some dopaminergic blockers, such as perphenazine,[105,132] chlorpromazine,[132] spiroperidol[105,132] (Fig. 7.5G), droperidol,[120] trifluperidol,[106] haloperidol[104-106,132-34] and domperidone.[108,124,125,135,136] The suppression of chemoreception by continuous superfusion of cat carotid bodies with haloperidol reported by Nolan et al[137] might have been due to a nonspecific anesthetic effect of the accumulated drug or its diluents. Furthermore, the variability of interspike intervals in single chemosensory fibers increased after haloperidol administration.[138] These observations suggest that endogenous DA exerts a tonic inhibition on chemosensory discharges under normoxic conditions. It is possible that modulation of chemosensory activity in carotid bodies in situ may depend on endogenous DA, locally released from glomus cells or diffused from plasma, since significant levels of plasmatic DA are detected under resting conditions[139] and they increase during exercise.[140]

As a consequence of the above, i.v. injections of dopaminergic antagonists (spiroperidol, haloperidol, perphenazine and chlorpromazine) increased resting ventilation in cats, the intensity and duration of the effects being dependent on the doses of the blocker[132] (Fig. 7.5F). This ventilatory enhancement is absent when applying the blockers after section of the carotid and aortic nerves. Intracarotid injections of haloperidol are also known to enhance ventilation in rabbits, as well as to block the ventilatory depressant effects of intracarotid injections of DA.[141] In mice, ventilation is enhanced at all levels of F_IO_2 after treatment with the dopaminergic blockers droperidol, chlorpromazine and prochlorperazine.[142] In humans, resting ventilation and the ventilatory response to asphyxia are augmented after treatment with prochlorperazine,[143] as well as the slope of the ventilatory response to hypoxia after droperidol.[101]

Haloperidol treatment has been found to potentiate chemosensory responses to both hypoxia and hypercapnia,[104] but another study has shown that haloperidol increases the chemosensory responses to hypoxia but not those to hypercapnia.[133] This may explain why the ventilatory responses to NaCN were enhanced after domperidone treatment in rats.[144] Domperidone increases carotid chemosensory activity in adult cats in hypoxia, normoxia, hyperoxia, normocapnia and hypercapnia, but such increase is observed only during hypoxia or hypercapnia in neonatal (4-7 days) cats,[108,135] suggesting that the low level of chemosensory activity observed in neonatal animals is not due to a tonically enhanced dopaminergic inhibition of arterial chemoreceptors.

INDOLAMINERGIC AGONISTS AND ANTAGONISTS

Serotonin (5-Hydroxy-Tryptamine, 5-HT)

The presence of 5-HT in the carotid bodies of humans,[145] cats[146] and rats,[147] and its colocalization with chromogranin in 95% of glomus cells of cat carotid bodies[28] (see also chapters 1 and 3 by Verna and González et al, respectively) prompted the study of its effects upon chemosensory activity.

Intracarotid injections of 5-HT into rats[148] and dogs[88] produced tachypnea and hyperpnea, respectively, which were abolished by section of the carotid nerves. However, in the cat,[88] they provoked apnea, bradycardia and hypotension, still present after carotid nerve section, but prevented by excision of the nodose ganglion, which sensory neurons are known to be excited by 5-HT.[149]

Intracarotid or i.v. injections of 5-HT provoked chemosensory excitation in rats,[148,150] and excitation followed by inhibition in cats[151,152] and dogs,[50] but similar effects were exerted on barosensory discharges.[151]

Intrastream injections of 5-HT did not produce excitation of cat carotid bodies superfused in vitro, except in 1 out of 35 trials,[20] suggesting that most effects observed in situ were vascularly mediated.

Serotoninergic Antagonists

The serotoninergic antagonists methysergide and gramine, applied in doses preventing 5-HT systemic vascular effects, did not block 5-HT excitatory effects on carotid chemosensory activity in cats[151] and rats,[148] nor the chemosensory responses to asphyxia and NaCN in cats.[151] The 5-HT_3 receptor antagonist MDL 72222 abolished the chemoexcitatory effect and reduced the chemodepressant effect of 5-HT.[152] The 5-HT_2 antagonist ketanserin had no effect on the transient chemoexcitation induced by 5-HT in cats, slightly reduced the following chemodepressant effect and abolished a delayed longer-lasting effect as well as the associated hypotension.[152] The 5-HT_3 antagonist 3-tropanyl-indole-3-carboxylate methiodide (ICS 205-930) blocked the 5-HT-induced increase in chemosensory discharges in rats.[150] Thus, at least two types of 5-HT-receptors appear to be involved in the chemosensory responses to 5-HT. However, neither MDL 72222 nor ketanserin—alone or in combination—had any effect upon chemosensory responses to hypoxia.[152]

The chemosensory excitation induced by 5-HT in dogs was blocked by d-tubocurarine[50] and that observed in rats was blocked by mecamylamine,[148] suggesting involvement of nicotinic cholinoceptors. However, 5-HT-induced chemosensory excitation in cats was unaffected by hexamethonium or atropine.[151]

PURINERGIC AGONISTS AND ANTAGONISTS

Adenosine Triphosphate (ATP)

Anichkov and Belen'kii[11] proposed that chemoreceptor excitability was lost by exhaustion of ATP stores and restored by adding ATP. They observed that ATP applied to the cat carotid body induced reflex hyperpnea. However, Matsumoto et al[92] observed ATP-evoked ventilatory depression in rabbits, prevented by sectioning their carotid nerves.

Jarisch et al[153] had in fact observed that intracarotid injections of ATP were immediately followed by heavy chemoreceptor discharges in cats and dogs. Krylov and Anichkov[154] also observed that ATP perfusion of the isolated carotid bifurcation region (species not mentioned) increased chemosensory activity, but Joels and Neil[130] observed that such perfusion reduced chemosensory responses to NaCN and 2,4-dinitrophenol in cats, instead of producing their potentiation.

Working on cat carotid bodies superfused in vitro, Spergel and Lahiri[155] observed that ATP and adenosine-5'-O-(3-thiotriphosphate) (ATPγS; a nonhydrolyzable analog of ATP) induced transient, dose-dependent increases in the frequency of chemosensory discharges, but prolonged infusions of ATP produced only an equivalent transient increase in chemosensory discharges followed by rapid return to baseline level. GTP, ADP and AMP were less effective stimulants of chemosensory activity.

ATP is contained within the dense-core granules of glomus cells[156,157] and should be released during hypoxia-induced exocytosis. Its degradation by ectonucleotidases yields adenosine.

Adenosine

The fact that hypoxia induces the release of adenosine from the coronary territory,[158] prompted the study of adenosine in chemotransmission. Intracarotid injections of adenosine in cats produced a rapid and dose-dependent increase in the frequency of carotid chemosensory discharges.[159,160] This dose-dependent excitatory effect was also observed in cat carotid bodies superfused in vitro,[161] an indication of its direct effects on chemotransmission. However, Spergel and Lahiri[155] failed to observe chemosensory excitation in cat carotid bodies superfused in vitro with Tyrode's solution without CO_2-HCO_3^-. The excitatory effects of adenosine on arterial chemoreceptors may explain the stimulatory effect of this substance upon ventilation in rats[162] and humans,[163,164] an effect potentiated by inhibition of adenosine uptake.[165] McQueen[166] studied the simultaneous effects of adenosine on chemosensory discharge of one carotid nerve and on ventilation in rats, concluding that the dose-related increases in ventilation were not explained by the slight increases in chemosensory discharges.

Intracarotid injections of adenosine analogues 2-CADO (2-chloro-adenosine), NECA (5'-N-ethyl-carboxamido-adenosine) and PIA (N^6-phenyl-isopropyl-adenosine) also caused dose-related increases in carotid chemosensory discharges in cats.[160,167] However, i.p. injections of PIA in awake rats produced a dose-dependent decrease of ventilation, attaining its maximum at 30-80 min, an effect still observed in chemodenervated animals.[168] The adenosine antagonists theophylline and 8-phenyltheophylline (8-PT) partially blocked the chemoexcitatory actions of NECA and adenosine, respectively.[167] Both theophylline and aminophylline transiently decreased the frequency of spontaneous chemosensory discharges.[159] The sensitivity of carotid chemoreceptors to hypoxia was also reduced by 8-PT.[167] The rank order of potency of analogues and the blocking activity of antagonists classifies as A_2 the adenosine receptors involved in chemoexcitation.

There are two classes of purinoceptors: with higher affinity for adenosine (P_1) or for ATP (P_2). Two categories of P_1 receptors (A_1 and A_2) and at least four of P_2 receptors (P_{2X}, P_{2Y}, P_{2Z} and P_{2T}) have been described.[169]

EICOSANOIDS AND THEIR ANTAGONISTS

Prostaglandins

The well known role of prostaglandins in the sensitization of nociceptive nerve endings prompted studies on its actions on carotid barosensory and chemosensory fibers. Thus, McQueen and Belmonte[170] recorded the changes in electrical activity produced by prostaglandins E_2, A_2 and $F_{2\alpha}$ in preparations in situ and in vitro from cats. In the first condition, they observed changes in baro- and chemo-sensory activities that were concomitant or secondary to changes in systemic arterial pressure. However, the isolated and superfused carotid bodies in vitro failed to show any effect of prostaglandins, leading to the conclusion that effects observed in situ were of vascular origin.

Salicylates

The action of salicylates is discussed here since they inhibit prostaglandin synthesis, although they also uncouple oxidative phosphorylation.

As hyperventilation is a salient sign of salicylate toxicity, central and peripheral sites of action have been searched for. McQueen et al[171] observed in rats that a single i.v. injection of sodium salicylate caused a rapid and transient hyperventilation, not shown after bilateral section of the carotid nerves, although a delayed hyperventilation could still be evoked after carotid sensory denervation. Intracarotid injections of salicylate also led to increased respiration only when the ipsilateral carotid nerve was intact. Thus, it was concluded that the carotid bodies were the exclusive origin of the early (reflex) phase of salicylate-induced hyperventilation.

Recordings of chemosensory discharges from the carotid nerves of rats[171] provided direct evidence that sodium salicylate induced dose-dependent increases in their frequency, beginning within 10 s of i.v. injections and lasting for 1-2 min. The dose-response curves for chemosensory and ventilatory effects were broadly similar. On the other hand, carotid sinus barosensory discharges were unaffected by salicylate injections.

The above observations may explain the persistent hyperventilation and enhancement of the hypoxic ventilatory response in men treated daily with nearly 4 g of aspirin.[172]

PEPTIDERGIC AGONISTS AND ANTAGONISTS

Substance P

Substance P (SP) and neurokinin A (NKA) belong to the group of tachykinins. Substance P-like immunoreactivity was initially found in a network of fine nerve fibers distributed throughout these organs,[173,174] probably corresponding to chemosensory nerve fibers. However, SP was later found in glomus cells directly apposed to sensory nerve endings,[175] being colocalized with met-enkephalin (78%), TH (78%) and 5-HT (78%) in glomus cells of cat carotid bodies.[28] In the same preparation, many glomus cells and a sparse plexus of fine fibers also exhibit NKA-immunoreactivity.[176] The involvement of SP in chemoreception is suggested by the finding that its level in rabbit carotid bodies was reduced by nearly 40% after 1 h of hypoxic exposure,[177] while the same challenge increased by nearly 150% its level in cat carotid bodies[176] (see chapters 1 and 3). Also, it must be mentioned that intracellular recordings from sliced carotid bodies of cats and mice revealed that SP depolarized 69% of glomus cells, hyperpolarized 17% of them and was without effect on membrane potential on the rest.[178]

Intracarotid injections of SP initially increased (first 15-s) and then decreased (for up to 5 min) the frequency of basal chemosensory discharges recorded from cat carotid bodies in situ; they also potentiated the chemosensory excitation evoked by NaCN.[179] The excitatory effect of SP was observed even in cats breathing hyperoxic or hyperoxic-hypercapnic mixtures.[180] Working on cat carotid bodies superfused in vitro, Monti-Bloch and Eyzaguirre[181] observed that SP produced excitation in 17 instances, inhibition in 16 instances and no effect in 3 instances. The excitatory effects of SP on carotid chemosensory discharges have also been observed in rats.[182]

The chemosensory excitation induced by intracarotid injections of SP in cats was very similar to that induced by equimolar injections of NKA[176] and physalaemin, while eledoisin was without chemosensory effects,[183] in spite of previously reported excitatory effects of eledoisin.[184] On the contrary, intracarotid administration of D-Arg-D-Trp,^{7,9} Leu^{1,2}-SP, D-Pro,^{2} D-Trp^{7,9}-SP, spantide and CP-96,345 blocked the excitatory responses of exogenous SP and markedly attenuated the chemosensory responses to hypoxia in cats[180,185,186] and rats.[182] The effectiveness of SP analogues and antagonists on carotid chemosensory activity suggests that SP effects are mediated by NK-1, but not NK-2 or NK-3 receptors.

Opioids

The presence of *leucine-enkephalin* and *methionine-enkephalin* immunoreactive substances has been shown in the glomus cells of cat carotid bodies.[173,174] Met-enkephalin is colocalized with 5-HT (91%), TH (90%) and SP (78%) in glomus cells of cat carotid bodies.[28] Furthermore, 1-h hypoxic stimulation of rabbits decreases by 40% enkephalin levels within their carotid bodies[177] (see also chapter 3). Intracellular recordings from sliced carotid bodies of cats and mice revealed that met-enkephalin depolarized 88% of glomus cells, hyperpolarized 8% of them and had no effect on the rest.[178]

Experiments on cat carotid bodies in situ[187,188] reveal that intracarotid injections of met-enkephalin cause a rapid inhibition of spontaneous chemosensory discharges, which intensity and duration were dose-dependent. Inhibitory effects for leu-enkephalin had also been reported.[189,190] McQueen and Ribeiro[187] also observed that *morphine* provokes a less intense inhibition than met-enkephalin, and that both substances slightly reduce the chemosensory excitation induced by ACh and NaCN injections. A later report[191] showed that *β-endorphin* also transiently decreased the frequency of spontaneous chemosensory discharges.

It must be noted that previous observations had shown that morphine caused transient increases in the frequency of chemosensory discharges recorded from cat carotid bodies in situ[31] and in vitro.[30] In the last preparation, met-enkephalin produced transient inhibition followed by enhancement of basal chemosensory discharges, as well as reduction of chemosensory responses to hypoxia, hypercapnia and acidosis.[181]

The opiate antagonist *naloxone* slightly increased the spontaneous chemosensory discharges recorded from cat carotid bodies in situ.[187] Although another study[188] reported that naloxone did not affect basal chemosensory activity in cats under normoxic conditions, it increased their ventilation even under hyperoxia and potentiated the carotid chemosensory response to hypoxia. Intravenous injections of naloxone and naltrexone in rats caused dose-dependent increases in ventilation and antagonized the ventilatory depressant effects of morphine.[192] Naloxone reduced the chemosensory inhibition caused by met-enkephalin and morphine,[187] as well as that induced by β-endorphin.[191]

Kirby and McQueen[190] observed that met-enkephalin, leu-enkephalin, D-Ala,[2] D-Leu[5]-enkephalin and D-Pen[5]-enkephalin were more potent chemodepressants than D-Ala[2].Me-Phe[4], Gly-ol[5]-enkephalin, dynorphin(1-8) and ethyl-keto-cyclazocine, while morphiceptine was inactive. On the other hand, ICI-154129 and ICI-174864 antagonized the chemosensory inhibition caused by met-enkephalin and other opioids, and increased the chemosensory excitation induced by hypoxia. These results indicate that the chemosensory depression induced by these substances is mediated by a δ-opioid receptor and that endogenous opioids may restrain the chemosensory excitation evoked by hypoxia.

Endothelins (ETs)

They constitute a family of peptides with at least four distinct isoforms (ET-1, ET-2, ET-3 and VIC -vasoactive intestinal contractor) and two receptor subtypes identified and sequenced (ET_A and ET_B).[193] They can be released from endothelial and other cells by different stimuli, hypoxia among them. ET-binding sites have been demonstrated in the cat carotid body,[194] a binding displaceable by ET_A antagonist FR139317 (see reference 195; see also chapter 3).

Intracarotid injections of ET-1, ET-2 and ET-3 induce delayed (45-90 s) dose-related increases in the frequency of carotid chemosensory discharges in cats.[194] Intravenous administration of ET-1 has been found to increase carotid chemosensory activity concomitantly with an augmentation of respiratory frequency and minute ventilation in the rat.[195] The ventilatory effect is partially blocked by administration of FR139317 and abolished by sectioning of both carotid nerves,[195] indicating that it is a reflex effect initiated by activation of ET_A receptors at the level of the carotid bodies.

Vasoactive Intestinal Polypeptide (VIP)

Intracarotid infusion or i.v. injection of VIP induced hyperventilation in dogs, an effect abolished after section of the carotid nerves.[196] Later it was found that intracarotid injections of low doses of VIP decrease the spontaneous chemosensory discharge recorded from cat carotid bodies in situ while that of larger doses produce delayed, long-lasting increases in chemosensory activity.[191,197]

VIP-like immunoreactivity has not been found in the glomus cells of cat carotid bodies, but it is present in their varicose nerve fibers, mostly concentrated around blood vessels.[173,174] That they probably correspond to sympathetic nerve fibers was confirmed by the disappearance of VIP-positive fibers in the carotid body after excision of the superior cervical ganglion in the guinea pig.[198]

Cholecystokinin (CCK)

Cholecystokinin-like immunoreactivity has been shown in carotid bodies of cats[199] and infant humans.[200] Intracarotid injections of cholecystokinin octapeptide (CCK-8) caused a brief decrease followed by an increase of the spontaneous chemosensory discharge recorded from cat carotid bodies in situ.[191]

Atrial Natriuretic Peptide (ANP)

Immunocytochemical studies have shown that the glomus cells of cat carotid bodies exhibit ANP-like immunoreactivity.[201] Studies on cat carotid bodies superfused in vitro with Tyrode's solution equilibrated with 100% O_2 showed that while an infusion of atriopeptin III—a synthetic ANP analogue—did not alter basal chemosensory activity, the chemosensory response to superfusion with 20% equilibrated Tyrode's solution was slowed and diminished.[201] This inhibition was dose-dependent and completely reversible after washout of the drug. Further studies on rabbit carotid bodies superfused in vitro confirmed that submicromolar concentrations of atriopeptin III inhibited the chemosensory responses to hypoxia and nicotine, without modifying basal chemosensory activity or the response to high K^+ media.[202]

The effects of ANP seem to be mediated by activation of guanylate cyclase and cGMP formation. In fact, dibutyryl-cGMP and 8-bromo-cGMP (cell-permeant analogues of cGMP) were also able to inhibit the chemosensory responses to hypoxia and nicotine, without modifying basal chemosensory activity[202] (see chapter 8).

Other Polypeptides

Working on cat carotid bodies in situ, McQueen[184] observed that intracarotid injections of *bradykinin*, *angiotensin II* and *vasopressin* (ADH) produced increases and/or decreases in chemosensory nerve discharges, while neurotensin induced only excitatory effects and somatostatin only inhibitory effects. *Somatostatin* also reduces carotid body neural activity in Pekin ducks.[203] Intravenous infusion of angiotensin depresses ventilation in humans.[70]

ANALEPTICS

Intracarotid injections of the analeptics *nikethamide* (pyridinoyl-diethylamide, Coramine) and *pentylenetetrazol* (1,5-pentamethylene-tetrazole, Leptazol, Metrazole, Cardiazole) have failed to modify carotid chemosensory discharges,[43] suggesting that the respiratory stimulant properties of these substances are mediated by effects on the respiratory centers. This was confirmed by the finding that the ventilatory responses to i.v. injections of pentylenetetrazol in decerebrate cats were not reduced by sectioning the carotid or vagus nerves.[204] Similarly, the ventilatory stimulant effect of *aminophylline* persists after section of the glossopharyngeal nerves and removal of the carotid bodies in rats.[205]

It has been found that the ventilatory stimulating effects of *doxapram* (1-ethyl-4 (2-morpholino-ethyl)-3,3-diphenyl-2-pyrrolidinone hydrochloride hydrate), injected i.v. or intracarotidally in decerebrated or chloralose-anesthetized adult cats, are decreased or abolished by bilateral section of the carotid nerves.[204,206] Similar observations were performed on rats.[207] Intravenous injections of this drug in doses of from 0.5 to 10 mg/kg increased the chemosensory activity of the carotid nerve in adult cats, with a mean latency of 8 s and a peak response at 15 s, the effect subsiding within 2-20 min.[208] In chloralose anesthetized cats, the increases in chemosensory activity caused by doxapram were of the same magnitude at all levels of P_aO_2 and P_aCO_2, while the ventilatory effects were more than additive to concomitant stimulation by hypoxia or hypercapnia.[209] Furthermore, studies in kittens (1-11 days old) revealed that i.v. injections of doxapram counteracted the chemosensory depressant effects of hyperoxia, and potentiated the chemosensory responses to hypoxia and hypercapnia.[210] It must be noted that doxapram inhibits K^+ currents in glomus cells of neonatal rat carotid bodies.[211]

It has also been reported that *almitrine* (S-2620) causes long lasting hyperventilation in mammals, through prolonged excitation of arterial chemoreceptors.[212-214] Interestingly, although a blunted ventilatory response to transient hypoxia is observed after chronic hypoxia, a vigorous ventilatory response to almitrine is maintained in that condition.[215] Almitrine does indeed increase the frequency of chemosensory discharges recorded from carotid nerves of rabbits[216] and cats.[217] The carotid chemosensory excitation induced by almitrine in dogs takes 2-5 min to reach the peak and the effect persists for 20-30 min, being augmented by hypoxia and reduced by hyperoxia.[218] Contrarily, the chemosensory response to hypoxia was markedly potentiated by almitrine.[216] It was found in cats that the stimulating effect of almitrine on basal carotid chemosensory activity—as well the potentiation of chemosensory responses to hypoxia and hypercapnia—were more intense when the ganglioglomerular nerves were intact.[219] Intravenous infusion of almitrine in man causes a large and dose-dependent increase in hypoxic chemosensitivity.[220] It has recently been shown that almitrine decreases the opening probability of the O_2-sensitive K^+_{Ca} channels in isolated rat chemoreceptor cells (López-López et al, personal communication).

CENTRAL DEPRESSANTS

Intracarotid injections of *morphine* produced a transient increase in chemosensory nerve discharges.[31] In cat carotid bodies superfused in vitro, the addition of morphine to the superfusing solution also produced a transient increase of chemosensory discharges.[30] These excitatory effects on chemoreflex afferences are quite opposite to the well-known depressing effects of morphine on respiratory centers.

Intracarotid injections of barbitone (diethyl-barbituric acid), *pentobarbitone* (Nembutal), diallyl-barbituric acid (dial) and ethyl-methyl-butyl-barbituric acid (pentothal) had been found without effects on cat carotid chemosensory discharges, except for slight increases in chemosensory activity temporally associated to falls in systemic arterial pressure.[131] We have also observed that the changes in chemosensory activity produced by i.v. injections of pentobarbitone in cats may be entirely ascribed to the changes in arterial pressure and ventilation induced by this drug, the overdoses used to sacrifice these animals at the end of experiments resulting in apneusis, and pronounced and prolonged increases in carotid chemosensory discharges.

Anesthesia of rabbits and cats by the volatile agents *halothane*, *enflurane* and *isoflurane* in concentrations of up to 1% resulted in mild depression of carotid chemosensory activity and downward shifts of O_2 and CO_2 chemosensory response curves, but this depression was overcome by reducing P_aO_2 below 40 Torr.[221]

CARDIAC GLYCOSIDES

It has been proposed that the respiratory effects of digoxin and *ouabain* (strophanthin-G) are mediated by stimulation of arterial chemoreceptors.[222] McQueen and Ribeiro[223] observed that intracarotid and i.v. injections of ouabain in cats produced a marked increase in the frequency of chemosensory discharges followed by desensitization; the drug also potentiated the chemosensory responses to hypoxia and NaCN.

ACKNOWLEDGMENTS

Thanks are due to Mrs. Carolina Larrain for her continuous help in the laboratory as well as in the preparation of manuscripts. The work of the author has been supported by grants from FONDECYT (National Fund for Scientific and Technological Development) and DIPUC (Research and Postgraduate Division, Catholic University of Chile).

References

1. Eyzaguirre C, Zapata P. Perspectives in carotid body research. J Appl Physiol 1984; 57:931-957.
2. Zapata P, Eyzaguirre C Bioelectric potentials in the carotid body. Brain Res 1985; 331:39-50.
3. Kondo H. Innervation of the carotid body of the adult rat. Cell Tiss Res 1976; 173: 1-15.
4. McDonald DM, Mitchell RA. The innervation of glomus cells, ganglion cells and blood vessels in the rat carotid body: a quantitative ultrastructural analysis. J Neurocytol 1975; 4:177-230.
5. McDonald DM, Larue DT. The ultrastructure and connections of blood vessels supplying the rat carotid body and carotid sinus. J Neurocytol 1983; 12: 117-153.
6. Eyzaguirre C, Uchizono K. Observations on the fibre content of nerves reaching the carotid body of the cat. J Physiol, London 1961; 159:268-281.
7. Verna A. Ultrastructural localization of postganglionic sympathetic nerve endings in the rabbit carotid body. In: Belmonte C, Pallot D, Acker H, Fidone S, eds. Arterial Chemoreceptors. Leicester, UK: Leicester University Press. 1981; 336-343.
8. Hess A. Electron microscopic observations of normal and experimental cat carotid bodies. In: Torrance RW, ed. Arterial Chemoreceptors. Oxford, UK: Blackwell. 1968; 51-56.
9. Woods IR. Penetration of horseradish peroxidase between all elements of the carotid body. In: Purves MJ, ed. The Peripheral Arterial Chemoreceptors. London: Cambridge University Press. 1975; 195-205.
10. de Castro F. Nuevas observaciones sobre la inervación de la región carotídea. Los quimio- y preso-receptores. Trab Inst Cajal Invest Biol 1940; 32:297-384.
11. Anichkov SV, Belen'kii ML. Pharmacology of the Carotid Body Chemoreceptors. (Translated from Russian). Oxford: Pergamon; New York: Macmillan. 1963: 225.
12. Heymans C, Neil E. Reflexogenic Areas of the Cardiovascular System. London: Churchill. 1958:271.
13. Euler US von, Liljestrand G, Zotterman Y. Über den Reizmechanismus der Chemorezeptoren im Glomus Caroticum. Acta Physiol Scand 1941; 1:383-385.
14. Schweitzer A, Wright S Action of prostigmin and acetylcholine on respiration. Quart J Exp Physiol 1938; 28:33-47.
15. Heymans C. Action of drugs on carotid body and sinus. Pharmacol Rev 1955; 7:119-142.
16. Eyzaguirre C, Koyano H, Taylor JR. Presence of acetylcholine and transmitter release from carotid body chemoreceptors. J Physiol, London 1965; 178:463-476.
17. Fidone SJ, Weintraub S, Stavinoha WB. Acetylcholine content of normal and denervated cat carotid bodies measured by pyrolysis gas chromatography/mass fragmentometry. J Neurochem 1976; 26:1047-1049.
18. Metz B. Release of acetylcholine from the carotid body by hypoxia and hypoxia plus hypercapnia. Respir Physiol 1969; 6:386-394.
19. Fitzgerald RS, Shirahata M. Release of acetylcholine from the in vitro cat carotid body. Adv Exp Med Biol 1996; 410: 227-232.
20. Eyzaguirre C, Koyano H. Effects of some pharmacological agents on chemoreceptor discharges. J Physiol, London 1965; 178:410-437.
21. Fidone S, Sato A, Eyzaguirre C. Acetylcholine activation of carotid body chemoreceptor A fibers. Brain Res 1968; 9:374-376.
22. Docherty RJ, McQueen DS. Inhibitory effect of acetylcholine and dopamine on rabbit carotid chemoreceptors. J Physiol, London 1978; 277:64P-66P.
23. Docherty RJ, McQueen DS. The effects of acetylcholine and dopamine on carotid chemosensory activity in the rabbit. J Physiol, London 1979; 288:411-423.
24. Ponte J, Sadler CL. Interactions between hypoxia, acetylcholine and dopamine in the carotid body of rabbit and cat. J Physiol, London 1989; 410:395-410.
25. Monti-Bloch L, Eyzaguirre C. A comparative physiological and pharmacological study of cat and rabbit carotid body chemoreceptors. Brain Res 1980; 193: 449-470.

26. Hayashida Y, Koyano H, Eyzaguirre C. An intracellular study of chemosensory fibers and endings. J Neurophysiol 1980; 44:1077-1088.
27. Eyzaguirre C, Leitner LM, Nishi K, Fidone S. Depolarization of chemosensory nerve endings in carotid body of the cat. J Neurophysiol 1970; 33:685-696.
28. Wang Z-Z, Stensaas LJ, Dinger B, Fidone SJ. The coexistence of biogenic amines and neuropeptides in the type I cells of the cat carotid body. Neuroscience 1992; 47:473-480.
29. Eyzaguirre C, Zapata P. The release of acetylcholine from carotid body tissues. Further study on the effects of acetylcholine and cholinergic blocking agents on the chemosensory discharge. J Physiol, London 1968; 195:589-607.
30. Eyzaguirre C, Zapata P. Pharmacology of pH effects on carotid body chemoreceptors in vitro. J Physiol, London 1968; 195: 557-588.
31. Landgren S, Liljestrand G, Zotterman Y. The effect of certain autonomic drugs on the action potentials of the sinus nerve. Acta Physiol Scand 1952; 26:264-290.
32. McQueen DS. A quantitative study of the effects of cholinergic drugs on carotid chemoreceptors in the cat. J Physiol, London 1977; 273:515-532.
33. Nishi K, Eyzaguirre C. The action of some cholinergic blockers on carotid body chemoreceptors in vivo. Brain Res 1971; 33:37-56.
34. Pokorski M, Lahiri S. Presynaptic neurotransmitter and chemosensory responses to natural stimuli. J Appl Physiol 1984; 56:447-453.
35. Heymans C, Bouckaert JJ, Dautrebande L. Sinus carotidien et réflexes respiratoires; sensibilité des sinus carotidiens aux substances chimiques. Action stimulante respiratoire réflexe du sulfure de sodium, du cyanure de potassium, de la nicotine et de la lobéline. Arch Intl Pharmacodyn Thér 1931; 40:54-91.
36. Euler US von, Liljestrand G, Zotterman Y. The excitation mechanism of the chemoreceptors of the carotid body. Skand Arch Physiol 1939; 83:132-152.
37. Zapata P, Zuazo A, Llados F. Respiratory and circulatory reflexes induced by nicotine injections: role of carotid body chemoreceptors. Arch Intl Pharmacodyn Thér 1976; 219:128-139.
38. Zapata P, Zuazo A, Llados F. Acute changes in ventilation and blood pressure induced by inhalation of tobacco smoke. Arch Intl Pharmacodyn Thér 1976; 219:116-127.
39. Main RJ. Acute effects of smoking on respiration and circulation. Proc Soc Exp Biol Med 1941; 48:495-500.
40. Yamamoto H, Inaba S, Nishiura Y, et al. Acute inhalation of cigarette smoke augments hypoxic chemosensitivity in humans. J Appl Physiol 1985; 58:717-723.
41. McQueen DS. Effects of suberyldicholine on carotid baroreceptors and chemoreceptors. Neuropharmacology 1974;13: 829-835.
42. Nishi K, Iwasaki K, Kase Y. Actions of piperidine and dimethyl-phenyl-piperazinium (DMPP) on afferent discharge of the cat's carotid body. Eur J Pharmacol 1979; 54:141-152.
43. Gernandt B, Zotterman Y. The effect of some drugs on the chemoreceptive fibre activity in the carotid sinus nerve. Acta Physiol Scand 1945; 9:362-366.
44. Philippot E. Action respiratoire et circulatoire reflexes de quelques derivés de la choline. Arch Intl Pharmacodyn Thér 1937; 57:357-368.
45. McQueen DS Effects of methacholine on the carotid chemoreceptors. Quart J Exp Physiol 1978; 63:171-178.
46. Sampson SR, Aminoff MJ, Jaffe RA, Vidruk EH. A pharmacological analysis of neurally induced inhibition of carotid body chemoreceptor activity in cats. J Pharmacol Exp Ther 1976; 197:119-125.
47. Eyzaguirre C, Zapata P. A discussion of possible transmitter or generator substances in carotid body chemoreceptors. In: Torrance RW, ed: Arterial Chemoreceptors. Oxford: Blackwell. 1968: 213-251.
48. Zapata P. Arterial chemoreceptors: searching for transmitter and modulator substances. In: S Kalsner, ed: Trends in Autonomic Pharmacology. vol. 2. Baltimore, MD: Urban & Schwarzenberg. 1982:343-361.
49. Sampson SR. Effects of mecamylamine on responses of carotid body chemoreceptors in vivo to physiological and phar-

macological stimuli. J Physiol, London 1971; 212:655-666.
50. Bisgard GE, Mitchell RA, Herbert DA. Effects of dopamine, norepinephrine, and 5-hydroxytryptamine on the carotid body of the dog. Respir Physiol 1979; 37:61-80.
51. Moe Gk, Capo LR, Peralta B. Action of tetraethylammonium on chemoreceptor and stretch receptor mechanisms. Am J Physiol 1948; 153:601-605.
52. Douglas WW. The effect of a ganglionic-blocking drug, hexamethonium, on the response of the cat's carotid body to various stimuli. J Physiol, London 1952; 118:373-383.
53. McQueen DS. Effects of dihydro-b-erythroidine on the cat carotid chemoreceptors. Quart J Exp Physiol 1980; 65:229-237.
54. Mulligan E, Lahiri S. Cat carotid body chemoreceptor responses before and after nicotine receptor blockade with α-bungarotoxin. J Auton Nerv Syst 1987; 18:25-31.
55. Eyzaguirre C, Lewin J. Chemoreceptor activity of the carotid body of the cat. J Physiol, London 1961; 159:222-237.
56. Iturriaga R, Larrain C, Zapata P. Phrenic nerve activity during artificial ventilation at different body temperatures and its relationships with carotid chemosensory activity. Biol Res 1994; 27:145-157.
57. Granit R, Skoglund S, Thesleff S. Activation of muscle spindles by succinylcholine and decamethonium. The effects of curare. Acta Physiol Scand 1953; 28:134-151.
58. Fitzgerald RS, Shirahata M. Acetylcholine and carotid body excitation during hypoxia in the cat. J Appl Physiol 1994; 76:1566-1574.
59. Flandrois R, Favier R, Pequignot JM. Role of adrenaline in gas exchanges and respiratory control in the dog at rest and exercise. Respir Physiol 1977; 30:291-303.
60. Whelan RF, Young MI. The effect of adrenaline and noradrenaline infusion on respiration in man. Br J Pharmacol Chemother 1953; 8:98-102.
61. Yasuhara H, Nakayama S, Mayahara T. Depressed respiration induced by intravenously administered dopamine in anesthetized dogs. Jap J Pharmacol 1980; 30:251-255.
62. Joels N, White H. The contribution of the arterial chemoreceptors to the stimulation of respiration by adrenaline and noradrenaline in the cat. J Physiol, London 1968; 197:1-23.
63. Young MI. Some observations on the mechanism of adrenaline hyperpnea. J Physiol, London 1957; 137:374-395.
64. Zapata P, Hess A, Bliss EL, Eyzaguirre C. Chemical, electron microscopic and physiological observations on the role of catecholamines in the carotid body. Brain Res 1969; 14:473-496.
65. Matsumoto S, Ibi A, Nagao T, Nakajima T. Effects of carotid body chemoreceptor stimulation by norepinephrine, epinephrine and tyramine on ventilation in the rabbit. Arch Intl Pharmacodyn Thér 1981; 252:152-161.
66. Wang Z-Z, Stensaas LJ, Dinger B, Fidone SJ Coexistence of tyrosine hydroxylase and dopamine β-hydroxylase immunoreactivity in glomus cells of the cat carotid body. J Auton Nerv Syst 1991; 32: 259-264.
67. O'Regan RG. Responses of carotid body chemosensory activity and blood flow to stimulation of sympathetic nerves in the cat. J Physiol, London 1981; 315:81-88.
68. Prabhakar NR, Kou Y-R, Cragg PA, Cherniack NS. Effects of arterial chemoreceptor stimulation: role of norepinephrine in hypoxic chemotransmission. Adv Exp Med Biol 1993; 337:301-306.
69. Cunningham DJC, Hey EN, Patrick JM, Lloyd BB. The effect of noradrenaline infusion on the relation between pulmonary ventilation and the alveolar PO_2 and PCO_2. Ann NY Acad Sci 1963; 109: 756-771.
70. Heistad DD, Wheeler RC, Mark AL Schmid PG, Abboud FM. Effects of adrenergic stimulation on ventilation in man. J Clin Invest 1972; 51:1469-1475.
71. Eclache JP, Favier R, Flandrois R. Commande chémoréflexe de la ventilation et stimulus nor-adrénaline chez l'homme. Arch Intl Physiol Biochim 1979; 87: 969-979.
72. Zapata P, Zuazo A. Respiratory effects of dopamine-induced inhibition of chemosensory inflow. Respir Physiol 1980; 40:79-92.

73. Milsom WK, Sadig T. Interaction between norepinephrine and hypoxia on carotid body chemoreception in rabbits. J Appl Physiol 1983; 55:1893-1898.
74. Llados F, Zapata P. Effects of adrenoceptor stimulating and blocking agents on carotid body chemosensory inhibition. J Physiol, London 1978b; 274: 501-509.
75. Neil E, Joels N. The carotid glomus sensory mechanism. In: Cunningham DJC, Lloyd BB, eds. The Regulation of Human Respiration. Oxford: Blackwell. 1963; 163-171.
76. Zapata P. Effects of dopamine on carotid chemo- and baroreceptors in vitro. J Physiol, London 1975; 244:235-251.
77. Folgering H, Ponte J, Sadig T. Adrenergic mechanisms and chemoreception in the carotid body of the cat and rabbit. J Physiol, London 1982; 325:1-21.
78. Bisgard G, Warner M, Pizarro J, Niu W, Mitchell G. Noradrenergic inhibition of the goat carotid body. Adv Exp Med Biol 1993; 337:259-263.
79. Cobbold AF, Ginsburg J, Paton A. Circulatory, respiratory and metabolic responses to isopropylnoradrenaline in man. J Physiol, London 1960; 151: 539-550.
80. Keltz H, Samortin T, Stone DJ. Hyperventilation: a manifestation of exogenous β-adrenergic stimulation. Am Rev Respir Dis 1972; 105:637-640.
81. Eldridge FL, Gill-Kumar P. Mechanisms of hyperpnea induced by isoproterenol. Respir Physiol 1980; 40:349-363.
82. Wasserman K, Mitchell RA, Berger AJ, Casaburi R, Davis JA. Mechanisms of isoproterenol hyperpnea in the cat. Respir Physiol 1979;38:359-376.
83. Winn R, Hildebrandt JR, Hildebrandt J. Cardiorespiratory responses following isoproterenol injection in rabbits. J Appl Physiol 1979; 47:352-359.
84. Lahiri S, Pokorski M, Davies RO. Augmentation of carotid body chemoreceptor responses by isoproterenol in the cat. Respir Physiol 1981; 44:351-364.
85. Gonsalves SF, Smith EJ, Nolan WF, Dutton RE. β-Adrenoceptor blockade spares chemoreceptor responsiveness to hypoxia. Brain Res 1984; 324:349-353.
86. Heymans C, De Schaepdryver A, De Vleeschhouwer G. Catecholamines and chemoreceptors. In: Torrance RW, ed. Arterial Chemoreceptors. Oxford: Blackwell. 1968:263-266.
87. Biscoe TJ. Some effects of drugs on the isolated superfused carotid body. Nature, London 1965; 208:294-295.
88. Black AMS, Comroe JH Jr, Jacobs L. Species difference in carotid body response of cat and dog to dopamine and serotonin. Am J Physiol 1972; 223: 1097-1102.
89. Jacobs L, Comroe JH Jr. Stimulation of the carotid body chemoreceptors of the dog by dopamine. Proc Natl Acad Sci USA 1968; 59:1187-1193.
90. Okajima Y, Nishi K. Analysis of inhibitory and excitatory actions of dopamine on chemoreceptor discharges of carotid body of cat in vivo. Jap J Physiol 1981; 31:695-704.
91. Silva-Carvalho L, Silva-Carvalho J, Moniz De Bettencourt J. Les réflexes carotidiens déclenchés par la dopamine et leurs modifications par la phentolamine et le sulpiride. C R Soc Biol, Paris 1983; 177:708-711.
92. Matsumoto S, Nagao T, Ibi A, Nakajima T. Effects of carotid body chemoreceptor stimulation by dopamine on ventilation. Arch Intl Pharmacodyn Thér 1980a; 245:145-155.
93. Cardenas H, Zapata P. Dopamine induced ventilatory depression in the rat, mediated by carotid nerve afferents. Neurosci Lett 1981; 24:29-33.
94. Bisgard GE, Forster HV, Klein JP, Manohar M, Bullard VA. Depression of ventilation by dopamine in goats-effects of carotid body excision. Respir Physiol 1980;41:379-392.
95. Mayock DE, Standaert TA, Guthrie RD, Woodrum DE. Dopamine and carotid body function in the newborn lamb. J Appl Physiol 1983; 54:814-820.
96. Welsh MJ, Heistad DD, Abboud FM. Depression of ventilation by dopamine in man. Evidence for an effect on the chemoreceptor reflex. J Clin Invest 1978; 61:708-713.
97. Bainbridge CW, Heistad DD. Effect of haloperidol on ventilatory responses to

dopamine in man. J Pharmacol Exp Ther 1980; 213:13-17.
98. Olson LG, Hensley MJ, Saunders NA. Ventilatory responsiveness to hypercapnic hypoxia during dopamine infusion in humans. Am Rev Respir Dis 1982a; 126:783-787.
99. Sabol SJ, Ward DS. Effect of dopamine on hypoxic-hypercapnic interaction in humans. Anesth Analg 1987; 66:619-624.
100. Ward DS, Belville JW. Reduction of hypoxic ventilatory drive by dopamine. Anesth Analg 1982; 61:333-337.
101. Ward DS. Stimulation of hypoxic ventilatory drive by droperidol. Anesth Analg 1984; 63:106-110.
102. Ward DS, Belville JW. Effect of intravenous dopamine on hypercapnic ventilatory response in humans. J Appl Physiol 1983; 55:1418-1425.
103. Docherty RJ, McQueen DS. Inhibitory action of dopamine on cat carotid chemoreceptors. J Physiol, London 1978b; 279:425-436.
104. Lahiri S, Nishino T, Mokashi A, Mulligan E. Interaction of dopamine and haloperidol with O_2 and CO_2 chemoreception in carotid body. J Appl Physiol 1980; 49:45-51.
105. Llados F, Zapata P Effects of dopamine analogues and antagonists on carotid body chemosensors in situ. J Physiol, London 1978; 274:487-499.
106. Nishi K. A pharmacologic study on a possible inhibitory role of dopamine in the cat carotid body chemoreceptor. In: Acker H, Fidone S, Pallot D, Eyzaguirre C, Lübbers DW, Torrance RW, eds. Chemoreception in the Carotid Body. Berlin: Springer-Verlag. 1977:145-151.
107. Sampson SR, Aminoff MJ, Jaffe RA, Vidruk EH. Analysis of inhibitory effect of dopamine on carotid body chemoreceptors in cats. Am J Physiol 1976; 230:1494-1498.
108. Tomares SM, Bamford OS, Sterni LM, Fitzgerald RS, Carroll JL. The role of endogenous dopamine as an inhibitory neuromodulator in neonatal and adult carotid bodies. Adv Exp Med Biol 1994; 360:321-323.
109. Zapata P. Modulatory role of dopamine on arterial chemoreceptors. Adv Biochem Psychopharmacol 1977; 16:291-298.
110. Sampson SR, Vidruk EH. Hyperpolarizing effects of dopamine on chemoreceptor nerve endings from cat and rabbit carotid bodies in vitro. J Physiol, London 1977; 268:211-221.
111. Goldman WF, Eyzaguirre C. The effect of dopamine on glomus cell membranes in the rabbit. Brain Res 1984; 321: 337-340.
112. Mir AK, McQueen DS, Pallot DJ, Nahorski SR. Direct biochemical and neuropharmacological identification of dopamine D_2-receptors in the rabbit carotid body. Brain Res 1984; 291:273-283.
113. Leitner L-M, Roumy M. Effects of dopamine superfusion on the activity of rabbit carotid chemoreceptors in vitro. Neuroscience 1985; 16:431-438.
114. Cardenas H, Zapata P. Dual effects of dopamine upon chemosensory responses to cyanide. Neurosci Lett 1980; 18: 317-322.
115. Zapata P, Larrain C. Antagonism of dopamine-induced chemosensory inhibition by ergot alkaloids. Neurosci Lett 1978; 8:131-136.
116. Goldstein M, Lew JY, Nakamura S, Battista AP, Lieberman A, Fuxe K. Dopaminophilic properties of ergot alkaloids. Fed Proc 1978; 37:2202-2206.
117. Zuazo A, Zapata P Effects of 6-hydroxy-dopamine on carotid body chemosensory activity. Neurosci Lett 1978; 9:323-328.
118. Leitner L-M, Roumy M, Verna A. In vitro recording of chemoreceptor activity in catecholamine-depleted rabbit carotid bodies. Neuroscience 1983; 10: 883-891.
119. Leitner L-M, Roumy M. Chemoreceptor response to hypoxia and hypercapnia in catecholamine depleted rabbit and cat carotid bodies in vitro. Pflügers Arch 1986; 406:419-423.
120. Aminoff MJ, Jaffe RA, Sampson SR, Vidruk EH. Effects of droperidol on activity of carotid body chemoreceptors in cat. Br J Pharmacol 1978; 63:245-250.
121. Zapata P, Llados F. Blockade of carotid body chemosensory inhibition. In: Acker H, Fidone S, Pallot D, Eyzaguirre C, Lübbers DW, Torrance RW, eds. Chemoreception in the Carotid Body. Berlin: Springer-Verlag. 1977:152-159.

122. Mitchell RA, McDonald DM. Adjustment of chemoreceptor sensitivity in the cat carotid body by reciprocal synapses. In: MJ Purves, ed. The Peripheral Arterial Chemoreceptors. London: Cambridge Univ Press 1975:269-291.
123. Zapata P, Serani A, Lavados M. Inhibition in carotid body chemoreceptors mediated by D-2 dopaminoceptors: antagonism by benzamides. Neurosci Lett 1983; 42:179-184.
124. Zapata P, Torrealba F. Blockade of dopamine-induced chemosensory inhibition by domperidone. Neurosci Lett 1984; 51:359-364.
125. Zapata P, Torrealba F. Interference by domperidone on chemosensory and ventilatory responses to dopamine. In: Ribeiro JA, Pallot DJ, eds. Chemoreceptors in Respiratory Control. London: Croom Helm 1987:322-333.
126. Iturriaga R, Larrain C, Zapata P. Effects of dopaminergic blockade upon carotid chemosensory activity and its hypoxia-induced excitation. Brain Res 1994; 663:145-154.
127. McQueen DS, Mir AK, Brash HM, Nahorski SR. Increased sensitivity of rabbit carotid body chemoreceptors to dopamine after chronic treatment with domperidone. Eur J Pharmacol 1984; 104: 39-46.
128. Lahiri S, Nishino T. Inhibitory and excitatory effects of dopamine on carotid chemoreceptors. Neurosci Lett 1980; 20:313-318.
129. Cools AR, VAN Rossum JM. Excitation-mediating and inhibition-mediating dopamine-receptors: a new concept towards a better understanding of electrophysiological, biochemical, pharmacological, functional and clinical data. Psychopharmacologia 1976; 45:243-254.
130. Joels N, Neil E. The idea of a sensory transmitter. In: Torrance RW, ed. Arterial Chemoreceptors. Oxford: Blackwell. 1968:153-178.
131. Landgren S, Liljestrand G, Zotterman Y. Impulse activity in the carotid sinus nerve following intracarotid injections of sodium iodo-acetate, histamine hydrochloride, lergitin, and some purine and barbituric acid derivatives. Acta Physiol Scand 1954; 30:149-160.
132. Zapata P, Zuazo A. Reversal of respiratory responses to dopamine after dopamine antagonists. Respir Physiol 1982; 47:239-255.
133. Donnelly DF, Smith EJ, Dutton RE. Neural response of carotid chemoreceptors following dopamine blockade. J Appl Physiol 1981; 50:172-177.
134. Chow CM, Winder C, Read DJC. Influence of endogenous dopamine on carotid body discharge and ventilation. J Appl Physiol 1986; 60:370-375.
135. Tomares SM, Bamford OS, Sterni LM, Fitzgerald RS, Carroll JL. Effects of domperidone on neonatal and adult carotid chemoreceptors in the cat. J Appl Physiol 1994; 77:1274-1280.
136. Lahiri S, Hsiao C, Zhang R, Mokashi A, Nishino T. Peripheral chemoreceptors in respiratory oscillations. J Appl Physiol 1985; 58:1901-1908.
137. Nolan WF, Donnelly DF, Smith EJ, Dutton RE. Haloperidol-induced suppression of carotid chemoreception in vitro. J Appl Physiol 1985; 59:814-820.
138. Donnelly DF, Nolan WF, Smith EJ, Dutton RE. Effect of dopamine antagonism on carotid chemoreceptor interspike intervals. Brain Res 1987; 407: 195-198.
139. Bühler HU, Da Prada M, Haefely W, Picotti GB. Plasma adrenaline, noradrenaline and dopamine in man and different animal species. J Physiol, London 1978; 276:311-320.
140. VAN Loon GR, Schwartz L, Sole MJ. Plasma dopamine responses to standing and exercise in man. Life Sci 1979; 24:2273-2278.
141. Matsumoto S, Nishimura Y, Kohno M, Nakajima T. Effects of haloperidol on chemoreceptor reflex ventilatory response in the rabbit. Arch Intl Pharmacodyn Thér 1980; 247:234-242.
142. Olson LG, Saunders NA. Structure and function of the carotid body. Austr N Z J Med 1985; 15:775-781.
143. Olson LG, Hensley MJ, Saunders NA. Augmentation of ventilatory response to asphyxia by prochlorperazine in humans. J Appl Physiol 1982; 53:637-643.
144. Lagneaux D, Lecomte J. Dopamine et chémorégulation de la ventilation chez le rat. Arch Intl Physiol Biochim 1984; 92:263-265.

145. Steele RH, Hinterberger H. Catecholamines and 5-hydroxytryptamine in the carotid body in vascular, respiratory, and other diseases. J Lab Clin Med 1972; 80:63-70.
146. Chiocchio SR, Biscardi AM, Tramezzni JH. 5-Hydroxytryptamine in the carotid body of the cat. Science 1967; 158: 790-791.
147. Hellström S. Putative neurotransmitters in the carotid body. Mass fragmentographic studies. Adv Biochem Psychopharmacol 1977; 16:257-263.
148. Sapru HN, Krieger AJ. Effects of 5-hydroxtryptamine on the peripheral chemoreceptors in the rat. Res Commun Chem Pathol Pharmacol 1977; 16: 245-250.
149. Sampson SR, Jaffe RA. Excitatory effects of 5-hydroxytryptamine, veratridine and phenyldiguanide on sensory ganglion cells of the nodose ganglion of the cat. Life Sci 1974; 15:2157-2165.
150. Yoshioka M, Matsumoto M, Togashi H, Abe M, Tochihara M, Saito H. The 5-hydroxytryptamine-induced increase in chemoreceptor afferent nerve discharge and its blockade by ICS 205-930 in the rat. Res Commun Psychol Psychiat Behav 1987; 12:215-220.
151. Nishi K. The action of 5-hydroxytryptamine on chemoreceptor discharges of the cat's carotid body. Br J Pharmacol 1975; 55:27-40.
152. Kirby GC, McQueen DS. Effects of the antagonists MDL 72222 and ketanserin on responses of cat carotid body chemoreceptors to 5-hydroxytryptamine. Br J Pharmacol 1984; 83:259-269.
153. Jarisch A, Landgren S, Neil E, Zotterman Y. Impulse activity in the carotid sinus nerve following intracarotid injection of potassium chloride, veratrine, sodium citrate, adenosine-triphosphate and α-dinitrophenol. Acta Physiol Scand 1952; 25:195-211.
154. Krylov SS, Anichkov SV. The effect of metabolic inhibitors on carotid chemoreceptors. In: Torrance RW, ed. Arterial Chemoreceptors. Oxford: Blackwell. 1968:103-113.
155. Spergel D, Lahiri S. Differential modulation by extracellular ATP of carotid chemosensory response. J Appl Physiol 1993; 74:3052-3056.
156. Bock P. Adenine nucleotides in the carotid body. Cell Tiss Res 1980; 206: 279-290.
157. Bock P. Histochemical demonstration of adenine nucleotides in carotid body type I cells. Adv Biochem Psychopharmacol 1980; 25:235-239.
158. Berne RM. The role of adenosine in the regulation of coronary blood flow. Circ Res 1980; 47:807-813.
159. McQueen DS, Ribeiro JA. Effect of adenosine on carotid chemoreceptor activity in the cat. Br J Pharmacol 1981; 74:129-136.
160. McQueen DS, Ribeiro JA. On the specificity and type of receptor involved in carotid body chemoreceptor activation by adenosine in the cat. Br J Pharmacol 1983; 80:347-354.
161. Runold M, Cherniack NS, Prabhakar NR. Effect of adenosine on isolated and superfused cat carotid body activity. Neurosci Lett 1990; 113:111-114.
162. Monteiro EC, Ribeiro JA. Ventilatory effects of adenosine mediated by carotid body chemoreceptors in the rat. Naunyn-Schmiedeberg's Arch Pharmacol 1987; 335:143-148.
163. Watt AH, Routledge PA. Adenosine stimulates respiration in man. Br J Clin Pharmacol 1985; 20:503-506.
164. Watt AH, Reid PG, Stephens MR, Routledge PA. Adenosine-induced respiratory stimulation in man depends on site of infusion. Evidence for an action on the carotid body? Br J Clin Pharmacol 1987; 23:486-490.
165. Monteiro EC, Ribeiro JA. Adenosine deaminase and adenosine uptake inhibitions facilitate ventilation in rats. Naunyn-Schmieberg's Arch Pharmacol 1989; 340:230-238.
166. McQueen DS. Does adenosine stimulate rat carotid body chemoreceptors? Adv Exp Med Biol 1993; 337:289-293.
167. McQueen DS, Ribeiro JA. Pharmacological characterization of the receptor involved in chemoexcitation induced by adenosine. Br J Pharmacol 1986; 88: 615-620.

168. Burr D, Sinclair JD. The effect of adenosine on respiratory chemosensitivity in the awake rat. Respir Physiol 1988; 72:47-58.
169. Olsson RA, Pearson JD. Cardiovascular purinoceptors. Physiol Rev 1990; 70: 761-845.
170. McQueen DS, Belmonte C. The effects of prostaglandins E_2, A_2 and $F_{2\alpha}$ on carotid baroreceptors and chemoreceptors. Quart J Exp Physiol 1974; 59:63-71.
171. McQueen DS, Ritchie IM, Birrell GJ. Arterial chemoreceptor involvement in salicylate-induced hyperventilation in rats. Br J Pharmacol 1989; 98:413-424.
172. Riley DJ, Legawiec BA, Santiago TV, Edelman NH. Ventilatory responses to hypercapnia and hypoxia during continuous aspirin ingestion. J Appl Physiol 1977; 43:971-976.
173. Lundberg JM, Hökfelt T, Fahrenkrug J, Nilsson G, Terenius L. Peptides in the cat carotid body (glomus caroticum): VIP-, enkephalin-, and substance P-like immunoreactivity. Acta Physiol Scand 1979; 107:279-281.
174. Wharton J, Polak JM, Pearse AGE, et al. Enkephalin-, VIP- and substance P-like immunoreactivity in the carotid body. Nature 1980; 284:269-271.
175. Chen IV, Yates RD, Hansen JT. Substance P-like immunoreactivity in rat and cat carotid bodies: Light and electron microscopic studies. Histol Histopathol 1986; 1:203-212.
176. Prabhakar NR, Landis SC, Kumar GK, Mullikin-Kilpatrick D, Cherniack NS, Leeman S. Substance P and neurokinin A in the cat carotid body: Localization, exogenous effects and changes in content in response to arterial PO_2. Brain Res 1989; 481:205-214.
177. Hanson G, Jones L, Fidone S. Physiological chemoreceptor stimulation decreases enkephalin and substance P in the carotid body. Peptides 1986; 7:767-769.
178. Eyzaguirre C, Monti-Bloch L, Woodbury JW. Effects of putative transmitters of the carotid body on its own glomus cells. Eur J Neurosci 1990; 2:77-88.
179. McQueen DS. Effects of substance P on carotid chemoreceptor activity in the cat. J Physiol, London 1980b; 302:31-47.
180. Prabhakar NR, Mitra J, Cherniack NS. Role of substance P in hypercapnic excitation of carotid chemoreceptors. J Appl Physiol 1987; 63:2418-2425.
181. Monti-Bloch L, Eyzaguirre C. Effects of methionine-enkephalin and substance P on the chemosensory discharge of the cat carotid body. Brain Res 1985; 338: 297-307.
182. Cragg PA, Runold M, Kou YR, Prabhakar NR. Tachykinin antagonists in carotid body responses to hypoxia and substance P in the rat. Respir Physiol 1994; 95:295-310.
183. Prabhakar NR, Kou YR, Runold M. Chemoreceptor responses to substance P, physalaemin and eledoisin: evidence for neurokinin-1 receptors in the cat carotid body. Neurosci Lett 1990; 120:183-186.
184. McQueen DS. Effects of some polypeptides on carotid chemoreceptor activity. In: Belmonte C, Pallot DJ, Acker H, Fidone S, eds. Arterial Chemoreceptors. Leicester: Leicester Univ Press. 1981: 299-308.
185. Prabhakar NR, Runold M, Yamamoto Y, Lagercrantz H, Von Euler C. Effect of substance P antagonist on the hypoxia-induced carotid chemoreceptor activity. Acta Physiol Scand 1984; 121:301-303.
186. Prabhakar NR, Cao H, Lowe JA III, Snider RM. Selective inhibition of the carotid body sensory response to hypoxia by the substance P receptor antagonist CP-96,345. Proc Natl Acad Sci USA 1993; 90:10041-10045.
187. McQueen DS, Ribeiro JA. Inhibitory actions of methionine-enkephalin and morphine on the cat carotid chemoreceptors. Br J Pharmacol 1980; 71: 297-305.
188. Pokorski M, Lahiri S. Effects of naloxone on carotid body chemoreception and ventilation in the cat. J Appl Physiol 1981; 51:1533-1538.
189. McQueen DS, Ribeiro JA. Comparison of the depressant effects of leucine- and methionine-enkephalin on spontaneous chemoreceptor activity in cats. Br J Pharmacol 1981; 72:544P-545P.
190. Kirby GC, McQueen DS. Characterization of opioid receptors in the cat carotid body involved in chemosensory depression in vivo. Br J Pharmacol 1986; 88: 889-898.

191. McQueen DS, Ribeiro JA. Effects of b-endorphin, vasoactive intestinal polypeptide and cholecystokinin octapeptide on cat carotid chemoreceptor activity. Quart J Exp Physiol 1981; 66:273-284.
192. Mauser PJ, Chapman RW. Role of endogenous opioids on ventilation and chemical control of breathing in pentobarbitone-anesthetized rats. Pharmacology 1987; 35:317-326.
193. Thomas CP, Simonson MS, Dunn MJ. Endothelin: receptors and transmembrane signals. News Physiol Sci 1992; 7:207-211.
194. Spyer KM, McQueen DS, Dashwood MR, Sykes RM, Daly M De B, Muddle JR. Localisation of [^{125}I]endothelin binding sites in the region of the carotid bifurcation and brainstem of the cat: possible baro- and chemoreceptor involvement. J Cardiovasc Pharmacol 1991;17(suppl 7): S385-S389.
195. McQueen DS, Dashwood MR, Cobb VJ, Marr CG. Effects of endothelins on respiration and arterial chemoreceptor activity in anaesthetized rats. Adv Exp Med Biol 1994; 360:289-291.
196. Said SI, Mutt V. Polypeptide with broad biological activity: isolation from small intestine. Science 1970; 169:1217-1218.
197. Fitzgerald R, Raff H, Garger P, Fechter L, Anand A, Said S. Vasoactive intestinal polypeptide (VIP) and the carotid body. In: Belmonte C, Pallot DJ, Acker H, Fidone S, eds. Arterial Chemoreceptors. Leicester: Leicester Univ Press. 1981; 289-298.
198. Kummer W. Three types of neurochemically defined autonomic fibres innervate the carotid baroreceptor and chemoreceptor regions in the Guinea-pig. Anat Embryol 1990; 181:477-489.
199. Kummer W, Addicks K, Henkel H, Heym C. Cholecystokinin-like immunoreactivity in cat extra-adrenal paraganglia. Neurosci Lett 1985; 55:207-210.
200. Wang YY, Perrin DG, Cutz E Localization of cholecystokinin-like and calcitonin-like peptides in infant carotid bodies: a light- and electron-microscopic immunohistochemical study. Cell Tiss Res 1993; 272:169-174.
201. Wang Z-Z, He L, Stensaas LJ, Dinger BG, Fidone SJ. Localization and in vitro actions of atrial natriuretic peptide in the cat carotid body. J Appl Physiol 1991a; 70:942-946.
202. Wang W-J, He L, Chen J, Dinger B, Fidone S Mechanisms underlying chemoreceptor inhibition induced by atrial natriuretic peptide in rabbit carotid body. J Physiol, London 1993; 460: 427-441.
203. Powell FL, Hempleman SC. The effect of somatostatin on carotid body neural activity. Physiologist 1985; 28:338[Abstract].
204. Hirsch K, Wang SC. Selective respiratory stimulating action of doxapram compared to pentylenetetrazol. J Pharmacol Exp Ther 1974; 189:1-11.
205. Lundberg DB, Breese GR, Mueller RA. Aminophylline may stimulate respiration in rats by activation of dopaminergic receptors. J Pharmacol Exp Ther 1981; 217:215-221.
206. Folgering H, Vis A, Ponte J. Ventilatory and circulatory effects of doxapram, mediated by carotid body chemoreceptors. Bull Eur Physiopath Respir 1981; 17: 237-241.
207. Sapru HN, Krieger AJ. Carotid and aortic chemoreceptor function in the rat. J Appl Physiol 1977; 42:344-348.
208. Mitchell RA, Herbert DA. Potencies of doxapram and hypoxia in stimulating carotid-body chemoreceptors and ventilation in anesthetized cats. Anesthesiology 1975; 42:559-566.
209. Nishino T, Mokashi A, Lahiri S. Stimulation of carotid chemoreceptors and ventilation by doxapram in the cat. J Appl Physiol 1982; 52:1261-1265.
210. Bairam A, Marchal F, Hannhart B, Crance J-P, Lahiri S. Carotid chemosensory response to doxapram in the newborn kitten. Adv Exp Med Biol 1993; 337:381-385.
211. Peers C. Effects of doxapram in ionic currents recorded in type I cells of the neonatal rat carotid body. Brain Res 1991; 568:116-122.
212. Gautier H, Bonora M, Milic-Emili J, Siafakas NM. Effets de différents stimulants respiratoires sur la ventilation du chat éveillé. Bull Eur Physiopathol Respir 1979; 15:183-193.

213. Laubie M, Schmitt H. Long lasting hyperventilation induced by almitrine: evidence for a specific effect on carotid and thoracic chemoreceptors. Eur J Pharma 1980; 61:125-136.
214. Maskrey M. Changes in ventilation, breathing pattern and acid-base balance of conscious rabbits following intravenous almitrine. Aust J Exp Biol Med Sci 1986; 64:389-395.
215. Lagneaux D. Ventilatory responses to histotoxic chemostimulation in hypoxia adapted rats. Adv Exp Med Biol 1994; 360:265-267.
216. Roumy M, Leitner L-M. Stimulant effect of almitrine (S 2620) on the rabbit carotid chemoreceptor afferent activity. Bull Eur Physiopathol Respir 1981; 17: 255-259.
217. O'Regan RG, Majcherczyk S, Przybyszewski A. Effects of almitrine bismesylate on activities recorded from nerves supplying the carotid bifurcation in the cat. Eur J Respir Dis 1983; 64 (suppl 126):197-202.
218. Bisgard GE. The response of few-fiber carotid chemoreceptor preparations to almitrine in the dog. Can J Physiol Pharmacol 1981; 59:396-401.
219. McQueen DS, Evrard Y, Gordon BH, Campbell DB. Ganglioglomerular nerves influence responsiveness of cat carotid body chemoreceptors to almitrine. J Auton Nerv Syst 1989; 27:57-66.
220. Stanley NN, Galloway JM, Gordon B, Pauly N. Increased respiratory chemosensitivity induced by infusing almitrine intravenously in healthy man. Thorax 1983; 38:200-204.
221. Ponte J, Sadler CL. Effects of halothane, enflurane and isoflurane on carotid body chemoreceptor activity in the rabbit and the cat. Br J Anaesth 1989; 62:33-40.
222. Viana AP The role of carotid body chemoreceptors in the respiratory effects of digoxin. Arch Intl Pharmacodyn Thér 1974; 208: 94-101.
223. McQueen DS, Ribeiro JA. Effects of ouabain on carotid body chemoreceptor activity in the cat. J Physiol, London 1983; 335:221-235.

CHAPTER 8

Neurotransmitter Mediation of Carotid Chemoreceptor Efferent Inhibition

Laura Almaraz, Zuo-Zhong Wang, Bruce Dinger and Salvatore J. Fidone

INTRODUCTION

Neil and O'Regan,[1] and Fidone and Sato[2,3] were the first to establish that stimulation of the peripheral cut end of the carotid sinus nerve (CSN) inhibited chemoreceptor discharge recorded from single or few fiber filaments split off from the main nerve trunk (Fig. 8.1). Biscoe and Sampson[4] had earlier described spontaneous centrifugal neural activity in the central cut end of the CSN, so consequently it became generally accepted that the CSN contained an efferent inhibitory pathway, presumably of parasympathetic origin. However, McDonald and Mitchell later showed that this so-called "efferent" inhibition persisted 10 days after intracranial section of the glossopharyngeal and vagus nerves, together with removal of both the nodose and SCG;[5,6] these surgical procedures should collectively have eliminated all efferent neuronal projections to the carotid body. McDonald therefore considered that "efferent" inhibition might involve primary afferent depolarization (PAD) of sensory nerve terminals in the brainstem, with subsequent "backfiring" of these axons.[7] The consequent antidromic invasion of sensory nerve endings in the carotid body, together with reciprocal synapses between nerve endings and type I cells, would provide a logical basis for antidromic inhibition of the chemoresponse. It mostly escaped attention, however (but see refs. 8,9), that the extensive surgical denervations described above would not have eliminated a group of neurons, first described by de Castro in his 1926 treatise[10] but rarely cited in modern literature, which are found dispersed along the glossopharyngeal and CSN between the petrosal ganglion and carotid body.

Thus, while chemoreceptor inhibition via the CSN was well documented physiologically as a negative feedback to chemoreceptor drive, the identity of the inhibitory neurons remained

The Carotid Body Chemoreceptors,
edited by Constancio González.

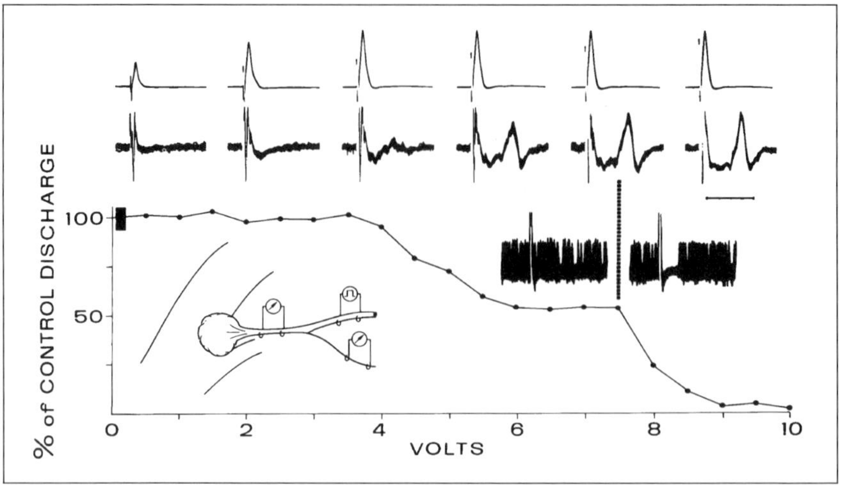

Fig. 8.1. Chemoreceptor inhibition by carotid nerve C-fibers. Effect of increasing voltage on spontaneous chemoreceptor activity during electrical stimulation of carotid nerve at 20/sec. Resting discharge of unit, 4/sec; each point on graph measured over 10 sec period of stimulation. Bar at left of graph represents semi-interquartile range for preceding twenty-five 10 sec measurement periods. At top of figure, multiple storage oscilloscope sweeps of compound action potential of carotid nerve C-fibers is shown for increasing stimulus voltages (from left to right, 0.5, 2.0, 4.0, 5.0, 7.0 and 9.0 V). Compound A-fiber potential reached maximal amplitude at about 3 V (not shown). Note parallel growth of inhibitory effect and compound C-fiber potential. Multiple sweeps of spontaneous activity obtained at 7.5 and 9.0 V. Time marker: 5.0 and 25.0 msec, respectively, for compound C-potential and multiple sweeps of spontaneous activity. (from ref. 3.)

an unsettled and hotly debated issue. Whether the inhibition derived from mechanisms directed at the type I cell/nerve ending complex or from changes in organ blood flow also remained controversial.[11] Virtually nothing was known regarding neurotransmitters which might mediate these inhibitory effects, and how they might interact with the plethora of putative sensory transmitters contained in type I cells.

This chapter reviews recent studies which have revealed neurons associated with the IXth cranial nerve, as well as cellular elements within the carotid body, which appear to participate in chemosensory "efferent" inhibition. In addition, some of the neurotransmitter and biochemical mechanisms possibly mediating this inhibitory phenomenon will be discussed. Specifically considered here are two agents recently described in the carotid body which we believe modulate chemoreceptor excitation: 1) a diffusible gas, nitric oxide (NO); 2) a hormone first described in the heart, called atrial natriuretic peptide (ANP). A third substance, dopamine (DA), the catecholamine contained in high concentrations in type I chemoreceptor cells and perhaps in CSN fibers as well, may also be involved in mediating this inhibitory effect.[12] More comprehensive and historically detailed treatments of the efferent control of carotid body activity, including influences conveyed by the sympathetic innervation of the organ, can be found elsewhere[13] (see also ref. 14).

NITRIC OXIDE AND EFFERENT CONTROL OF CAROTID CHEMORECEPTOR ACTIVITY

Known for decades as an air pollutant, nitric oxide (NO) has recently been shown to be a cellular messenger important for many bodily functions. Its activity as endothelium-derived relaxing factor (EDRF) helps maintain blood pressure,[15] while its role as a mediator for macrophage cytotoxicity is important for eliminating invading pathogens.[16] Additionally, NO is now recognized as a novel transmitter agent with an essential role in a diverse assortment of neural functions, including hippocampal long-term potentiation, cerebral signal transmission, and the nonadrenergic, noncholinergic (NANC) mediation of smooth muscle relaxation throughout the gastrointestinal tract and penis.[17,18] These various actions of NO appear to arise from its ability to activate soluble guanylate cyclase, thereby stimulating the production of cGMP in neurons and other cells receiving input from NO-synthesizing elements.[19]

Several earlier findings indicated that NO may participate in the receptor mechanisms of the mammalian carotid body. Previous neurochemical and immunocytochemical studies have shown that sodium nitroprusside, a well-known donor of NO, activates guanylate cyclase in the carotid body, leading to the production of cGMP.[20,21] Cyclic GMP has been found to be an important second messenger that potentially inhibits chemoreceptor discharge evoked by hypoxia.[22] These findings prompted immunocytochemical and histochemical studies designed to localize the synthetic enzyme for NO, nitric oxide synthase (NOS) in the carotid body, and in addition, to investigate the actions of endogenous NO using pharmacological and physiological techniques.

Immunocytochemical and histochemical experiments utilizing a rabbit anti-NOS IgG,[23,24] and the NADPH-diaphorase technique,[24-27] demonstrated an extensive plexus of NOS-positive fibers which penetrates the parenchyma of the cat and rat carotid body and innervates blood vessels and lobules of type I cells. The plexus consists of small caliber axons ($\leq$ 1 mm, presumably nonmyelinated), which branch to give rise to even thinner, sinuous processes with multiple, bead-like enlargements or varicosities. Some of these axons branch within the parenchymal cell lobules to encircle type I cells, while others can be observed in proximity to both large ($\approx$30-100 μm) and small ($\approx$10-30 μm) blood vessels, where they lie in association with the vascular adventitial layer. NOS immunoreactivity (NOS-IR) can occasionally be observed in endothelial cells lining the larger vessels, but is not seen in the sinusoidal capillaries surrounding the lobules.[25,28] Parenchymal type I cells, as well as sustentacular type II cells, fibroblasts and vascular smooth muscle cells were found to be devoid of NOS-IR.

High levels of NOS-IR were found in some large neurons ($\approx$15-30 μm) located near the connective tissue capsule at the periphery of the organ in both the cat and rat.[25,28] Similar neurons were also found dispersed along the CSN, and were particularly numerous near the CSN/glossopharyngeal nerve branch point. The somata of these neurons show short dendritic, tapering processes which resemble autonomic microganglial neurons, as first described by de Castro in 1926.[10] These neurons also display a single NOS-IR axon which projects towards the carotid body.

The majority of NOS-IR nerve fibers in the CSN arise from neurons concentrated in the proximal (central) part of the petrosal ganglion.[25] Unlike the strongly immunoreactive autonomic neurons described above, levels of NOS-IR in petrosal ganglial cells varied considerably.[25,28] The spectrum of immunoreactivity ranged from almost undetectable to extremely high levels. Most NOS-IR petrosal neurons were small cells (15-20 mm), lacking dendrites and having the smooth contour of sensory neurons. Such elements are absent, for example, from the superior cervical ganglion, where NOS-IR was found confined exclusively to preganglionic sympathetic axons (but see ref. 27). In addition, it has been shown recently[27] that NOS-positive fibers of the CSN terminate in the nucleus tractus solitarius (commissural nucleus) where they might contribute to the maintenance of hypoxia-induced increase in respiratory output.[29]

In addition to these immunocytochemical data, biochemical studies confirmed the presence of NOS activity in the carotid body, by showing that rat and cat carotid bodies incubated in the NO precursor, ^{3}H-arginine, produced ^{3}H-citrulline, the byproduct of NO synthesis.[25,28] Likewise, superfusion of cat carotid bodies in vitro in the presence of L-arginine inhibited the chemoreceptor response (recorded from CSN) evoked by superfusion media equilibrated with low O_2. This inhibition was marked by a delay in the elevation of nerve activity, and by a reduction in both the peak and sustained nerve discharges.[28] This inhibition of stimulus-evoked CSN activity by L-arginine was dose-dependent, and preparations bathed in basic amino acids which are not NOS substrates (e.g., D-arginine [1 mM] and L-lysine [1 mM]) displayed only normal responses to low O_2 stimuli[28] (see also ref. 24). Furthermore, the inhibitory effects of L-arginine were completely reversed by the competitive NOS inhibitor, L-N^G-nitroarginine methylester (L-NAME, 1 mM), suggesting that the inhibition is NOS/NO related, and not due to nonspecific metabolic effects. NO donors, such as nitroglycerine and sodium nitroprusside (SNP), likewise inhibited evoked CSN activity,[28,30] and immunocytochemical studies with nitroglycerine demonstrated elevated levels of cGMP in lobules of type I cells and in vascular smooth muscle.[28]

Additional experiments demonstrated that L-NAME alone, even at relatively low concentrations (0.01 mM), augmented the chemosensory response to moderate low O_2 stimuli (40% O_2-equilibrated media; 5 min[28]). This excitatory effect was dose-related and could be reversed by simultaneous administration of excess L-arginine (1 mM). Basal chemoreceptor discharge in 100% O_2 equilibrated superfusion media was slightly enhanced by L-NAME at concentrations up to 1 mM,[28] and longer exposures to L-NAME or a related inhibitor, N^G-monomethyl-L-arginine acetate (L-NMMA), resulted in a gradual sustained increase in nerve activity which was incompletely reversed by low concentrations of L-arginine (50-500 μM;[30]). These experiments suggested that NO may be an endogenous neuroactive agent which tonically inhibits the chemoreceptor response to hypoxia. An interesting aspect of the action of L-NAME is that its ability to enhance basal activity is greatly augmented in preparations which are simultaneously perfused and superfused,[28] suggesting that NO released in proximity to vascular elements leads to vasodilation and increased blood flow to the chemoreceptor apparatus, resulting in inhibition of the chemoreceptor discharge.

The possibility that NOS mediates efferent chemosensory inhibition was further studied in experiments which examined ^{3}H-citrulline production during electrical stimulation of the CSN in superfused carotid body preparations.[31] The results demonstrated that NO production is elevated 2-fold by a 15 min period of electrical stimulation of the CSN (5 V, 1 msec, 20 Hz). Monitoring the stimulus-evoked compound action potentials from the CSN confirmed that this increased NO production occurred only with activation of CSN C-fibers; activation of A-fibers alone failed to alter ^{3}H-citrulline formation. Finally, C-fiber activation in the absence of Ca^{2+} also failed to elevate ^{3}H-citrulline production, a finding consistent with the known Ca^{2+} dependency of the neuronal form of the NOS enzyme.[19]

Experiments designed to assess the role of NO in mediating chemosensory inhibition again utilized the perfused/superfused preparation.[31] At first, it was found that a low O_2 stimulus delivered simultaneously with electrical stimulation of the CSN trunk did not diminish the hypoxic response. However, if CSN stimulation was begun 5-10 min before delivering the low O_2 stimulus, both the basal chemoreceptor discharge and the hypoxic response were significantly attenuated. It could be shown that the magnitude of the integrated response to the low O_2 stimulus was inversely proportional to the length of the preceding period of CSN stimulation. Furthermore, moderate concentrations (0.1 mM) of the NOS antagonist, L-NAME, completely reversed the inhibitory effects of CSN stimulation. Similar experiments involving only superfusion of the carotid body (no simultaneous perfusion) revealed that prolonged electrical stimulation of the CSN inhibited the low O_2-evoked response without modifying basal chemoreceptor discharge. These findings suggest that basal chemoreceptor activity measured in perfused/superfused preparations is primarily influenced by flow through the organ's vasculature, while the low O_2-evoked response is controlled by NOS-IR afferent fiber innervation of the type I cell lobules, and probably also by the vasculature mechanism of NO action.

Parallel studies assessed changes in carotid body cGMP levels evoked by electrical stimulation of the CSN.[31] Immunocytochemical data demonstrated that brief (1 min) periods of CSN stimulation enhanced cGMP staining primarily in smooth muscle cells surrounding arterioles, while prolonged nerve stimulation (10 or 15 min) elevated cGMP levels in type I cells as well. These findings correlate well with the inhibition of basal and low O_2-evoked chemoreceptor activity observed with nerve stimulation. Furthermore, the changes in cGMP levels evoked by CSN stimulation could be prevented by the addition of 0.1 mM L-NAME to the bathing media. Finally, these effects of L-NAME could be reversed by competing concentrations of L-arginine (1 mM), further confirming the involvement of NOS and NO in the chemosensory inhibition.[32]

The disposition of NOS and the plausible function of NO are summarized schematically in Figure 8.2. The available data are consistent with two functional roles for NO in the carotid body. First, NO appears to act as an anterograde transmitter released from the terminals of autonomic neurons located near vascular elements which control carotid body blood flow. Second, NO release resulting from antidromic activity invading sensory nerve terminals may depress the chemoreceptor nerve discharge via an elevation of cGMP in type I cells. It appears that the vasomotor neuronal pathway modulates the steady-state activity, while NOS containing sensory neurons inhibit the dynamic response to hypoxic stimuli.

ATRIAL NATRIURETIC PEPTIDE AS A MEDIATOR OF CHEMORECEPTOR INHIBITION

DeBold first described the correlative relationship between the incidence of distinct storage granules in atrial cardiocytes and body water/electrolyte balance.[33] In later studies, DeBold and colleagues[34] showed that the injection of atrial granular extracts initiated a rapid and extensive diuresis and natriuresis, and they identified the active substituent as the 29 amino acid peptide, atrial natriuretic peptide (ANP), which is released from the atria by distension or local hypoxia (see refs. 35,36). Receptors for ANP have been localized in the renal glomerular vasculature, suggesting that the circulating peptide directly modulates kidney function.[37] The unique physiologic role of ANP as a regulator of volume and electrolyte levels in the periphery led others to postulate parallel functions for this peptide in the central nervous system (CNS). In fact, studies have revealed the presence of ANP[38,39] and ANP receptors[40,41] in specific CNS sites associated with cardiovascular control. In addition, central administration of ANP was shown to decrease the release of arginine vasopressin (AVP) in dehydrated animals[42,43] and to decrease salt-water intake following salt deprivation. Thus, ANP appears to act globally at specific targets both in the CNS and periphery to initiate coordinated adjustments in response to changes in systemic hydration and electrolyte balance.

Although classical views do not attribute a role for the carotid body in water and solute metabolism, the earlier work of Eyzaguirre and his colleagues,[44] and a more recent review by Honig,[45] established a relationship between carotid body function and water and electrolyte balance. In addition, like NO, many of the effects of ANP in other tissues have been shown to be mediated by cGMP. Consequently, we undertook a series of multidisciplinary studies to determine whether ANP (via cGMP) might play a role in modulating chemoreceptor activity.

Immunocytochemical studies revealed ANP immunostaining in virtually all lobules

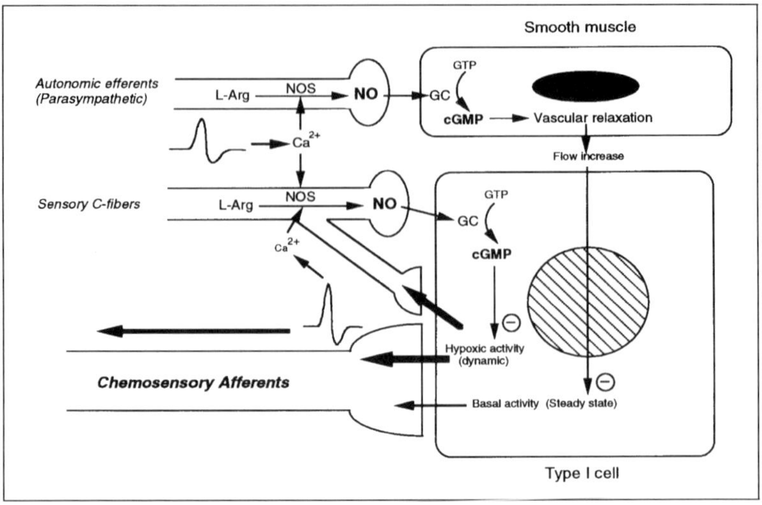

Fig. 8.2. Schematic diagram depicting the two NO-mediated efferent inhibitory neural pathways that control carotid body chemoreceptors. GC, guanylate cyclase. Chemosensory discharge generated in the afferent sensory A-fibers is influenced by two separate NO-synthesizing neural pathways. Centrifugal nerve activity activates NOS in nerve terminals in the carotid body via a Ca^{2+}-dependent mechanism. NO released from parasympathetic vasomotor fibers stimulates cGMP production in postsynaptic vascular smooth muscle and triggers vasodilation. The resultant flow increase attenuates the basal steady-state chemosensory activity. NO generated by axonal terminals of sensory C-fibers diffuses to adjacent type I cells and stimulates cGMP accumulation, which modulates the chemoreceptor response to hypoxia. Reproduced with permission from Wang et al.[31]

of type I cells of cat carotid body, where it was estimated that 80% of type I cells contained the natriuretic peptide.[46] Staining levels were relatively uniform amongst all identified type I cells, and appeared in the cells throughout the cytoplasm in accord with the known distribution of dense-cored vesicles. Later studies showed that incubation of cat and rat carotid bodies in submicromolar concentrations of the ANP analog, atriopeptin III (APIII), led to elevated levels of cGMP immunoreactivity in type I cells.[21,47] Moreover, cells with increased levels of cGMP were shown to contain ANP as well.[47] In parallel studies of rat and rabbit carotid bodies, radioimmunoassay techniques confirmed a dose-response relationship between the increase in tissue cGMP levels and the concentration of APIII in the incubation media.[22,47]

Correlative studies of the effects of APIII on CSN activity were first carried out in the in vitro superfused cat carotid body-CSN preparation,[46] and later more detailed studies utilized similar preparations obtained from rabbits.[22] Results in the cat chemoreceptor tissue showed that 1, 10 and 100 nM concentrations of APIII produced 26.17 ± 2.5% (X- ± SEM), 69.3 ± 1.3% and 86.1 ± 1.9% inhibition, respectively, of activity evoked by a moderate hypoxic stimulus (superfusion media equilibrated with 20% O_2). The presence of APIII did not alter basal CSN activity established in 100% O_2 media, but it delayed the onset and reduced the peak activity evoked by hypoxia. In rabbit preparations, it was shown that submicromolar concentrations of APIII inhibited activity evoked not only by hypoxia, but also by nicotine, a stimulus which is thought to act via receptors located on type I cells. In contrast, APIII did not alter CSN activity evoked by elevated levels of extracellular K^+ (20 mM), which purportedly causes direct nerve terminal depolarization even in the absence of extracellular Ca^{2+} (ref. 22). Additional data indicated that the effects of APIII may be mediated by specific ANP receptors because a modified version of the peptide, clearance-ANP (C-ANP), which in other tissues binds to a receptor not coupled to guanylate cyclase, did not affect either basal or evoked CSN activity.[22] In fact, preliminary immunocytochemical studies in our laboratory using an antibody directed against guanylate-cyclase-coupled-ANP receptors have revealed specific immunostaining in pig carotid body type I cells.[48]

Further electrophysiological experiments in the in vitro rabbit preparation revealed a role for cGMP in carotid body inhibition.[22] Cell permeant analogs of the cyclic nucleotide (dibutyryl-cGMP and 8-bromo-cGMP, 2 mM) inhibited CSN activity evoked by hypoxia or nicotine. As with APIII, basal CSN activity was not affected by the cGMP analogs. Similar concentrations of cGMP, which is nonpermeant, did not alter either basal or evoked chemoreceptor activity.

Other experiments in our laboratory have examined whether other neurotransmitters may also be involved in the ANP-mediated chemoreceptor inhibition. Our initial studies focused on a possible role for dopamine (DA), because this catecholamine has often been reported from pharmacological experiments to be inhibitory in the carotid body, although there remains a great deal of uncertainty with respect to physiological action of DA in the carotid body (see refs. 49,50). It is known that large amounts of DA are released from type I cells during hypoxia, so consequently our finding that the hypoxia-evoked release of DA is unaffected by concentrations of APIII which inhibit the hypoxia-evoked CSN discharge suggests that changes in DA release may not be involved in the ANP-mediated inhibitory effect.[22] It is especially true that any involvement of DA should be associated with substantial changes in its release, because previous studies showed that zero Ca^{2+} media reduced evoked DA release by more than 85%, while the concomitant CSN discharge decreased by only 50%; that is, there is a large 'safety factor' for DA action and a change in its release should be detected before a change in nerve discharge.[51] In preliminary experiments, we have found that opiate receptor antagonists such as naloxone and the specific delta receptor antagonist naltrindole, reverse the CSN inhibition produced by APIII.[52] These results suggest a possible role for met-enkephalin in ANP-mediated inhibition. It is well known that met-enkephalin is present in type I cells, and has been shown in pharmacological experiments to inhibit chemoreceptor discharge.[49,50]

Finally, consideration must be given to the important question of the mobilization and release of ANP from type I cells. Studies in the heart have shown that in addition to atrial distension, ANP release is also evoked by hypoxia,[35] and by calcitonin gene-related peptide (CGRP).[53] Morphological studies have demonstrated a plexus of CGRP/substance P-containing fibers in the carotid bodies of various species, and some of these fibers enter the glomus cell lobules where they come into close association with type I cells.[54] In preliminary experiments addressing the possible involvement of CGRP in ANP-mediated inhibition, we have found that submicromolar concentrations of CGRP evoke the release of ANP, and mimic the inhibitory effects of APIII on chemoreceptor discharge. Furthermore, ANP immunostaining in the carotid body is significantly diminished following 1-2 hr of hypoxia in vivo or in vitro,[55] but returns to normal levels when the tissue is allowed to recover for 2 hr in 100% O_2 media. These findings suggest that hypoxia evokes the release of ANP from chemosensitive type I cells, and that ANP synthesis occurs de novo in the carotid body.

DOPAMINE AND CAROTID BODY EFFERENT INHIBITION

As mentioned earlier, the role of endogenous DA in carotid body physiology remains controversial, because based on pharmacological and biochemical data, this catecholamine has been variously proposed as inhibitory or excitatory to chemoreceptor discharge (see refs. 49,50). Lahiri and his colleagues[56,57] were the first to suggest that DA may play a role in efferent inhibition of the carotid chemoreceptors. Specifically, these investigators documented the existence of an efferent inhibitory pathway which became active in chronically hypoxic, but not normoxic cats.[56] Their experiments involved recording chemoreceptor activity in vivo from a few fibers split off from an otherwise intact CSN. Upon transection of the CSN (central to the recording site), the nerve discharge was significantly increased, suggesting the presence of a tonic inhibition of chemoreceptor activity. They further showed that the dopaminergic antagonist, haloperidol, blocked the increased discharge which followed nerve transection.[57] However, they also observed an additional increase in nerve activity if haloperidol was instead given after cutting the nerve. Logically, it was suggested that increased efferent inhibition is associated with chronic hypoxia and appears to be mediated by DA, and that furthermore, endogenous DA in the carotid body can mediate an inhibitory effect independent of the efferent pathway[57] (Fig. 8.3A). It was implicit in their interpretation that the DA involved in efferent inhibition should be secreted by the type I cells. However, later observations suggested the existence of a subpopulation of catecholaminergic chemosensory neurons in the petrosal ganglia. In these latter studies, Katz and his colleagues[58] described petrosal sensory neurons in the rat which contained enzymatically active tyrosine hydroxylase (TH), the rate-limiting enzyme for catecholamine synthesis. From retrograde tracer studies, it was estimated that 80-90% of these neurons project peripherally in the CSN and that most innervate the carotid body where they form endings in close apposition to type I cells. Centrally these fibers terminate in the commissural subnucleus of the tractus solitaires[59] (see chapter 9). These TH-positive neurons also contain DOPA decarboxylase, but not dopamine beta hydroxylase, suggesting that they are dopaminergic and not adrenergic.[58] Katz and his colleagues also demonstrated that these TH-positive neurons were a subpopulation separate from the ganglion's substance P-containing neurons, which were later shown to express NOS.[25] These findings were confirmed and extended by Almaraz et al[60] who observed that TH-positive nerve fibers innervate the cat carotid body and establish extensive contacts with type I cells. The source of these fibers was examined in denervation experiments which demonstrated that chronic CSN section, but not sympathectomy, eliminated all TH-positive intralobule nerve profiles. Neurochemical studies showed that DA is the predominant catecholamine in the CSN, and although both DA and norepinephrine (NE) are synthesized by the nerve at similar rates, NE synthesis was completely abolished by chronic sympathectomy, suggesting that DA is not present in the nerve as a mere precursor of NE (Fig. 8.3B). Moreover, following a 3 hr incubation of carotid bodies with their attached nerves in media containing the radiolabeled catecholamine precursor ^{3}H-tyrosine (20 μM), electrical stimulation of CSN fibers provoked the release of ^{3}H-catecholamines.[12,60] Following chronic sympathectomy, this ^{3}H-catecholamine release consisted primarily of ^{3}H-DA (Fig. 8.3C). Importantly, this phenomenon was observed only at stimulus intensities capable of recruiting C-fibers to the nerve's compound action potential. Although numerous intralobular terminals appear to contain high levels of TH, consistent with a detectable release of DA, it was impossible in these experiments to assign ^{3}H-DA release to either the nerve terminals or the type I cells (perhaps mediated via the action of reciprocal synapses), or some combination of the two. Nevertheless, the morphological and neurochemical data obtained in the cat are consonant with the observations of Katz et al (in the rat) and Lahiri et al,[56-58] in that both suggest the possible existence of a dopaminergic efferent pathway to the carotid body.

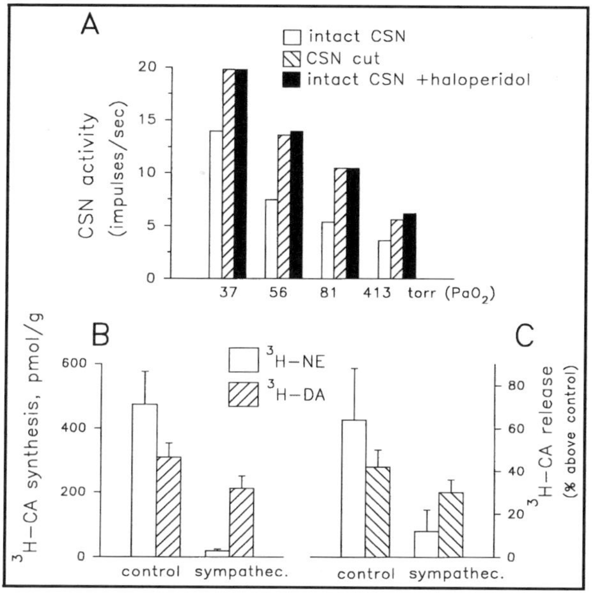

Fig. 8.3. (A) Evidence for efferent inhibition in chronically hypoxic cat carotid bodies, and the apparent involvement of a dopaminergic mechanism (see text for details). (B) ^{3}H-catecholamine (^{3}H-CA) synthesis in the carotid sinus nerve from control and chronically sympathectomized cat carotid bodies. (C) ^{3}H-CA release in response to supramaximal stimulation of the carotid sinus nerve of control and chronically sympathectomized cat. ^{3}H-NE and ^{3}H-DA, tritiated norepinephrine and dopamine, respectively. (Redrawn with data from references 57(A) and 60(B)).

CONCLUSIONS AND PERSPECTIVES

The available data suggest that multiple neuronal and neurotransmitter mechanisms may mediate "efferent" inhibition in the carotid body. Nitric oxide appears to produce inhibition via dual neuronal pathways involving: 1) cholinergic autonomic efferent neurons regulating vascular tone; and 2) substance P-containing sensory neurons whose production of NO may be triggered by axon reflexes or central primary afferent depolarization (PAD). NO derived from sensory neurons might act as a retrograde transmitter modulating the chemosensory activity of type I cells by controlling intracellular levels of cGMP. The activation of ANP-mediated inhibition may likewise involve the tachykininergic sensory neurons because these substance P/NOS-positive nerve fibers have also been shown to contain CGRP (see ref. 25,54). Membrane-bound ANP receptors are known to be coupled to a particulate form of guanylate cyclase, whereas NO acts via a soluble form of the enzyme. Consequently, a single set of peptidergic neurons may command two distinct and individually powerful inhibitory mechanisms. Unfortunately, virtually nothing is known at this time about the various physiological conditions which might initiate inhibition involving either NO or ANP, and whether these unique transmitters are regulated by different chemosensory stimuli, stimulus intensities, or durations.

The data of Lahiri and his colleagues[56,57] suggest that efferent inhibition is a dynamic phenomenon which develops as a consequence of extended hypoxia. The ability of haloperidol to abolish the emergent inhibition implicates the involvement of DA; however, the evidence implicating dopaminergic sensory neurons in this process is less than compelling. Although Lahiri et al showed that haloperidol abolished the efferent inhibition during both normoxia and hypoxia, it is well known that low O_2 stimuli evoke DA release from type I cells in amounts which far exceed that which could be released by maximal C-fiber stimulation of the CSN. On the other hand, because DA receptors are known to be associated with CSN endings, it is plausible that DA released from any source might depolarize peptidergic terminals, thereby activating the NO-ANP mechanisms. It also is possible that some sensory fibers containing DA and originating in the CB vasculature contribute to the inhibition of CSN via producing vasodilation via DA_1 receptors tentatively located in blood vessels.[61] Certainly our understanding of the roles of DA, NO, ANP and other putative neurotransmitters in chemoreceptor inhibition is incomplete and requires further experimental studies.

References

1. Neil E, O'Regan RG. The effects of electrical stimulation of the distal end of the cut sinus and aortic nerves on peripheral arterial chemoreceptor activity in the cat. J Physiol London 1971; 215:15-32.
2. Fidone SJ, Sato A. A study of chemoreceptor and baroreceptor A and C-fibres in the cat carotid nerve. J Physiol 1969; 205:527-548.
3. Fidone SJ, Sato A. Efferent inhibition and antidromic depression of chemoreceptor A-fibers from the cat carotid body. Brain Res 1970; 22:181-193.
4. Biscoe TJ, Sampson SR. Rhythmical and non-rhythmical spontaneous activity recorded from the central cut end of the sinus nerve. J Physiol 1968; 196:327-338.
5. McDonald DM, Mitchell RA. The neural pathway involved in "efferent inhibition" of chemoreceptors in the cat carotid body. J Comp Neurol 1981; 201: 457-476.
6. Mitchell RA, McDonald DM. Adjustment of chemoreceptor sensitivity in the cat carotid body by reciprocal synapses, In: Purves MJ, ed. The Peripheral Arterial Chemoreceptors. London: Cambridge Univ Press 1975:269-291.
7. McDonald DM. Regulation of chemoreceptor sensitivity in the carotid body: the role of presynaptic sensory nerves. Fed Proc 1980; 39:2627-2635.
8. McAllen RM, Willshaw P. Sinus nerve efferent activity survives suprapetrosal section. J Physiol 1979; 295:58P.
9. Willshaw P, McAllen RM. Sinus nerve efferent activity originates outside the brain. In: Belmonte C, Pallot D, Acker H, Fidone S, eds. Arterial Chemoreceptors. Proc 6th Int'l Mtg, United Kingdom: Leicester Univ Press 1981:440-447.
10. deCastro F. Sur la structure et l'innervation de la glande intercarotidienne (glomus caroticum) de l'homme et des mammiferes, et sur un nouveau systeme d'innervation autonome du nerf glossopharyngien. Trab Lab Invest Biol Univ Madrid 1926; 24:365-432.
11. Belmonte C, Eyzaguirre C. Efferent influences on carotid body chemoreceptors. J Neurophysiol 1974; 37:1131-1143.
12. Almaraz L, Fidone S. Carotid sinus nerve C-fibers release catecholamines from the cat carotid body. Neurosci Lett 1986; 67:153-158.
13. O'Regan RG, Majcherczyk S. Control of peripheral chemoreceptors by efferent nerves. In: Acker H, O'Regan RG, eds. Physiology of the Peripheral Arterial Chemoreceptors. Amsterdam: Elsevier Science Publishers BV 1983:257-298.
14. Almaraz L, Perez-Garcia MT, Gomez-Niño A, González C. Mechanisms of α-adrenoceptor-mediated inhibition in the rabbit carotid body. Am J Physiol 1997; 272:C628-C637.
15. Palmer RMJ, Ferrige AG, Moncada S. Nitric oxide release accounts for the biological activity of endothelium-derived relaxing factor. Nature 1987; 327: 524-526.
16. Hibbs JR, Jr., Taintor RR, Vavrin Z. Macrophage cytotoxicity: Role for L-arginine deiminase and imino nitrogen oxidation to nitrite. Science 1987; 235: 473-476.
17. Garthwaite J. Glutamate, nitric oxide and cell-cell signaling in the nervous system. Trends Neurosci 1991; 14:60-67.
18. Burnett AL, Lowenstein CJ, Bredt DS, Chang TSK, Snyder SH. Nitric oxide: A physiological mediator of penile erection. Science 1992; 257:401-403.
19. Bredt DS, Snyder SH. Nitric oxide, a novel neuronal messenger. Neuron 1992; 8:3-11.
20. Wang W-J, Cheng G-F, Dinger BG, Fidone SJ. Effects of hypoxia on cyclic nucleotide formation in rabbit carotid body in vitro. Neurosci Lett 1989; 105: 164-168
21. Wang Z-Z, Stensaas LJ, de Vente J, Dinger B, Fidone SJ. Immunocytochemical localization of cAMP and cGMP in cells of the rat carotid body following natural and pharmacological stimulation. Histochem 1991; 96:523-530
22. Wang W-J, He L, Chen J, Dinger B, Fidone S. Mechanisms underlying che-

moreceptor inhibition induced by atrial natriuretic peptide in rabbit carotid body. J Physiol 1993; 460:427-441.
23. Bredt DS, Hwang PM, Snyder SH. Localization of nitric oxide synthase indicating a neural role for nitric oxide. Nature 1990; 347:768-770.
24. Prabhakar NR, Kumar GK, Chang CH, Agani FH, Haxhiu MA. Nitric oxide in sensory function of the carotid body. Brain Res 1993; 625:16-22.
25. Wang Z-Z, Bredt DS, Fidone SJ, Stensaas LJ. Neurons synthesizing nitric oxide innervate the mammalian carotid body. J Comp Neurol 1993; 336:419-432.
26. Grimes PA, Lahiri S, Stone R, Mokashi A, Chug D. Nitric oxide synthase occurs in neurons and nerve fibers of the carotid body, In: O'Regan RG, Nolan P, McQueen DS, Patterson DJ, eds. Arterial Chemoreceptors, Advances in Experimental Medicine and Biology. New York: Plenum Press 1994:221-224.
27. Grimes PA, Mokashi A, Stone RA, Lahiri S. Nitric oxide synthase in autonomic innervation of the cat carotid body. J Auton Nerv Syst 1995; 54:80-86.
28. Wang Z-Z, Stensaas JJ, Bredt DS, Dinger B, Fidone SJ. Localization and actions of nitric oxide in the cat carotid body. Neurosci 1994; 60:275-286.
29. Haxhiu MA, Chang CH, Dreshaj IA, Erokwu B, Prabhakar NR, Cherniack NS. Nitric oxide and ventilatory response to hypoxia. Respir Physiol 1995; 101: 257-266.
30. Chugh DK, Katayama K, Mokashi A, Bebout DE, Ray DK, Lahiri S. Nitric oxide-related inhibition of carotid chemosensory nerve activity in the cat. Resp Physiol 1994;97:147-156.
31. Wang Z-Z, Stensaas LJ, Dinger BG, Fidone SJ. Nitric oxide mediates chemoreceptor inhibition in the cat carotid body. Neurosci 1995; 65:217-229.
32. Wang Z-Z, Dinger BG, Stensaas LJ, Fidone SJ. The role of nitric oxide in carotid chemoreception. Biol Signals 1995; 4:109-116.
33. DeBold AJ. Heart atria granularity. Effects of changes in water and electrolyte balance. Proc Soc Exp Biol Med 1979; 161:508-511.
34. DeBold AJ, Borenstein HB, Veress AJ, Sonnenberg H. A rapid and potent natriuretic response to intravenous injection of atrial myocardial extract in rats. Life Sci 1981; 28:89-94.
35. Baertschi AJ, Hausmaninger C, Walsh RS, Mentzer RM, Wyatt DA, Pence RA. Hypoxia-induced release of atrial natriuretic factor (ANF) from the isolated rat and rabbit heart. Biochem Biophys Res Commun 1986; 140:427-433.
36. Genest J, Cantin M, Anand-Srivastava MB et al. The atrial natriuretic factor: its physiology and biochemistry. Rev Physiol Biochem Pharmacol 1988; 110: 1-145.
37. Bianchi C, Gutkowska J, Thibault G et al. Distinct localization of atrial natriuretic factor and angiotensin II binding sites in the glomerulus. Am J Physiol 1986; 251: F594-F602
38. Kawata M, Nakao K, Morii N et al. Atrial natriuretic polypeptide: topographical distribution in the rat brain by radioimmunoassay and immunocytochemistry. Neurosci 1985; 16:521-546.
39. Skofitsch G, Jacobowitz DM, Eskay RL, Zamir N. Distribution of atrial natriuretic factor-like neurons in the rat brain. Neurosci 1985; 16:917-948.
40. Quirion R, Dalpe M, Dam T-V. Characterization and distribution of receptors for atrial natriuretic peptides in mammalian brain. Proc Natl Acad Sci USA 1986; 83:174-178.
41. Saavedra JM, Correa FM, Plunkett LM et al. Binding of angiotensin and strial natriuretic peptide in brain of hypertensive rats. Nature 1986; 320:758-760.
42. Samson WK. Atrial natriuretic factor inhibits dehydration and hemorrage-induced vasopressin release. Neuroendocrinology 1985; 40:277-279.
43. Samson WK, Aguila MC, Martinovic J et al. Hypothalamic action of atrial natriuretic factor to inhibit vasopressin secretion. Peptides 1987; 8:449-454.
44. Gallego R, Eyzaguirre C, Monti-Bloch L. Thermal and osmotic responses of arterial receptors. J Neurophysiol 1979; 42:665-680.
45. Honig A. Peripheral arterial chemoreceptors and reflex control of sodium and water homeostasis. Am J Physiol 1989; 257:R1282-R1302.

46. Wang Z-Z, He L, Stensaas LJ, Dinger BG, Fidone SJ. Localization and in vitro actions of atrial natriuretic peptide in the cat carotid body. J Appl Physiol 1991; 70:942-946.
47. Wang Z-Z, Stensaas LJ, Wang W-J et al. Atrial natriuretic peptide increases cyclic guanosine monophosphate immunoreactivity in the carotid body. Neurosci 1992; 49:479-486.
48. Wang Z-Z, Hirose S, Dinger B et al. Localization of atrial natriuretic peptide receptors in the carotid body. Soc Neurosci Abstr 1991; 17:118(abstr).
49. Fidone SJ, González C. Initiation and control of chemoreceptor activity in the carotid body, In: Fishman AP, ed. Handbook of Physiology - The Respiratory System II, Vol. II, Part I, Bethesda: Am Physiol Soc, 1986:247-312.
50. Fidone SJ, González C, Dinger B, Gomez-Niño A, Obeso A, Yoshizaki K. Cellular aspects of peripheral chemoreceptor function, In: Crystal RG, West JB, eds., The Lung: Scientific Foundations, New York, Raven Press, Ltd., 1991: 1319-1332.
51. Fidone S, González C, Yoshizaki K. Effects of low oxygen on the release of dopamine from the rabbit carotid body in vitro. J Physiol 1982; 333:93-110.
52. He L, Chen J, Dinger B, Fidone S. Mechanism of action of atrial natriuretic peptide (ANP) in rabbit carotid body. Soc Neurosci Abstr 1991; 17:117 (abstr).
53. Yamamoto A, Kimura S, Hasui K et al. Calcitonin gene-related peptide (CGRP) stimulates the release of atrial natriuretic peptide (ANP) from isolated rat atria. Biochem Biophys Res Comm 1988; 155: 1452-1458.
54. Kummer W, Fischer A, Heym C. Ultrastructure of calcitonin gene-related peptide- and substance P-like immunoreactive nerve fibres in the carotid body and carotid sinus of the guinea pig. Histochem 1989; 92:433-439.
55. Stensaas LJ, Wang Z-Z, Dinger B, Fidone S. Alteration of atrial natriuretic peptide (ANP) immunostaining in the rat carotid body evoked by hypoxia. Soc Neurosci Abstr 1991; 17:118 (abstr).
56. Lahiri S, Smatresk N, Pokorski M et al. Efferent inhibition of carotid body chemoreception in chronically hypoxic cats. Am J Physiol 1983; 245:R678-R683.
57. Lahiri S, Smatresk N, Pokorski M et al. Dopaminergic efferent inhibition of carotid body chemoreceptors in chronically hypoxic cats. Am J Physiol 1984; 247: R24-R28.
58. Finley JCW, Polak J, Katz DM. Transmitter diversity in carotid body afferent neurons: Dopaminergic and peptidergic phenotypes. Neurosci 1992; 51:973-987.
59. Massari VJ, Shirahata M, Johnson TA, Gatti PJ. Carotid sinus nerve terminals which are tyrosine hydroxylase immunoreactive are found in the commissural nucleus of the tractus solitarius. J Neurocytol 1996; 25:197-208.
60. Almaraz L, Wang Z-Z, Stensaas LJ, Fidone SJ. Release of dopamine from carotid sinus nerve fibers innervating type I cells in the cat carotid body. Biol Signals 1993; 2:16-26.
61. Almaraz L, Pérez-García MT, González C. Presence of D_1 receptors in the rabbit carotid body. Neurosci Lett 1991; 132: 259-262.

CHAPTER 9

Organization and Development of Chemoafferent Input to the Brainstem

David M. Katz, James C.W. Finley, Jeffrey T. Erickson and Theresa Brosenitsch

INTRODUCTION

Primary sensory neurons associated with the glossopharyngeal nerve provide the afferent link between carotid body chemoreceptors and cardiorespiratory pathways in the brainstem. Studies conducted over the last decade have revealed an unexpected degree of phenotypic heterogeneity within this afferent population, leading to new opportunities and challenges for understanding the physiology and development of chemoafferent transmission. This heterogeneity is particularly apparent with respect to neurotransmitter phenotype, and is also evident in the synaptic interactions between carotid body afferent (CBA) neurons and their peripheral and central targets. Application of neuroanatomic tracing methods, as well as more recent activity-dependent mapping techniques, have made it possible to begin defining higher-order neurons in the chemoafferent pathway with greater precision than previously possible. This chapter reviews these recent advances in our understanding of the organization of the chemoafferent pathway and also discusses new insights into genetic mechanisms of chemoafferent development.

ANATOMIC LOCALIZATION OF CAROTID BODY AFFERENT NEURONS

The carotid sinus nerve (CSN), a branch of the glossopharyngeal trunk, provides sensory innervation to the carotid body and carotid sinus. This dual innervation has made it difficult to identify CSN neurons that selectively innervate the carotid body using standard neuroanatomic tracing strategies. We found, however, that CBA neurons can be selectively

The Carotid Body Chemoreceptors,
edited by Constancio González.

identified using retrograde tracers, such as fluorogold or wheat germ agglutinin-conjugated horseradish peroxidase (WGA-HRP), introduced directly into the carotid body isolated in situ.[1-3] Tracers are introduced by either microinjection or by a cannula placed in the carotid body artery.[1] These techniques label a restricted subset of afferents compared to the population of neurons labeled following application of tracers to the entire CSN (compare Finley and Katz, 1992[2] and Housley et al, 1987[5]).

Results from our laboratory, using the carotid body microinjection procedure, demonstrated that approximately 250 afferent neurons innervate each carotid body in the rat.[3] These data are in good agreement with those of Claps and Torrealba[6] in the cat, but may underestimate the true number of CBA neurons since the efficiency of retrograde labeling is likely to be less than 100%. The rat CSN contains between 450 and 750 (mean, 625) axons.[7] Based on these observations, CBA neurons may account for only 40-50% of the fibers in the entire nerve. In addition to CBA neurons, other populations known to project in the CSN include sinus afferents, a small number of peripheral autonomic fibers, and, in some species, efferent fibers that arise from neurons in the brainstem.[8]

Approximately 75% of CBA neurons are located in the distal third of the petrosal ganglion (PG).[2] In contrast, 14% are located in the jugular ganglion (JG), 10% in the proximal PG and 1-2% in the proximal nodose ganglion (NG). In addition to these ganglionic cell populations, a variable number of labeled neurons (approximately 10-50 per animal) are also found in the glossopharyngeal nerve itself.[3] Recent studies indicate that at least some of these cells are autonomic neurons that terminate in the carotid body.[9]

The vast majority of CBA neurons in the distal PG are small or medium in size (mean diameters, 14.98 and 20.52 mm, respectively), whereas the majority of those in the JG, proximal PG, and NG are relatively large (mean diameter, 29.29 mm).[3] This heterogeneity in perikaryal diameters raises the possibility that CBA neurons localized to different cranial sensory ganglia may exhibit distinguishing functional properties as well.

NEUROCHEMICAL ORGANIZATION OF CAROTID BODY AFFERENT NEURONS

To specifically define transmitter properties expressed by CBA neurons, studies in our laboratory combined retrograde labeling with immunocytochemical localization of transmitter-related proteins. The largest population of neurochemically distinct CBA neurons in the rat PG express dopaminergic (DA) transmitter properties, including catalytically active tyrosine hydroxylase (TH),[10] the rate-limiting enzyme in catecholamine biosynthesis, dopa-decarboxylase, the dopamine-synthesizing enzyme,[3] formaldehyde-induced catecholamine fluorescence,[10] and a monoamine oxidase-like pathway for catecholamine metabolism.[10] In the rat, DA sensory neurons account for at least 42% of the entire CBA population. However, DA properties are only rarely seen in cells that project to other ganglion targets.[1] This phenotype, therefore, provides a highly selective marker for CBA neurons in the PG. Subsequent studies in other laboratories demonstrated that catecholaminergic properties are also expressed by CBA neurons in guinea pig[11] and cat.[12]

Using immunocytochemical localization of tyrosine hydroxylase at the electron microscopic level we found that approximately 40% of all afferent terminals on glomus cells exhibit TH immunoreactivity.[3,13] These analyses were performed on both intact carotid bodies and following sympathetic denervation to avoid inclusion of sympathetic TH-immunoreactive fibers. Most afferent terminals were postsynaptic to glomus cells, supporting the view that the dopaminergic CBA neurons are part of the chemotransductive unit in the carotid body. In addition, however, some DA afferent terminals exhibited reciprocal synapses, raising the possibility that, in addition to transmitting chemoreceptor input to the brainstem, these fibers may also play a role in local modulation of glomus cell function.

TH immunoreactivity has also been localized to the central terminals of CSN afferents within the brainstem nucleus tractus solitarius (nTS) in the cat (Massari et al, 1996). Using HRP tracing combined with TH immunostaining and electron microscopy, Massari and colleagues found that approximately half of all CSN terminals in the nTS are TH^+, consistent with a role for catecholaminergic transmission between CBA neurons and their postsynaptic targets in the brainstem.

Despite these anatomic findings, the physiologic actions of dopamine synthesized by CBA neurons remain undefined. Studies by Almaraz and colleagues[14,15] have shown that dopamine is present in the peripheral processes of CSN fibers in the cat and that nerve stimulation at strengths sufficient to excite small caliber fibers evokes peripheral release of dopamine. These data suggest that dopamine can be released from afferent terminals within the carotid body. It is also possible, however, that CSN stimulation leads to dopamine release from cells within the carotid body itself, rather than from CBA fibers. Similarly, Lagercrantz and colleagues[16] demonstrated dopamine release within the brainstem nucleus solitarius, the central target of CBA neurons, during hypoxia or CSN stimulation; here too, however, the source of the dopamine could not be identified with precision. Thus, although both peripheral and central roles have been proposed, the function of dopamine in the CSN pathway remains undefined.

To date, there is little evidence to suggest that dopaminergic CBA neurons coexpress other transmitter properties. TH is not colocalized with either the neurokinin substance P (SP) or nitric oxide synthase (NOS), both of which are found within a small subset of CBA neurons (see below).[2,9] The only exception to this observation is the occasional colocalization of TH and the neuropeptide galanin.[17] Interestingly, galanin expression in adult CBA neurons is markedly upregulated following fluorogold injection into the carotid body. Given the fact that upregulation of galanin is common following sensory nerve injury, we suspect this finding reflects a subtle neurotoxic effect of fluorogold on the CBA neurons. This effect is selective, however, in that TH expression in PG neurons is unchanged in these same animals. Although the role of galanin in CBA neurons is unknown, these data indicate that CSN fibers retain a degree of neurochemical plasticity well into adulthood.

Although PG cells express several neuroactive peptides,[3,11,18-22] none, in contrast to dopamine, is selectively associated with the CBA population. Approximately 7% of CBA neurons contain SP.[3] This peptide is also expressed, however, by PG neurons that innervate other targets, such as lingual taste buds.[23] The majority of SP-containing CBA neurons are located within the proximal PG (54%) and JG (30%), with the remainder found in the distal PG and proximal NG. As noted above, SP-containing CBA neurons are distinct from those that express dopamine.[3] However, SP is colocalized with calcitonin gene-related peptide (CGRP) in PG neurons.[24-26] Despite the presence of SP within CBA neurons, a direct role for these peptidergic cells in chemoafferent transmission has been questioned (reviewed by González, et al 1994[27]). This is based on observations that in some species, SP-containing carotid body afferents terminate in the vicinity of blood vessels, and not in contact with type I glomus cells.[28] In the human carotid body, a small number of close, nonsynaptic appositions between SP-containing fibers and glomus cells have been observed.[25] Whether or not any of these fibers are chemoafferents, SP could be released from CBA terminals and influence chemosensory output indirectly by regulating blood flow within the carotid body.[25,28] Although other peptides, including somatostatin[29] and enkephalin[30] have been identified within fibers in the carotid body, the cells of origin of these peptidergic fibers have not been precisely defined.

A third transmitter synthesized by a small subset of CBA neurons is nitric oxide.[9,31-36] Immunocytochemical studies demonstrated that less than 10% of fibers in the rat CSN stain positively for NOS, and NOS enzymatic activity can be detected in the

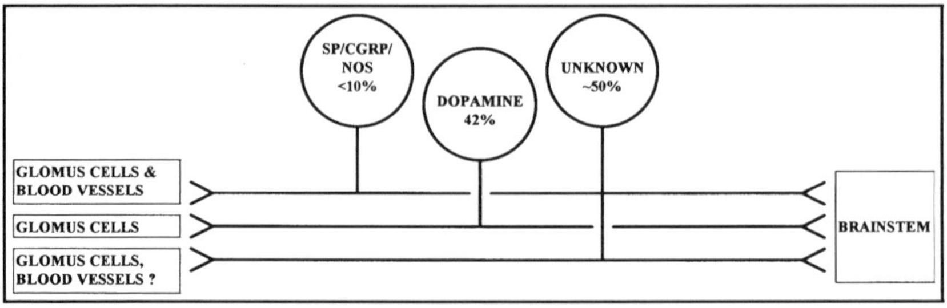

Fig. 9.1. Schematic diagram illustrating transmitter heterogeneity in carotid body afferent (CBA) neurons in the rat petrosal ganglion. Boxes at left indicate the presumed targets of the different CBA subpopulations within the carotid body. SP, substance P; NOS, nitric oxide synthase; CGRP, calcitonin gene-related peptide.

CSN, PG and carotid body. Approximately 50% of NOS-positive PG neurons can be retrogradely labeled from the CSN. At least some of these fibers terminate in the carotid body, which contains a dense plexus of NOS-positive fibers that disappears following CSN section.[9] Physiologic studies indicate that nitric oxide has an inhibitory effect on chemosensory output, raising the possibility that NOS-positive PG afferents provide an anatomic substrate for so-called "efferent" inhibition of carotid body glomus cells[32-34] (see chapter 8). However, the CSN also contains postganglionic parasympathetic neurons that express NOS and project to the carotid body.[9] Moreover, virtually all NOS-positive neurons in the rat PG also express SP[9] and, as noted above, SP-positive CBA afferents do not innervate type I glomus cells in this species. Therefore, it still seems unclear whether the primary targets of the NOS-positive CBA neurons are glomus cells or blood vessels within the carotid body.

In aggregate, immunocytochemical studies to date can account for the neurochemical profile of approximately 50% of all primary afferents that innervate the carotid body in the rat (Fig. 9.1), the only species in which transmitter properties expressed by identified CBA neurons have been characterized in detail. The largest subpopulation (42% of all CBA neurons) synthesize dopamine and do not normally co-express detectable levels of SP, NOS or other known markers. The second population (7% of all CBA neurons) identified thus far appear to co-express SP, CGRP and NOS. These data illustrate the neurochemical heterogeneity of the CBA population and indicate that multiple transmitters are likely to be involved in regulating chemoafferent input to second-order neurons within the chemoafferent pathway.

CENTRAL PROJECTIONS OF CAROTID BODY AFFERENT NEURONS

The central projections of CBA neurons have been mapped in the rat and cat using transganglionic transport of WGA-HRP.[2,6,37] Studies in our laboratory demonstrated that, in the rat, CBA fibers enter the lateral aspect of the medulla 1.30 mm rostral to the obex and course dorsomedially to enter the ipsilateral tractus solitarius (TS). The fibers run caudally within the TS and then leave the tract at multiple levels between 0.36 mm and 1.50 mm caudal to the obex to enter the intermediate and caudal portions of the nucleus of the solitary tract (nTS). These fibers terminate ipsilaterally within the intermediate, interstitial, medial, dorsolateral and ventrolateral subnuclei, and bilaterally in the commissural subnucleus (Fig. 9.2). The densest projection was found within the ipsilateral commissural and medial subnuclei. These data are supported by the findings of Massari, et al (1996) in the cat that a large contingent of TH^+ CSN fibers terminate in the commissural subnucleus. Moreover, these authors found that although the TH^+ CSN terminals make frequent axo-axonic contacts with central TH^+ terminals,

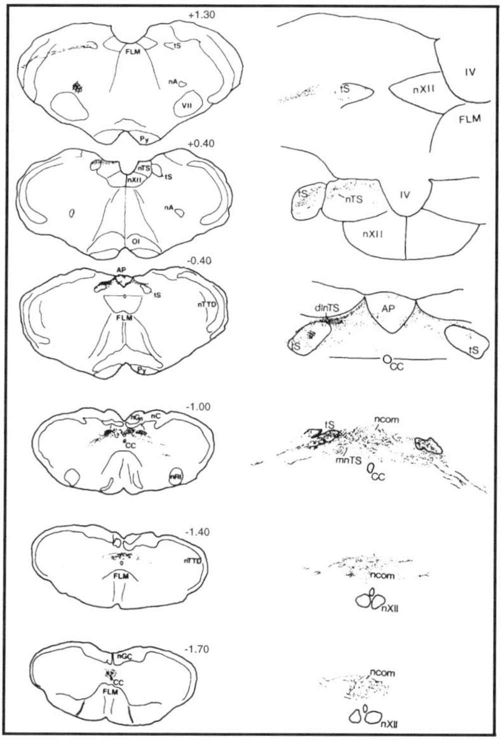

Fig. 9.2. Camera lucida drawings at low (left column) and high (right column) magnification showing the distribution of labeled fibers and efferent cell bodies within the rat brainstem following WGA-HRP microinjection into the right carotid body. The numbers above each low magnification drawing indicate approximate distance in millimeters from the obex. Reprinted from Finley and Katz[2], with permission.

no synaptic contacts were observed between CSN terminals and TH^+ positive perikarya or dendrites. We also observed labeled fibers in the ipsilateral dorsal parasolitary region described by Kalia and Sullivan.[38] Additional fibers crossed the midline at the level of the commissural subnucleus to terminate in the contralateral intermediate, interstitial, medial and dorsolateral subnuclei. These contralateral projections were, however, less dense than those ipsilateral to the injection site. Ciriello et al[37] have seen a similar pattern of projections in a more recent study. CBA projections to the rat nTS are similar to those described in the cat by Claps and Torrealba,[6] with the exception that the latter authors did not observe CBA fibers terminating within the ipsilateral ventrolateral nucleus or the contralateral interstitial, intermediate and medial subnuclei.

The finding that CBA fibers terminate most densely in the ipsilateral medial and commissural subnuclei of the nTS is consistent with the importance of this relatively restricted region in mediating hypoxic ventilatory responses. For example, Housley and Sinclair[39] found that kainic acid lesions of the caudal, but not the rostral, nTS in rats significantly reduced ventilatory drive during hypoxia.

In addition to these inputs to nTS, we and others observed a bilateral projection of CBA afferents into the caudal ventrolateral medulla (cVLM) in the rat, approximately 1 mm caudal to the obex.[2,37] This projection was first described by Davies and Kalia[40] in the cat, although they only observed an ipsilateral input to the cVLM. The precise target(s) of these fibers are unknown, however, they are found in close proximity to areas of the ventrolateral medulla known to contain neurons with cardiorespiratory-related activity. We also found sparse fibers that appeared to terminate bilaterally in the dorsal motor nuclei of the vagus nerve (DMNX) and the area postrema. Ciriello et al[37] did not report CBA projections to the DMNX proper, but rather, coursing around the medial surface of the nucleus *en route* to a region between the central canal and the DMNX. Finally, our experiments documented the presence of efferent neurons in the ipsilateral rostral nucleus ambiguous projecting to the carotid body.[2] The long-standing controversy regarding the existence of such a pathway has recently been reviewed[27] (see also chapter 8).

Several studies suggest a role for excitatory amino acids in the chemoreflex pathway at the level of nTS, including as mediators of some primary afferent inputs. Thus, Zhang and Mifflin (1995) reported that inotophoretic application of kynurenate, a broad spectrum antagonist of excitatory amino acids, in the rat nTS reduced by nearly 50% the mono- and polysynaptic CSN-evoked responses in nTS neurons. These data are consistent with earlier studies by Vardhan et al (1993) showing that microinjections of NMDA and non-NMDA receptor antagonists in the midline commissural nucleus of nTS blocked responses to carotid chemoreceptor stimulation. Similarly, Dogas et al (1995) found that the NMDA receptor antagonist AP5 inhibited carotid body-mediated activation of bulbospinal expiratory neurons in the dog. Consistent with these electrophysiological studies, Mizuzawa et al (1994) found that hypoxic episodes in vivo elicited release of glutamate in the nTS in the rat.

HIGHER-ORDER NEURONS IN THE CHEMOAFFERENT PATHWAY

Although neuroanatomic tracing studies have provided a map of CBA projections within the brainstem, precise identification of second-order neurons in the chemoafferent pathway remains elusive (see also chapter 12). The CBA projection zones are cytoarchitecturally complex, and the postsynaptic targets of primary afferent inputs from the carotid body have not been defined. In the last few years, several groups have attempted to approach this issue with a strategy that identifies neurons on the basis of their level of activation following physiologic or electrical stimulation.

In 1987, Hunt and colleagues demonstrated that noxious stimulation of cutaneous nerve fibers leads to increased expression of the proto-oncogene *c-fos* in the spinal cord dorsal horn, as well as in higher-order neurons that respond to peripheral nociceptive input.[41] The Fos protein is a transcription factor involved in activity-dependent regulation of many neuronal genes, including some required for neurotransmitter synthesis.[42] Since that time, Fos immunocytochemistry has been used to identify activated neurons in pathways throughout the neuraxis. Erickson and Millhorn[43,44] demonstrated that exposure to systemic hypoxia, or electrical stimulation of the CSN, induces similar patterns of Fos protein expression in several medullary regions, including the nTS, area postrema and the cVLM (Fig. 9.3). Within nTS, labeled neurons were localized primarily to the commissural subnucleus and medial aspects of the nTS, with fewer but significant numbers of neurons found ventral and ventrolateral to the TS. In addition, Fos-positive neurons were observed in both the caudal and rostral ventrolateral medulla, as well as nucleus raphe pallidus, nucleus raphe magnus and the parapyramidal cell group along the ventral medullary surface. Similar results have been reported in cat using systemic hypoxia as a stimulus.[45]

Although the stimulus protocol used by Erickson and Millhorn[43,44] to activate CSN afferents (25 or 50 Hz, 0.05 ms pulse duration, 1-4 V) could not guarantee selective stimulation of CBA neurons, it is likely that the pattern of labeling they observed was due predominantly to activation of the chemoreflex rather than the baroreflex pathway. First, the overall pattern of labeling observed following either CSN stimulation at 25 and 50 Hz, or following hypoxia, was the same. Second, during electrical stimulation, phrenic nerve discharge (an index of central inspiratory drive) increased briskly with little or no change in mean arterial pressure (see Fig. 9.1[43]), suggesting that arterial baroreceptors were activated minimally, if at all. Moreover, studies aimed at selectively activating baroreceptors by intravenous infusion of phenylephrine[46-48] resulted in a substantially different and reduced pattern of Fos labeling, particularly in the cVLM. Finally, the pattern of labeling observed by Erickson and Millhorn[43,44] is unlikely to have resulted from a direct effect

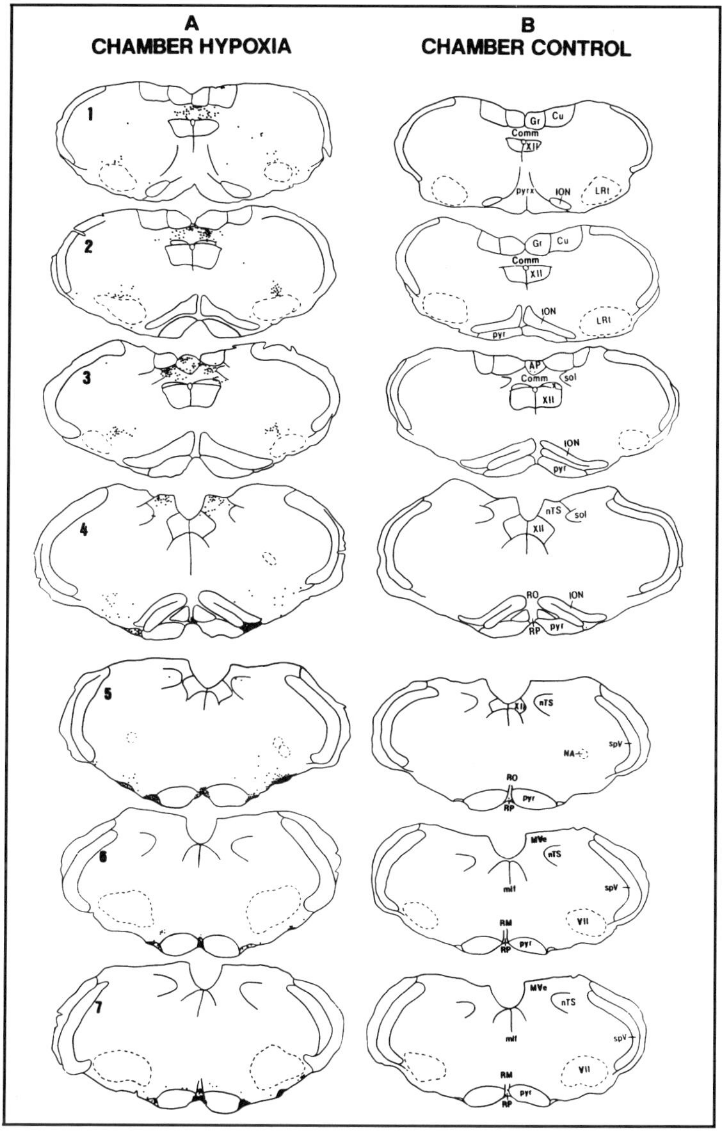

Fig. 9.3. Camera lucida drawings (x125) of single transverse sections of the rat medulla oblongata illustrating the distribution of Fos-like immunoreactivity (Fos-LI) at selected caudal (1) to rostral (7) levels. Each black dot represents one labeled cell nucleus. (A) chamber hypoxia. Animal was placed within an environmental chamber and exposed to 8-10% O_2 (hypoxia) for 3 h. (B) chamber control. Animal was placed within an environmental chamber and exposed to 21% O_2 (normoxia) for 3 h. AP, area postrema; Comm, commissural nucleus; Cu, cuneate nucleus; Gr, gracile nucleus; ION, inferior olivary nucleus; LRt, lateral reticular nucleus; mlf, medial longitudinal fasciculus; MVe, medial vestibular nucleus; NA, nucleus ambiguus; nTS, nucleus of the solitary tract; pyr, pyramidal tract; pyrx, pyramidal decussation; RM, nucleus raphe magnus; RO, nucleus raphe obscurus; RP, nucleus raphe pallidus; sol, solitary tract; spV, spinal trigeminal tract: VII, facial nucleus; X, dorsal motor nucleus of vagus; XII, hypoglossal nucleus. Reprinted from Erickson JT, Milhorn DE,[43] with permission.

of low oxygen since electrically-stimulated animals were maintained on a hyperoxic breathing mixture throughout the experiment.

As expected, the overall distribution of Fos-labeled neurons observed following hypoxia or electrical CSN stimulation[43,44] is more extensive than the distribution of CBA afferent projections alone.[2] It is striking, however, that within nTS and the cVLM, the pattern of CBA afferent projections described by Finley and Katz[2] is virtually superimposable on the pattern of Fos labeling within these regions following hypoxia- or CSN stimulation (compare Figs. 9.2 and 9.3). This overlap indicates that at least some of the Fos-labeled neurons within nTS and the cVLM are likely to be second-order neurons in the chemosensory pathway. The more extensive distribution of Fos labeling undoubtedly reflects polysynaptic activation of multiple populations of higher-order neurons following CSN afferent stimulation. The sequence of connections between these populations, however, remains to be defined.

The neurochemical content of second- and higher-order neurons in the chemoafferent pathway are largely unknown. Recently, however, Erickson and Millhorn[44] found that a significant percentage of neurons in the intermediate and caudal nTS and cVLM that express Fos following CSN afferent stimulation are catecholaminergic. Specifically, 20-65% of the TH-positive neurons in the intermediate and caudal portions of the nTS and greater than 80% of the TH-positive neurons in the cVLM expressed Fos following hypoxia in unanesthetized rats. In agreement with these findings, Dumas et al (1996) found that in rats acclimatized to hypoxia (10% O_2, 14 days) there was a marked increase in TH mRNA and protein in the caudal part of the nTS.

TROPHIC MECHANISMS OF CHEMOAFFERENT NEURON DEVELOPMENT

Definition of transmitter properties expressed by CBA neurons has provided a new tool for investigating the functional maturation of chemoafferent inputs to the brainstem. This is important because development of chemoreflex function involves not only maturation of neurotransmission between carotid body glomus cells and chemoafferent terminals, but between CBA neurons and the brainstem as well. Until recently, maturation of this critical component of the chemoafferent pathway has been largely ignored in studies of chemoreflex development and plasticity.

During early embryonic development (E11.5-15.5), neurons in many sensory ganglia, including the PG, transiently express TH, as well as selected peptidergic traits.[49,50] However, on embryonic day 16.5, stable expression of TH-immunoreactivity is first detectable in CBA neurons.[49] This occurs after the arrival of PG axons in the carotid body,[51,52] suggesting that target innervation and CBA transmitter development may be linked at this stage. After E16.5, the number of TH-immunoreactive (TH^+) cells in the PG gradually increases and peaks approximately one day after birth.

The close temporal correlation between dopaminergic phenotypic expression in CBA neurons, and the development of carotid body innervation, suggested a role for target-derived influences in CBA development. This possibility was supported by our finding that coculture of the fetal PG and carotid body led to an increase in PG neuron survival that was not mimicked by other tissues.[53] Thus, the carotid body exerts a trophic effect on development of fetal CBA neurons in culture. We subsequently found that CBA maturation in vivo is regulated by a similar trophic mechanism. Specifically, unilateral removal of the carotid body (glomectomy) in newborn rat pups results in a dramatic 73% decrease in the number of TH^+ neurons in the ipsilateral PG three weeks after birth.[53] This decrease in TH^+ cell number is accompanied by a corresponding reduction in the total number of PG neurons, indicating that CBA neurons are dependent on the carotid body for survival after birth. These data demonstrate, therefore, that in addition to its role as a sensory receptor, the carotid body also plays a trophic role in regulating CBA development in newborn animals.

Subsequent studies in our laboratory demonstrated that trophic regulation of CBA development is mediated primarily by brain-derived neurotrophic factor (BDNF), a member of the neurotrophin gene family, acting through the TrkB neurotrophin receptor. For example, initial studies in culture found that treatment of E16.5 PG explants with BDNF led to a striking 14-fold increase in the number of TH^+ cells, and an accompanying increase in total neuronal survival.[53] Similar results were obtained following treatment with the closely related neurotrophin-4 (NT-4), also a ligand for the TrkB receptor. Cell numbers were unaffected however, by treatment with the neurotrophins nerve growth factor (NGF) or neurotrophin-3 (NT-3) or the cytokine Leukemia Inhibitory Factor (LIF), all of which support survival of other populations of sensory neurons.[54] In BDNF- and NT-4-treated explants, TH^+ cells were segregated within the distal pole of the PG, as is typical of catecholaminergic neurons in vivo, indicating that TrkB ligands can support survival of the CBA population normally present in the PG. This possibility was confirmed by subsequent experiments demonstrating that BDNF supports survival of TH^+ PG neurons in vivo. Specifically, BDNF rescues TH^+ neurons in the PG that would otherwise die following carotid body removal.[53]

Recently, analyses of transgenic mice carrying disrupted *bdnf*, *nt-4* or *trkB* alleles established that CBA neurons are absolutely dependent on TrkB ligands for survival during development.[56] In particular, over 50% of TH^+ PG neurons die in mice carrying the *bdnf null* mutation (*bdnf -/-*), and over 80% are lost in mice lacking either TrkB or *both* BDNF and NT. Moreover, *bdnf -/-* mice exhibit a severe developmental deficit in control of breathing characterized by a 70% depression in minute ventilation and the absence of a ventilatory response to hyperoxia.[56] Interestingly, TrkB- and BDNF-deficient mice die within a few weeks after birth, and we suspect that the lethality of these mutations is linked to deficits in ventilatory control.

CONCLUSIONS

The past decade has seen considerable progress in defining the development, neurochemistry and central targets of peripheral chemosensory neurons. These advances enable us to pose exciting new questions, including:

1) What is the full range of transmitters expressed by chemoafferent neurons and what is the functional significance of transmitter heterogeneity among these cells? For example, is chemoafferent drive shaped by a balance between excitatory and inhibitory transmitters released by peripheral chemosensory inputs to the brainstem?

2) Do functionally and/or neurochemically distinct populations of chemosensory fibers project to different central targets, i.e., nucleus tractus solitarius vs. the caudal ventrolateral medulla? Can we define the location and phenotypes of second-order neurons with precision and map their subsequent projections?

3) What is the role of chemoafferent development in shaping functional maturation of peripheral chemoreflexes and central respiratory drive?

4) Do derangements of trophic regulation and/or transmitter expression play a role in developmental disorders such as Sudden Infant Death syndrome (SIDS) or chronic hypoventilation syndromes?

In the coming years, multidisciplinary approaches, including molecular genetics and in vitro analysis, combined with classical anatomic and physiologic methods, should yield significant new insights into these questions.

Acknowledgements

This work was supported by U.S. Public Health Service Grants and by the Francis Families Foundation.

References

1. Katz DM, Black IB. Expression and regulation of catecholaminergic traits in primary sensory neurons: relationship to target innervation in vivo. J Neurosci 1986; 6:983-9.

2. Finley JC, Katz DM. The central organization of carotid body afferent projections to the brainstem of the rat. Brain Res 1992; 572:108-16.
3. Finley JC, Polak J, Katz DM. Transmitter diversity in carotid body afferent neurons: dopaminergic and peptidergic phenotypes. Neuroscience 1992; 51:973-87.
4. McDonald DM. Morphology of the rat carotid sinus nerve. I. Course, connections, dimensions and ultrastructure. J Neurocytol 1983; 12:345-72.
5. Housley GD, Martin Body RL, Dawson NJ et al. Brain stem projections of the glossopharyngeal nerve and its carotid sinus branch in the rat. Neuroscience 1987; 22:237-50.
6. Claps A, Torrealba F. The carotid body connections: a WGA-HRP study in the cat. Brain Res 1988; 455:123-33.
7. McDonald DM. Morphology of the rat carotid sinus nerve. II. Number and size of axons. J Neurocytol 1983; 12:373-92.
8. McDonald DM, Mitchell RA. The neural pathway involved in "efferent inhibition" of chemoreceptors in the cat carotid body. J Comp Neurol 1981; 201: 457-76.
9. Wang ZZ, Bredt DS, Fidone SJ et al. Neurons synthesizing nitric oxide innervate the mammalian carotid body. J Comp Neurol 1993; 336:419-32.
10. Katz DM, Markey KA, Goldstein M et al. Expression of catecholaminergic characteristics by primary sensory neurons in the normal adult rat in vivo. Proc Natl Acad Sci U S A 1983; 80:3526-30.
11. Kummer W, Gibbins IL, Stefan P et al. Catecholamines and catecholamine-synthesizing enzymes in guinea-pig sensory ganglia. Cell Tissue Res 1990; 261: 595-606.
12. Almaraz L, Wang ZZ, Stensaas LJ et al. Release of dopamine from carotid sinus nerve fibers innervating type I cells in the cat carotid body. Biol Signals 1993; 2:16-26.
13. Polak J, Finley JCW, Katz DM. Synaptic targets of dopaminergic chemoafferent fibers in the carotid body. In Preparation.
14. Almaraz L, Fidone S. Release of catecholamines by electrical stimulation of the cat carotid sinus nerve in vitro. In: Ribeiro JA, Pallot DJ, eds. Chemoreceptors in Respiratory Control. London & Sydney: Crrom Helm 1987:35-43.
15. Almaraz L, Fidone S. Carotid sinus nerve C-fibers release catecholamines from the cat carotid body. Neurosci Lett 1986; 67:153-8.
16. Goiny M, Lagercrantz H, Srinivasan M et al. Hypoxia-mediated in vivo release of dopamine in nucleus tractus solitarii of rabbits. J Appl Physiol 1991; 70: 2395-2400.
17. Finley JCW, Erickson JT, Katz DM. Galanin expression in carotid body afferent neurons. Neuroscience 1995; 68: 937-942.
18. Ayer-LeLievre CS, Seiger A. Development of substance-P immunoreactive neurons in cranial sensory ganglia of the rat. Int J Dev Neurosci 1984; 2:451-63.
19. Katz DM, Karten HJ. Substance P in the vagal sensory ganglia: localization in cell bodies and pericellular arborizations. J Comp Neurol 1980; 193:549-64.
20. Helke CJ, Hill KM. Immunohistochemical study of neuropeptides in vagal and glossopharyngeal afferent neurons in the rat. Neuroscience 1988; 26:539-51.
21. Ichikawa H, Helke CJ. Distribution, origin and plasticity of galanin-immunoreactivity in the rat carotid body. Neuroscience 1993; 52:757-67.
22. Czyzyk-Krzeska MF, Bayliss DA, Lawson EE et al. Expression of messenger RNAs for peptides and tyrosine hydroxylase in primary sensory neurons that innervate arterial baroreceptors and chemoreceptors. Neurosci Lett 1991; 129:98-102.
23. Nagy JI, Goedert M, Hunt SP et al. The nature of the substance P-containing nerve fibres in taste papillae of the rat tongue. Neuroscience 1982; 7:3137-51.
24. Kummer W. Retrograde neuronal labelling and double-staining immunohistochemistry of tachykinin- and calcitonin gene-related peptide-immunoreactive pathways in the carotid sinus nerve of the guinea pig. J Auton Nerv Syst 1988; 23:131-41.
25. Kummer W, Habeck JO. Substance P- and calcitonin gene-related peptide-like immunoreactivities in the human carotid

body studied at light and electron microscopical level. Brain Res 1991; 554: 286-92.
26. Kummer W, Fischer A, Heym C. Ultrastructure of calcitonin gene-related peptide- and substance P-like immunoreactive nerve fibres in the carotid body and carotid sinus of the guinea pig. Histochemistry 1989; 92:433-9.
27. González C, Almaraz L, Obeso A et al. Carotid body chemoreceptors: From natural stimuli to sensory discharges. Phys Rev 1994; 74:829-98.
28. Chen II, Yates RD, Hansen JT. Substance P-like immunoreactivity in rat and cat carotid bodies: light and electron microscopic studies. Histol Histopathol 1986; 1:203-12.
29. Kummer W, Gibbins IL, Heym C. Peptidergic innervation of arterial chemoreceptors. Arch Histol Cytol 1989; 52: 361-4.
30. Lundberg JM, Hokfelt T, Fahrenkrug J et al. Peptides in the cat carotid body (glomus caroticum): VIP-, enkephalin-, and substance P-like immunoreactivity. Acta Physiol Scand 1979; 107:279-81.
31. Hohler B, Mayer B, Kummer W. Nitric oxide synthase in the rat carotid body and carotid sinus. Cell Tissue Res 1994; 276:559-64.
32. Wang ZZ, Stensaas LJ, Bredt DS et al. Localization and actions of nitric oxide in the cat carotid body. Neuroscience 1994; 60:275-86.
33. Prabhakar NR, Kumar GK, Chang CH et al. Nitric oxide in the sensory function of the carotid body. Brain Res 1993; 625:16-22.
34. Wang ZZ, Stensaas LJ, Dinger BG et al. Nitric oxide mediates chemoreceptor inhibition in the cat carotid body. Neuroscience 1995; 65:217-29.
35. Tanaka K, Chiba T. Nitric oxide synthase containing neurons in the carotid body and sinus of the guinea pig. Micro Res and Tech 1994; 29:90-3.
36. Grimes PA, Lahiri S, Stone R et al. Nitric oxide synthase occurs in neurons and nerve fibers of the carotid body. Adv Exp Med Bio 1994; 360:221-4.
37. Ciriello J, Hochstenbach SL, Roder S. Central projections of baroreceptor and chemoreceptor afferent fibers in the rat. In: Robin I and Barraco A, eds. Nucleus of the Solitary Tract. Boca Raton: CRC Press, 1994:35-50.
38. Kalia M, Sullivan JM. Brainstem projections of sensory and motor components of the vagus nerve in the rat. J Comp Neurol 1982; 211:248-65.
39. Housley GD, Sinclair JD. Localization by kainic acid lesions of neurones transmitting the carotid chemoreceptor stimulus for respiration in rat. J Physiol 1988; 406:99-114.
40. Davies RO, Kalia M. Carotid sinus nerve projections to the brain stem in the cat. Brain Res Bull 1981; 6:531-41.
41. Hunt SP, Pini A, Evan G. Induction of c-fos-like protein in spinal cord neurons following sensory stimulation. Nature 1987; 328:632-4.
42. Morgan JI, Curran T. Stimulus-transcription coupling in the nervous system: involvement of the inducible proto-oncogenes *fos* and *jun*. Annu Rev Neurosci 1991; 14:412-51.
43. Erickson JT, Millhorn DE. Fos-like protein is induced in neurons of the medulla oblongata after stimulation of the carotid sinus nerve in awake and anesthetized rats. Brain Res 1991; 567:11-24.
44. Erickson JT, Millhorn DE. Hypoxia and electrical stimulation of the carotid sinus nerve induce fos-like immunoreactivity within catecholaminergicand serotonergic neurons of the rat brainstem. J Comp Neurol 1994; 348:161-82.
45. Larnicol N, Wallois F, Berquin P et al. c-fos-like immunoreactivity in the cat's neuraxis following moderate hypoxia or hypercapnia. J Physiol 1994; 88:81-8.
46. Li YW, Dampney RAL. Expression of fos-like protein in brain following sustained hypertension and hypotension in conscious rabbits. Neuroscience 1994; 61:613-34.
47. Murphy AZ, Ennis M, Shipley MT et al. Directionally specific changes in arterial pressure induce differential patterns of fos expression in discrete areas of the rat brainstem: A double-labeling study for fos and catecholamines. J Comp Neurol 1994; 349:36-50.
48. Chan RKW, Sawchenko PE. Spatially and temporally differentiated patterns of c-fos expression in brainstem catecholaminer-

gic cell groups induced by cardiovascular challenges in the rat. J Comp Neurol 1994; 348:433-60.
49. Katz DM, Erb MJ. Developmental regulation of tyrosine hydroxylase expression in primary sensory neurons of the rat. Dev Biol 1990; 137:233-42.
50. Katz DM, He H, White M. Transient expression of somatostatin peptide is a widespread feature of developing sensory and sympathetic neurons in the embryonic rat. J Neurobiol 1992; 23:855-70.
51. Kondo H. A light and electron microscopic study on the embryonic development of the rat carotid body. Am J Anat 1975; 144:275-93.
52. Rogers DC. The development of the rat carotid body. J Anat 1965; 99:89-101.
53. Hertzberg T, Fan G, Finley JCW et al. BDNF supports mammalian chemoafferent neurons in vitro and following peripheral target removal in vivo. Dev Biol 1994; 166:801-11.
54. Thaler CD, Suhr L, Ip N et al. Leukemia inhibitory factor and neurotrophins support overlapping populations of rat nodose sensory neurons in culture. Dev Biol 1994; 161:338-44.
55. Erickson JT, Smeyne RJ, Barbacid M et al. Visceral sensory neurons are severely depleted in mice lacking functional trkB protein tyrosine kinase receptors. [Abstract] Society for Neuroscience 1994.
56. JT Erickson, JC Conover, V Borday et al. Transgenic mice lacking BDNF exhibit visceral sensory neuron losses distinct from mice lacking NT4 and display a severe developmental deficit in control of breathing. J Neurosci 1996; 16: 5361-5371.

CHAPTER 10

Systemic Responses Elicited by Stimulating the Carotid Body: Primary and Secondary Mechanisms

Robert S. Fitzgerald and Machiko Shirahata

INTRODUCTION

The Nobel Prize for Physiology or Medicine was awarded to Corneille J.F. Heymans in 1938 "for the discovery of the role played by the sinus and aortic mechanisms in the regulation of respiration" (Fig. 10.1). Investigators of the 1920s and 1930s turned primarily to the systemic impact of this tiny taster of arterial blood, not to its mode of operation. Today, in addition to its physiological significance and role in maintaining organismal homeostasis, carotid body researchers are trying to uncover how it transduces decreases in arterial pH (pH_a) or partial pressure of oxygen in the arterial blood (P_aO_2), or increases in partial pressure of carbon dioxide (P_aCO_2) into increased neural output from the carotid body to the nucleus tractus solitarius (NTS) in the medulla via the glossopharyngeal nerve. It is this activity processed in the central nervous system which generates an impressive array of reflex responses (Fig. 10.2).

NEUROANATOMY

The NTS is like New York's Grand Central Station when it comes to the processing of information coming in from the periphery. Important for cardiopulmonary homeostasis, input via the ninth cranial nerve is accompanied by input from the vagus nerve. Such critically important information as arterial pressure, the status of the pulmonary receptors mediating airway stretch (as during the respiratory cycle), irritation (from environmental pollutants provoking cough), and interstitial pressure (signaling pulmonary edema) come to this station, as does information from the low pressure baroreceptors in the vena cava and right heart.

The Carotid Body Chemoreceptors,
edited by Constancio González.

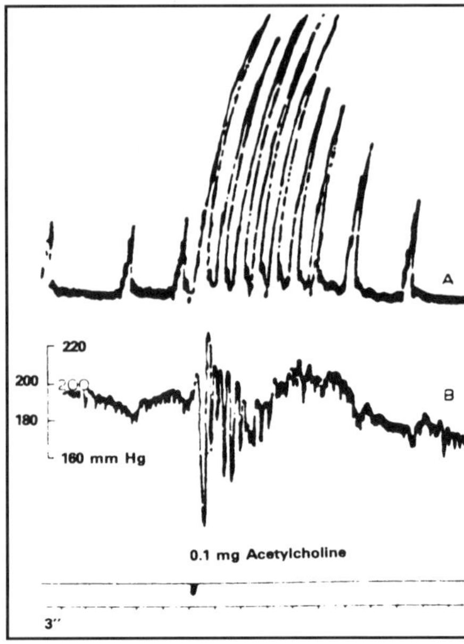

Fig. 10.1. Corneille Heymans received the 1938 Nobel Prize in Physiology or Medicine "for the discovery of the role played by the sinus and aortic mechanisms in the regulation of respiration." In his December 12, 1945 lecture he used this figure to show the respiratory (A) and the arterial pressure responses (B) to an injection of 0.1 mg of acetylcholine (marker at bottom). Timer at bottom marks 3 second intervals. Note the transient hyperpnea, bradycardia, and hypertension. (Adapted from Heymans[1]).

Input from the unmyelinated carotid chemoreceptor fibers enters the dorsomedial medulla going on to three subnuclei of the NTS, the medial, commissural, and lateral (see chapters 9 and 12). On the basis of antidromic mapping the ratio of ipsilateral/contralateral input into the three subnuclei is 6/1, 5/2 and 2/0, respectively. Some of this input is then projected down the cord to the motor neurons of the respiratory muscles. But it is also processed centrally for distribution to the sympathetic and parasympathetic systems. For the former five key areas innervate sympathetic preganglionic outflow: paraventricular hypothalamic nucleus, A5 noradrenergic cell group, caudal raphe region, rostral ventrolateral medulla, and ventromedial medulla. For the parasympathetic system input via the NTS is distributed to such nuclei as the Edinger-Westphal, superior and inferior salivatory, facial, dorsal vagal nuclei, and the nucleus ambiguus. The autonomic nervous system produces the changes in smooth and cardiac muscles, the glands responsible for the changes in hormonal and airways secretions, and in such mechanical variables as pump rate and volume, and flows, resistances and capacitances in the vessels and airways.

HISTORY

The initial report on the carotid body appears to have come from the laboratory of the great German physiologist Albrecht von Haller who presided at the thesis defense of his student Hartwig Wilhelm Louis Taube on January 31, 1743. The thesis was anatomical in content as were the subsequent descriptions of the carotid body up into the present century. Refining the neural relationships and the microscopic anatomy predominated research in this area until the early 20th century. But as these studies continued, other investigators were showing that reflex cardiovascular events occurred when the carotid sinus area was stimulated. Two very important contributors to this, preceding the prize-winning studies of Heymans, were G. Pagano and L. Siciliano. In 1900 they occluded the common carotid artery and observed tachycardia and hypertension. And when they injected blood into the central end of the common carotid artery, they observed hypotension and bradycardia. Siciliano also noted that occlusion of the carotid artery generated intense changes in respiration. Both of these early investigators thought the cardiopulmonary responses were reflexes

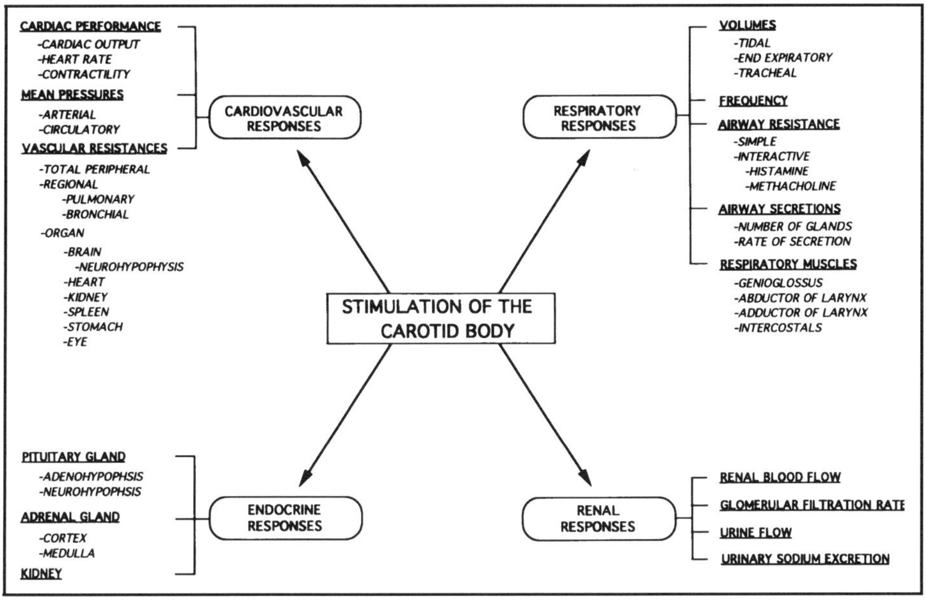

Fig. 10.2. Stimulation of the carotid body produces a remarkable array of reflex responses. What the carotid body produces when all other inputs are held constant is not always what is observed in the normally responding organism because of the interaction of inputs from more than one receptor.

whose origins were in the carotid region (Gallego[2] reviews this interesting period of carotid body studies.)

Ewald Hering in the mid-1920s showed that either electrical or mechanical stimulation at the bifurcation of the common carotid artery—known as the carotid sinus or bulb—generated cardiovascular changes which he called the "sinus reflex." He also demonstrated that a branch of the glossopharyngeal nerve innervated the carotid bulb. The nerve became known as the "sinus nerve" and later as "Hering's nerve." This is the same Hering after whom the Hering-Breuer reflex is named. Hering's name was put in candidacy to share the Nobel Prize with Heymans. The Committee, however, ultimately failed to include him for the award.

Heymans received many awards for his contributions to physiology. But in a very real sense he, too, "stood on the shoulders of giants". Certainly none more so than Fernando de Castro, an eminent Spanish histologist, who in 1928 speculated on the role of the carotid body: "organe sensoriel spécial dédié à percevoir quelques modifications qualitatives du sang, plutôt que d'un appareil destiné à recevoir les variations de la pression sanguine." Heymans considered de Castro's description of the carotid body's histology to be "very precise and detailed," and thought his speculation as to the role of the carotid body was especially valuable because it was data-based. Heymans acknowledged that de Castro's work formed the basis of his own working hypothesis. Indeed, he invited de Castro to come to Ghent to collaborate in some experiments, which de Castro never did.

Subsequent investigators, taking the lead of Heymans and his coworkers, initially emphasized the reflex effects—primarily respiratory and circulatory—of carotid body stimulation. But from the mid-1950s research efforts have also focused on determining the chemotransductive mechanisms in the carotid body; these are treated elsewhere in this volume (see chapter 5).

REFLEX RESPONSES—A CAUTION

Stimulation of the carotid body, while maintaining constant input from other receptors, can generate a very wide array of reflex responses (Fig. 10.2). However, at the outset it should be appreciated that in the in situ situation these reflexes may or may not be observed. Even though the "hard wiring" for a particular reflex can be demonstrated, the real-life reflex response may be masked by a more powerful receptor-afferent pathway-centers-efferent pathway-effector combination. Failure to appreciate this leads to data which appears to be contradictory, and sometimes to needless controversy.

RESPIRATORY RESPONSES

Resting Ventilation

Most obvious of the respiratory reflex responses of the respiratory system is the increased ventilation observed when the stimulus is either selectively applied to the carotid body or when it is in the form of systemic hypoxia. The increase in ventilation is frequently reported to be achieved by a larger increase in rate than in tidal volume. But the carotid body also responds to increased CO_2 or H^+ in the arterial blood. And hypoxia has been shown to increase the slope of the linear ventilatory response to hypercapnia in several species. This hypoxia-induced change in the CO_2-ventilation slope is also found in the carotid body neural output of the anesthetized cat.[3,4] Bisgard and his colleagues[5] have shown in the awake goat that selectively perfusing the carotid body with blood becoming progressively more hypoxic produced a larger increase in several ventilatory variables when the blood was hypercapnic than when it was normocapnic. Interaction at the carotid body was translated into the animal's ventilatory response as well. These ventilatory responses to carotid body stimulation (as well as the circulatory reflex responses) can be significantly altered by changing pressures in the neighboring carotid sinus.[6] The role of the carotid body in resting ventilation is significant, sometimes appraised as being responsible for between 20 and 40%. Daristotle recently showed that in goats selective perfusion of the carotid body with hypocapnic blood reduced resting ventilation by 70%.[7]

Resting ventilation during pregnancy increases. Though surely part of this is a central nervous system-based process, there are several studies which report that progesterone and estrogen increase the ventilatory response to hypoxia.[8,9] In pregnant cats the increased response to hypoxia was traced to increased sensitivity of the carotid bodies.[10] Testosterone also increases carotid body sensitivity to hypoxia.[11]

Ventilation During Exercise

The organism is either at rest or in some form of exercise. Mechanisms responsible for the increased ventilation during exercise remain only partially understood (Wasserman et al[12] and Dempsey et al[13] for review). Much evidence continues to support a significant role for the carotid body in the human ventilatory increase during exercise. But others[14] have felt that the carotid bodies work only minimally during submaximal exercise. However, there is good evidence that in humans they are singularly sensitive to and protective of variations in arterial pH encountered in the metabolic acidosis of heavy exercise. Additionally, they seem to be the first receptors to respond to the increased flow of CO_2 to the lungs.[15] If, in the laboratory, hypoxia is combined with exercise, the carotid bodies can account for as much as 75% of the increase in ventilation in humans.

In human subjects the exogenous administration of dopamine usually reduces ventilation. Plasma arterial potassium (K^+) increases in exercising human subjects; in one report changes in arterial plasma K^+ closely mirrored ventilatory changes both during exercise and recovery. But whereas dopamine diminished the ventilatory response to hypoxia, it had no effect on the ventilatory response during exercise.[16] Beta blockade in anesthetized cats reduced the sensitivity of the arterial chemoreceptors to increases in arterial K^+.[17] However, this is in contrast to humans and goats where there is evidence that beta adrenergic systems are not operating in the carotid body.[18,19]

Acclimatization

One of the most frequent nonlaboratory situations in which the carotid body plays a major role is in the acclimatization to altitude. Here the carotid body is paramount in the ventilatory response to the reduced partial pressure of oxygen. The work of Bisgard, Forster, Dempsey and their colleagues have contributed much to our current knowledge of how acclimatized ventilation evolves.[20] A feature of ventilatory acclimatization to hypoxia in goats, where the process occurs more rapidly than in other species, was an increase in hypoxic ventilatory sensitivity. This reinforces the key role of the carotid bodies in the process.[21] Indeed, at least part of this appears to be due to the carotid body increasing its sensitivity to hypoxia.[22] One could propose that this consists in the carotid body reducing its sensitivity to the inhibitory influences of dopamine or norepinephrine. However, this appears not to be the case.[23] Central nervous system mechanisms seem not to be involved in the acclimatization to hypoxia in goats.[24,25] Further, at least in goats, neither cerebral hypoxia nor hypocapnic alkalosis are needed to produce acclimatization.[26] Nor, finally, is the impact of systemic hypoxia anywhere else in the organism.[27] It is a phenomenon which appears to be solidly based in the carotid body. Acclimatization to both short-term and to long-term hypoxia remains a very complicated process, however, involving even the somewhat paradoxical (at least in this context) decline in ventilation that is observed after 10-15 minutes exposure to hypoxia in many species. An excellent review of the issues and concerning acclimatization is presented by Bisgard and Neubauer.[28]

Ventilation in the Newborn

That carotid bodies are important in the newborn is very clear (see chapter 11). Though subresponsive at birth, the carotid bodies quickly mature and play a major role in controlling ventilation in the newborn. If they are removed from the newborn, periods of extended apnea and frequently death ensue[29] (see Haddad et al[30] for review). Sudden Infant Death syndrome (SIDS) involves cardiorespiratory failure; and it seems reasonable to infer some form of carotid body malfunction (see chapter 12 by Pásaro and Ribas). However, a recent report[31] in which the carotid bodies from SIDS victims were compared to those of children who died of cystic fibrosis or congestive heart failure concluded that there were no significant findings to indicate that the carotid bodies play a direct role in the etiopathogenesis of SIDS.

Phillipson and his colleagues have explored the effect of aging on the carotid bodies of dogs,[32] and concluded that aging was accompanied by impairment of ventilatory and arousal responses to hypoxia during slow wave sleep. This effect was attributed to the aging of the carotid bodies as opposed to brainstem mechanisms or the respiratory neuromuscular system.

COPD

Surgical removal of the carotid bodies has been performed to alleviate the dyspnea encountered in chronic obstructive pulmonary disease (COPD). There is physiological rationale for such a procedure. For example, removing the carotid bodies removes the hypoxic drive to breathe in patients whose breathing is obstructed. Their "out-of-breathness" is reduced. Further, stimulation of the carotid bodies does increase airways resistance. Nonetheless, such surgery is extremely controversial because of attendant dangers due to the carotid body's proximity to the carotid sinus, so important in the regulation of blood pressure. And there has been no consistent pattern of improvement in the significant respiratory variables. Whipp and Ward recently concluded from their survey of 146 severely obstructed patients who had undergone bilateral carotid body resection (BCBR)[33] that the individual patient responses to the procedure were highly variable. The typical result was a small increase in hypoxemia and hypercapnia with no further impairment of pulmonary function. Almitrine bimesylate is a carotid body-stimulating drug frequently prescribed for COPD patients. DeBacker et al[34] found that in humans the well-documented almitrine-induced improvement in the ventilation/perfusion relationship is mediated only through carotid body stimulation, and that it had no effect in BCBR patients.

Static Respiratory Volumes

End expiratory volume (functional residual capacity)—a static lung volume—has also been reported to increase with either selective carotid body perfusion or systemic hypoxia in dogs, rabbits,[35] rats,[36] and human subjects.[37] Whipp and Ward in their study cited above reported that on average the patients' FRC decreased after BCBR.[33] In anesthetized dogs the volume of the trachea decreases when the carotid body is stimulated; it is a vagally mediated response.[38]

Airways Resistance

Stimulation of the carotid body provokes airway smooth muscle contraction, increasing airways resistance.[38] This reflex effect positively interacts with the local effect of either inhaled histamine[39] or methacholine[40] (Fig. 10.3). But the reflex response of the airways during hypoxia can be complicated since hypoxia relaxes airway smooth muscle in vitro. Hence when the intact organism is exposed to hypoxia, one might see a smaller increase in airways resistance due to the local effect of hypoxia counteracting the vagal response to carotid body stimulation.

Perhaps also contributing to an increase in resistance is the impact of carotid body stimulation on airways secretions, though so far this has been measured only in the trachea where the impact on resistance would seem to be negligible. However, the importance of airways secretions in the mucociliary transport of materials out of the airways cannot be overestimated. In anesthetized dogs carotid body stimulation significantly increased both the number of submucosal glands secreting and the rate at which they secreted[41] (Fig. 10.4). This effect may be the result of, or at least influenced by, the increase in bronchial blood flow also observed upon carotid body stimulation.[42]

Respiratory Muscles

Though carotid body stimulation in the laboratory setting produces an *increase* in airways resistance, presumably by provoking smooth muscle contraction, one generally finds that the contraction of the striated muscles of the upper airways produced by carotid body stimulation *reduces* airway resistance. Beginning with the alae nasi, van Lunteren and his colleagues[43] reported that in anesthetized dogs hypercapnia and hypoxia produced a shortening of the muscles during inspiration, an effect which was greater when airflow was obstructed, implying an inhibitory input from the pulmonary stretch receptors. Carotid body stimulation by sodium cyanide injection also induces an increase in nasal vascular resistance in anesthetized dogs with a simultaneous reduction in nasal airway resistance, an effect abolished by nasal sympathectomy.[44] England and her colleagues,[45] studying the pattern of laryngeal muscle contraction during wakefulness, slow wave sleep, and REM sleep in dogs, reported that hypercapnia and hypoxia generated significant contraction of laryngeal abductors, even during expiration when airflow was high, but only rare activation of the thyroarytenoid, a laryngeal adductor. The state of wakefulness made no difference. Consistent with this finding is the report that the carotid body provides a powerful excitatory input to inspiratory hypoglossal motoneurons during both inspiration and expiration.[46]

An interesting question has been raised as to whether the increased ventilation triggered by hypoxia and by hypercapnia was achieved with an identical use of the respiratory muscles. The study of Yasuma et al[47] in awake dogs reported that the EMGs of the external oblique and of the transversus abdominis, analyzed as a function of tidal volume, were the same for a given tidal volume whether it had been generated by hypercapnia or hypoxia. However, the diaphragmatic EMG was consistently greater

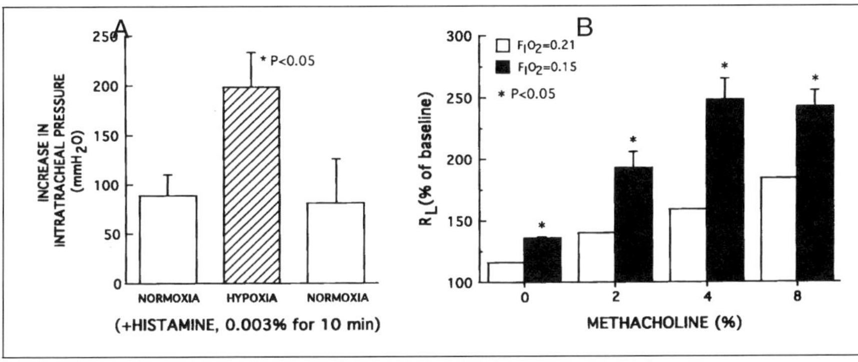

Fig. 10.3. Though the reflex hyperpnea in response to carotid body stimulation is well-known, less appreciated is the ability of the carotid body to amplify the response of the airways to histamine and methacholine challenges. (A) In anesthetized dogs; effect of hypoxia on mean (±SEM) reflex tracheal constriction induced by 10 minutes of inhaling 0.003% histamine solution; effect of hypoxia on response was abolished after bilateral sinus nerve section. Adapted from Tsuchiya et al.[39] (B) In awake normoxic or hypoxic sheep; mean (±SEM) response of total pulmonary resistance (RL) to aerosolized methacholine (% in phosphate buffered solutions). Adapted from Denjean et al.[40]

during hypoxia than during hypercapnia. This is consistent with Fitzgerald's study 20 years earlier in anesthetized cats[48] which demonstrated that there was much greater phrenic nerve output for a given tidal volume during hypoxia than during hypercapnia. However, this seems not to be the case in awake dogs.[49]

The behavior of the respiratory muscles during sleep is very much a concern in patients who suffer from Obstructive Sleep Apnea (OSA). Upper airway resistance is greater during sleep, and apnea produces hypoxemia and hypercapnia. If stimulation of the carotid body has a greater impact on activating muscles of the upper airways than on the diaphragm, then such activation would open the airways, overcoming the momentary subatmospheric pressure created by the contracting diaphragm. Using anesthetized rats, Oku et al[50] who had observed that carotid body stimulation produced preferential activation of upper airway respiratory muscles during both hypercapnia and hypoxemia, found that during hypoxia electrical activity in the hypoglossal nerve increased significantly more than phrenic nerve activity. This observation is consistent with that of Gauda et al in the anesthetized cat.[51] Further, using the neonatal pig, Martin et al[52] found the response of the diaphragm EMG to hypoxia to be biphasic, an increase followed by a decrease to prehypoxic levels after 10 minutes of 12% oxygen. On the other hand, the EMG of the muscles of the upper airways all remained significantly above control. In contrast to these findings Parisi et al[53] reported a more constant linkage of diaphragmatic and genioglossal EMG activation patterns in chronically instrumented goats during wakefulness, slow wave sleep and during REM sleep in response to hypoxia and hypercapnia.

CIRCULATORY RESPONSES

That the carotid body has significant impact on the cardiovascular as well as on the respiratory system is not surprising, given the involvement of each with tissue oxygenation. Many strategies are brought into play as the organism tries to cope with a hypoxic challenge. This overview will confine itself to what we shall call the "mechanical variables" of the cardiovascular system; i.e., the rate, volume, and contractility of the pump and the pressures, flows, resistances, and capacitances of the tubing. Initially the

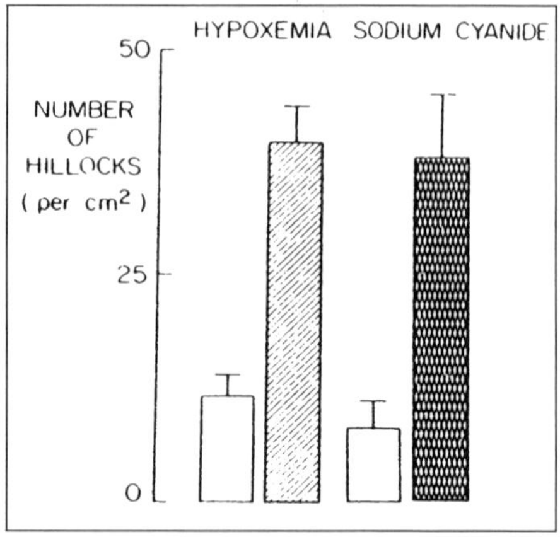

Fig. 10.4. In anesthetized dogs; Mean (±SEM) secretion from tracheal submucosal glands after 90 sec of normoxia ($PaO_2 = 99 \pm 6$ mmHg; open bar) vs 90 sec of hypoxemia ($PaO_2 = 27 \pm 4$ mmHg; cross-hatched bar), or an injection of saline (open bar) vs an injection of cyanide (25-75 mg in the carotid artery; cross-hatched bar). "Hillock" = small dark elevation on the tantalum-dusted trachea, indication of a gland secreting. From Davis et al.[41]

responses of these variables to selective stimulation of the carotid body will be presented, minimizing inputs from other receptors. However, as described above, stimulation of the carotid body evokes an increase in tidal volume. This stimulates pulmonary stretch receptors, which in turn have their own impact on the cardiovascular system. A sampling of such interactions will be presented at the end of this section. There are excellent, more detailed reviews of the impact of these factors.[54-56] Further complicating the picture are the perennial differences that frequently exist among species, and the differences due to the level of consciousness in the animal—awake, asleep, or anesthetized; in the last case, different anesthetics have different effects.

Cardiac Performance

If respiration and input from other neural influences are controlled, then selective stimulation of the carotid body produces bradycardia and an increase in systemic blood pressure.[57-61] Cardiac output is reported to decrease along with the bradycardia. The inotropic effect of carotid body stimulation, however, is not altogether clear. If heart rate, ventricular pre- and after-loads are kept constant, then one can observe a decrease in dP/dt_{max}, an index of cardiac contractility. Others have reported an increase in contractility, however.[62-66] If systemic blood pressure is held constant during a transient stimulation to the right carotid body in the anesthetized, paralyzed, ventilated cat, one observes an increase in activity of the left cardiac sympathetic nerve (and vice versa), simultaneously with a decrease in heart rate.[67] In the same preparation with constant heart rate systemic hypoxia, generated by providing either low PO_2 or carbon monoxide to the respirator, produces both an increase in cardiac output and an increase in dP/dt_{max} if the carotid body, aortic body, or both are operating. If they are not sending neural traffic to the NTS, then there is no increase in cardiac output and a decrease in contractility.[68]

Systemic Pressures

The increase in mean arterial pressure is due to vasoconstriction in many of the principal beds--skeletal muscle, splanchnic, kidney. So the increase in systemic blood pressure observed with carotid body stimulation selectively or with systemic hypoxia may arise from different sources—heart rate, stroke volume and/or peripheral resistance. Mean circulatory pressure—the pressure in the central veins of an animal with a fibrillating heart—also increases with carotid body stimulation, indicating contraction of the capacitance vessels.

It is pertinent to note here that the carotid bodies of borderline hypertensive patients have an increased sensitivity; these subjects show an exaggerated sympathetic response to hypoxic hypoxia.[69-71] The hypertension seen in patients with obstructive sleep apnea also seems attributable to carotid body pathology.[72]

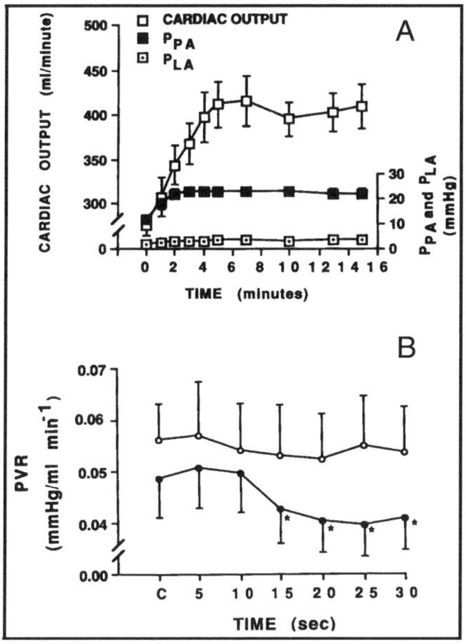

Fig. 10.5. (A) In anesthetized, paralyzed, aortic body-resected cats ventilated on 10% O_2 in N_2; mean (±SEM) cardiac output, pulmonary arterial and left atrial pressures (PPA, PLA). There is no significant increase in pressures after 1-2 min while cardiac output has not yet reached 50% of its maximum, suggesting an active vasodilation. (B) In anesthetized, paralyzed, room air-ventilated cats receiving a brief selective perfusion of the carotid bodies with cats's own arterial blood (open symbols) or with venous blood containing 0.3-0.5 mg NaCN (closed symbols). With no sustained significant change in cardiac output, there was a significant 17% decrease in the driving pressure (PPA minus alveolar pressure) generating this reduction in pulmonary vascular resistance (PVR); * = $p < 0.05$. Adapted from Fitzgerald et al.[80]

Vascular Resistances

As mentioned above, selective stimulation of the carotid bodies in the normoxic animal produces an increase in total peripheral resistance. As can be easily imagined, if systemic hypoxia is the stimulus, then there is a decrease in total peripheral resistance which is much less if the peripheral arterial chemoreceptors are intact; this seems to indicate a local vasodilatory effect of the hypoxia being offset somewhat by carotid body-stimulated sympathetic output to the vasculature.

Pulmonary

Investigations into a role for the carotid bodies in controlling the pulmonary vasculature have generated a significant amount of conflicting results. Daly first proposed that selective carotid body stimulation in the anesthetized dog induced a decrease in pulmonary vascular resistance.[73] In subsequent studies, in which he eliminated the bronchial circulation, however, the same procedure generated an increase in pulmonary vascular resistance.[74,75] The decrease reported in the earlier study was attributed to a parasympathetically mediated reflex bronchial vasodilatation. Others, using different techniques in anesthetized and unanesthetized dogs and cats,[76-80] have generated data which strongly suggests that carotid body stimulation blunts the well-known pulmonary vasoconstrictor response to alveolar hypoxia. For example, when the anesthetized, paralyzed, ventilated cat was exposed to hypoxic hypoxia for 15 minutes, cardiac output and the driving pressure (pulmonary arterial pressure minus left atrial pressure) both rose over the first minute. After that, the cardiac output continued to increase by another 80% over the control value, while the driving pressure changed little. This translates to a large decrease in pulmonary vascular resistance (Fig. 10.5). It is difficult to imagine how this large decrease could be attributed to changes in the bronchial circulation which receives, at least in sheep, only 1% of the total cardiac output.

Bronchial, Tracheal, Nasal

Like the pulmonary vasculature response to selective carotid body stimulation bronchial blood flow increases significantly with a decrease in bronchial vascular resistance.[42] In contrast to the bronchial and pulmonary vasodilatory response to carotid body stimulation, tracheal vascular resistance in the anesthetized dog and nasal vascular in the anesthetized sheep increased.[44,81]

Cerebral

Perhaps even more controversial than the effect of the carotid body on the pulmonary vasculature is the effect of carotid body stimulation on the cerebral vasculature. Again, there seems to be a discrepancy in the data which may be the result of the two different techniques used: (a) clearance of radiolabeled gases, or (b) localization of radiolabeled microspheres. The cerebral vasculature is innervated by the sympathetic and probably the parasympathetic systems. Selective carotid body stimulation in the dog has produced vasodilatation.[82-84] Sectioning of the carotid sinus nerves abolished the response. Others, using cat or dog with selective carotid body stimulation or systemic hypoxia, have found no influence of the carotid bodies.[85-90] In the unanesthetized dog with controlled ventilation selective carotid body stimulation increased and then decreased blood flow in the middle cerebral artery, signaling an increase in cerebral artery resistance. Carotid sinus nerve section abolished the effect as did cervical sympathectomy. The results were interpreted as supporting a cerebral vasoconstrictor role for the carotid body.[91,92] Studies in other conscious species suggest that the carotid body probably does play a role in the autonomic control of the cerebral vasculature[93,94] perhaps influencing one region more than another.

However, an interesting exception to those data suggesting that the carotid body does not influence the cerebral vasculature in the anesthetized dog is the study of Hanley and his colleagues[95] who observed that blood flow in the neurohypophysis increased during hypoxic hypoxia, but not during carbon monoxide hypoxia (carbon monoxide does not stimulate the carotid body, though it does stimulate the aortic body). The vasodilatation due to hypoxic hypoxia was abolished after sectioning the carotid sinus and vagus nerves (Fig. 10.6). A carotid body-mediated increase in total blood flow in the eye has also been reported in the anesthetized cat. Again, carbon monoxide hypoxia had no significant effect.[96]

Coronary

Carotid body stimulation in the anesthetized dog with controlled ventilation and heart rate reduces coronary vascular resistance. But there is also evidence that carotid body stimulation can produce both reflex a adrenoceptor-mediated constriction of large and small coronary arteries and a vagally-mediated dilatation to balance the small vessel constriction. Hence, both branches of the autonomic nervous system innervating the coronary vasculature are activated by carotid body stimulation in controlled conditions (see Kollai et al[67]).

Muscle

When investigators speak of the impact of carotid body stimulation on the vascular resistance of skeletal muscle, usually the reference is to limb muscle. In most species when ventilation is held constant, carotid body stimulation produces a vasoconstriction.

Splanchnic, Splenic

In most species tested carotid body stimulation under conditions of controlled ventilation provokes a generalized vasoconstriction in the splanchnic bed. Splanchnic veins also constrict in response to carotid body stimulation,[97] and in a different pattern than in the skeletal muscle veins, which do not. This may be due to the supply of sympathetic nerves to the splanchnic but not to the muscle veins. Splenic vasculature constricts under the conditions described above when the carotid body is stimulated. Interestingly, the spleen shows an increase in vascular resistance in the hypoxia-challenged, anesthetized, paralyzed, ventilated cat without input from either carotid or aortic bodies. The increase in resistance is even larger when the chemoreceptors are operating.[96]

Renal

Vasoconstriction in the kidney is the common result of carotid body stimulation

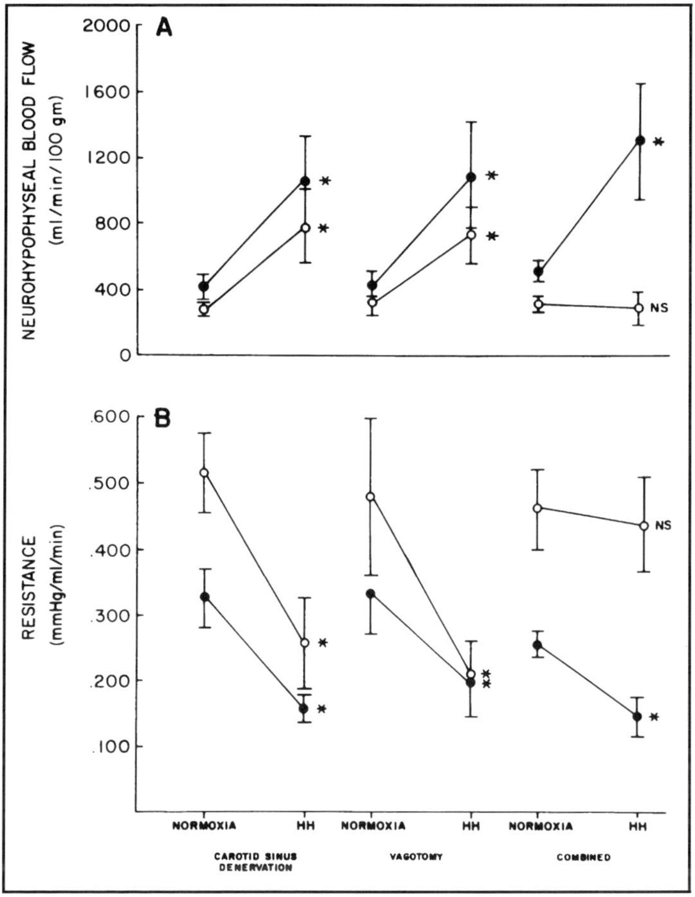

Fig. 10.6. In anesthetized, paralyzed, ventilated dogs, intact (closed dots) and post-denervation (open dots) mean (±SEM) responses in neurohypophyseal blood flow (A) and neurohypophyseal vascular resistance (B) under control conditions (Normoxia) and while being ventilated with 8% O_2 in N_2 (HH). * = $p < 0.05$, comparing Normoxia with HH. From Hanley et al.[95]

in a controlled preparation of most species. However, when another input, like local hypoxia, is present, the results can be different. In the anesthetized, paralyzed, ventilated cat, systemic hypoxia generated no change in the vascular resistance of the kidney, perhaps due to the strong vasodilatory effect of local hypoxia competing with the sympathetic input.[96]

CARDIOVASCULAR INTERACTIONS: EFFECTS OF CAROTID BODY INPUT INTERACTING WITH...

Up to this point we have only mentioned a few instances of the impact on the cardiovascular system when carotid body input interacts with other input into the NTS. It is both interesting and helpful to broaden one's appreciation of the extent to which afferent information from other receptors can modify carotid body input. A brief consideration of carotid body interactions with the carotid sinus baroreceptors, with the pulmonary stretch receptors, with laryngeal chemoreceptors, and with the "inspiratory drive" originating in the central nervous system will underline the complexity of the in situ cardiovascular responses to carotid body stimulation. For other influences on carotid body input (e.g., temperature, acid-base status) see Fitzgerald and Lahiri.[98]

Arterial Baroreceptors

The magnitude of the cardiovascular response elicited by carotid body stimulation depends on arterial pressure or on pressure in the carotid sinus.[6,99,100] The same statement could be made about the impact of the arterial baroreceptors on the respiratory responses elicited by carotid body stimulation. Stimulation of the baroreceptors per se evokes bradycardia, vasodilatation, and hypopnea. In several preparations the simultaneous stimulation of carotid body and carotid sinus abolished the carotid body-generated increase in vascular resistance in muscle, splanchnic bed and kidney.[99-102]

Pulmonary Stretch Receptors

During hyperpnea, pulmonary stretch receptors generate tachycardia and vasodilation. This is so strong in some species that when the hyperpnea is generated by carotid body stimulation, the tachycardia and vasodilation override the bradycardia and vasoconstriction of carotid body origin. The stretch receptor influence appears to be stronger in dogs than in cats, but it is also expression in rats.[103] In awake sheep the role of the stretch receptors is so powerful that it completely masks any effect of carotid body stimulation on several vascular resistances.[104] It is interesting to note that in cats pulmonary stretch receptors block the carotid body-induced bradycardia, but were ineffective against the bradycardia generated by pulmonary C fibers.[105]

Laryngeal Receptors

When the laryngeal area, sensitive to several chemicals, is stimulated, apnea is the response. This is especially well-developed in the newborn, where carotid body stimulation reduces the length of the apnea; carotid body inhibition, prolongs it. Also, it appears that in the newborn lamb normal carotid body function is important for the control of the laryngeal response to stimuli.[106] Carotid body-stimulated hindlimb vasoconstriction and bradycardia were enhanced by laryngeal input.[107]

Central Inspiratory Drive

The last influence on the cardiovascular responses to carotid body stimulation to be considered is that originating in the central nervous system. An example of this influence is seen in the normal respiratory sinus arrhythmia, an increase in heart rate during inspiration; decrease, during expiration. Carotid body input during the phases of respiration even in the absence of input from the pulmonary stretch receptors has different effects on vagal and sympathetic fibers to the heart and to the vasculature. The source of this difference comes from a complexus of nuclei located for the most part in the brainstem. The central pattern generator or central inspiratory activity is frequently described as if it was an autonomously operating neural source. Indeed, one theory of respiratory rhythm generation was the "Pacemaker Theory" in which cells in the brainstem were reported to have their own intrinsic firing pattern driving the respiratory cycle, like cardiac pacemaker cells are capable of driving the heart.

However, some later observations bring the real life efficacy of such "autonomous" centers into question. Kolobow and his colleagues[108] observed in unanesthetized lambs that if CO_2 was removed from the venous blood by an extracorporeal membrane "lung" (like a kidney dialyser) in the same amount as the lamb was producing it metabolically, and if a slight positive pressure was placed on a room air-containing spirometer connected to a chronic tracheostomy, the lamb stopped breathing completely. The lamb nonetheless remained conscious and alert during the experiment. Some of the lambs remained attached to the extracorporeal circuits for three days allowing for several observations in the same animal. Phillipson and his colleagues[109] have made essentially the same observations in sheep and in the dog. Arterial blood gases in these preparations remained normal during the period of apnea. Hence, one asks, "Where is the central pattern generator, the central inspiratory activity, the pacemaker cells?" It is conceivable that these "autonomous" centers need a certain level of input from the periphery which exceeds some threshold, allowing the centers to begin and maintain autonomous, periodic discharging. The mean arterial blood gases during apnea were normal in Phillipson's study; but during the apneic period the blood gases were presumably nonoscillatory. Perhaps the "threshold" to be crossed is not one of quantity but rather one of pattern. Answers to these questions are presently unavailable. What seems clear is that there is a central nervous system component which modifies carotid body input, but this component itself needs input, including metabolically produced CO_2 acting somewhere in the periphery.

What, then, is the impact of two simultaneous inputs on carotid body-generated bradycardia? The bradycardia results from increased activity in cardiac vagal fibers; this increase is attenuated when the stimulation takes place during the inspiratory phase of the nonbreathing preparation (as seen from a phrenic neurogram). Additionally, the greater the attention, the larger the phrenic activity. Not unexpectedly then, when laryngeal stimulation (input #1) abolishes central inspiratory activity (input #2), the bradycardia resulting from carotid body stimulation is intensified. It is apparent from that described above that the pulmonary stretch receptor influence would coalesce with the central inspiratory drive to block output to the heart in cardiac vagal fibers responding to carotid body stimulation. A large stimulus to the carotid body produces a large central inspiratory drive, generating large tidal volumes, flipping a carotid body stimulated bradycardia over to a tachycardia.

Turning from the modulation of carotid body stimulation of vagal influences on heart rate to the modulation of the sympathetic impact on heart rate, cardiac sympathetic fibers also show an input from the central inspiratory drive in the dog. The sinus arrhythymia in a preparation in which there is no longer feedback from the lungs' pulmonary stretch receptors, and in which vagal influence on the heart is blocked, is increased during inspiration and decreased during expiration most likely due to phasic input from cardiac sympathetic fibers. In a preparation in which the superior laryngeal nerves were stimulated, abolishing central inspiratory drive phasic activity in the sympathetic fibers ceased. There was a small decrease in heart rate and a significant vasodilatation in hindlimb muscles. Since stimulation of the carotid bodies will increase cardiac sympathetic nerve activity,[67] then if the central inspiratory activity is increased, the sympathetically mediated tachycardia is enhanced.

Clearly, the impact of the central nervous system components upon carotid body

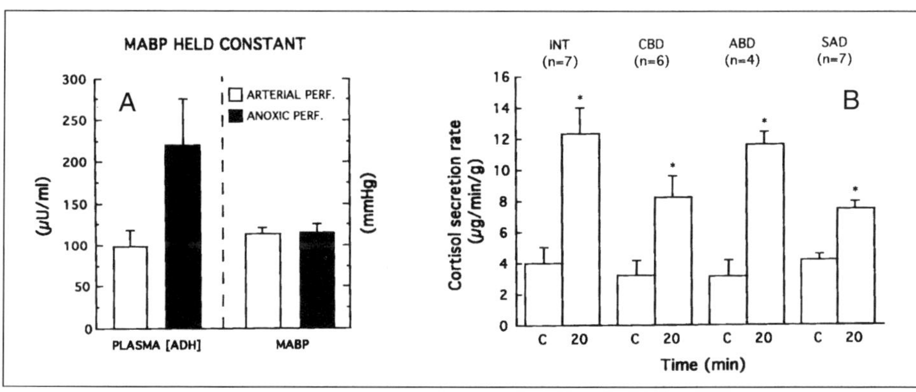

Fig. 10.7. (A) In anesthetized dogs, carotid bodies perfused with normal or deoxygenated blood mean (±SEM) response of plasma [ADH] and mean arterial pressure (MABP). Adapted from Share and Levy.[111] (B) In anesthetized, paralyzed, normocapnic dogs ventilated on room air (C) and after 20 minutes on 11% O_2 in N_2 mean (±SEM) cortisol secretion rate (CSR). Dogs were intact (INT), without carotid bodies (CBD), without aortic bodies (ABD), or without either (SAD). * = $p < 0.05$. During hypoxia (PaO_2=36mmHg) CSR increased significantly; INT = ABD > CBD = SAD. Data suggest that during hypoxia carotid body input, but not aortic body input, increases CSR. Adapted from Raff et al.[119]

stimulation of cardiac vagal and sympathetic fibers is extremely complex and any further detail is beyond the scope of this chapter.

ENDOCRINE RESPONSES

Five known endocrine structures are affected by carotid body stimulation: neurohypophysis, adenohypophysis, adrenal cortex, adrenal medulla and kidney.

Renin

In the kidney, at the juncture of the afferent arteriole to the glomerulus and the convoluted portion of the distal tubule, lies the juxtaglomerular apparatus made up of the macula densa and juxtaglomerular cells. Three stimuli promote the release of renin, responsible for the initiation of the angiotensin-aldosterone cascade: sodium load in the filtrate, blood pressure in the afferent arteriole, and sympathetic nerve activity. Though renin release in response to carotid body stimulation has not been measured, sympathetic activity to the macula densa has. Dorward et al[110] have reported that carotid body stimulation in the rabbit increased neural activity in sympathetic fibers proceeding to the macula densa. One could reasonably infer from this that renin secretion also increases with carotid body stimulation.

Vasopressin

An increase in the plasma levels of the neurohypophyseal antidiuretic hormone (ADH, vasopressin) in response to carotid body stimulation has been reported in the dog[111] (Fig. 10.7) as well as the firing of the supra-optic neurones responsible for its release in rats.[112-114] Additionally, plasma levels also rose in artificially ventilated dogs exposed to systemic hypoxic hypoxia; an effect which disappeared upon sinus and vagus nerve section.[95]

ACTH

Plasma levels of adrenocorticotrophic hormone (ACTH), released from the anterior pituitary gland (adenohypophysis), also increases with hypoxia in conscious rats[115] and in anesthetized dogs, but only when their ventilation is controlled.[116,117] Hyperventilation attenuated the response, as it does also in the case of ADH. The largest release of ACTH came in response to systemic hypoxia generated by carbon monoxide, which does not stimulate the carotid bodies.

Cortisol

Corticosteroids are released from the adrenal cortex when anesthetized dogs are exposed to systemic hypoxia, even when no peripheral arterial chemoreceptor is active (Fig. 10.7). The cortisol secretion rate is 47% of what it is in the intact dog.[118,119] With only the aortic body intact, systemic hypoxia reduces the rate to 69% of the intact value. The fact that the largest increase in plasma level of ACTH did not correlate with the largest increase in cortisol secretion rate plus the other data above were consistent with the hypothesis that under conditions of hypoxic stress corticosteroid secretion rate is the result of a multifactorial input. The arterial chemoreceptors seem to play the principal role, however.

Epinephrine, Norepinephrine

Finally the adrenal medulla releases significant amounts of both norepinephrine and epinephrine upon stimulation of the carotid bodies in rats, cats, and dogs though the ratio of catecholamines among the species is different.[120-123] This response was observed during both systemic hypoxia and during selective perfusion of the carotid bodies with hypoxic blood. The effect was not observed when the carotid sinus nerves were sectioned.

RENAL RESPONSES

Arterial chemoreceptor stimulation increases renal sodium and water excretion in normoxic mammals (Fig. 10.8). Bilateral carotid body denervation abolishes the natriuretic response to chemoreceptor stimulation in normoxic, anesthetized, vagotomized animals.[100,124-127] This natriuresis is thought to be due to decreased renal tubular sodium reabsorption. The fact that transecting the renal nerves prevents the vasoconstriction resulting from carotid body stimulation, but enhances the onset of

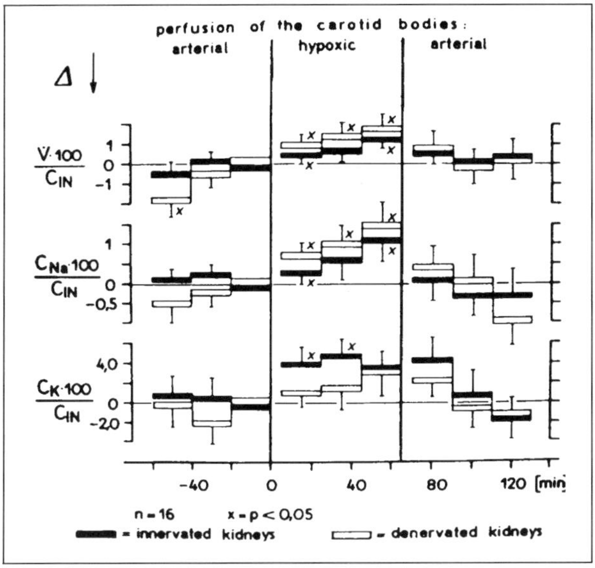

Fig. 10.8. In anesthetized, vagotomized, ventilated cats with vascularly isolated carotid bodies perfused with arterial or hypoxic blood; mean (±SEM) changes in fractional excretions of urine (top trace), sodium (middle trace), and potassium (bottom trace). Renal nerves were cut on left side. Osmotic diuresis was generated by intravenous infusion of mannitol in saline. Adapted from Honig.[125]

natriuresis suggests that the natriuresis may be mediated by a hormone. In human subjects challenged with isocapnic hypoxia the ventilatory drive correlated very well with hypoxic natriuresis and diuresis, while glomerular filtration rate remained constant.[128] Interestingly, carotid body stimulation also reduces the plasma levels of aldosterone in what appears to be teleologically a companion mechanism facilitating sodium loss.[129] Finally, the renal effects of carotid body stimulation in hypertensives appear to differ from those in normotensive subjects.[130-132]

CONCLUSIONS

The major effort in contemporary carotid body research is a clear description of mechanisms involved in the chemotransduction of hypoxia, hypercapnia and acidosis. Since the peripheral arterial chemoreceptors are the only receptors which signal hypoxemia, they function as a unique synapse between the organism and the most essential substrate the organism must capture from the environment, oxygen. Hence, any clear description of the mechanisms involved in the chemotransduction of hypoxia will be a major contribution to our understanding of what could be considered the most fundamental of all biological processes.

One can only say from the above brief review of the systemic reflex responses elicited by carotid body stimulation that the impact of carotid body input on the organism's survival, when confronted with the challenge of hypoxia, is extremely complex. The impact on respiration seems to be the most obvious and the most easily detected. Cardiovascular responses to carotid body stimulation seem more susceptible to being masked by input from other receptors, and being muted or even reversed as a consequence. The same could be said for both endocrine responses and kidney responses, a good number of which required ventilation to be kept constant in order for them to be seen. Even though complicated by multiple inputs in the in vivo situation, carotid body input seems to be of considerable significance in maintaining the organism's oxygen homeostasis. A better understanding of how that input is generated, besides being a major breakthrough in fundamental biology, would also allow the pursuit of pharmacological agents capable of upregulating or downregulating that input. In terms of infants at risk for SIDS, borderline hypertensives, and asthmatics who have experienced near-fatal episodes of asthma,[133] such agents would represent a significant contribution to their well-being.

References

1. Heymans CJF. The part played by vascular presso- and chemoreceptors in respiratory control. In: Nobel Lectures. Physiology of Medicine (1922-1941). Amsterdam: Elsevier 1965:460-81.
2. Gallego A. Fernando de Castro: contributions to the discovery and study of the vascular baroreceptors and blood chemoreceptors. In: Belmonte C, Pallot DJ, Acker H et al, eds. Arterial Chemoreceptors, Proceedings of the VI International Meeting. Leicester: Leicester University Press 1981:1-19.
3. Fitzgerald RS, Parks D. Effect of hypoxia on carotid chemoreceptor response to carbon dioxide in cats. Respir Physiol 1971; 12:218-29.
4. Fitzgerald RS, Dehghani GA. Neural responses of the cat carotid and aortic bodies to hypercapnia and hypoxia. J Appl Physiol 1982; 52:596-601.
5. Daristotle L, Berssenbrugge AD, Bisgard GE. Hypoxic-hypercapnic ventilatory interaction at the carotid body of awake goats. Respir Physiol 1987; 70:63-72.
6. Brunner MJ, Wallace A, MacAnespie CL. Interaction of carotid chemoreceptor and baroreceptor reflexes in anesthetized dogs. Am J Physiol 1988; 254:R1-10.
7. Daristotle L, Berssenbrugge AD, Engwall MJ et al. The effects of carotid body hypocapnia on ventilation in goats. Respir Physiol 1990; 79:123-35.
8. Tatsumi K, Mikami M, Kuriyama T et al. Effects of a synthetic progestin on ventilatory response to hypoxia in awake male rats. Jpn J Thorac Dis 1993; 31:563-8.
9. Hannhart B, Pickett CK, Moore LG. Effects of estrogen and progesterone on carotid body neural output responsiveness to hypoxia. J Appl Physiol 1990; 68:1909-16.
10. Hannhart B, Pickett CK, Weil JV et al. Influence of pregnancy on ventilatory and carotid body neural output responsiveness to hypoxia in cats. J Appl Physiol 1989; 67:797-803.
11. Tatsumi K, Hannhart B, Pickett CK et al. Effects of testosterone on hypoxic ventilatory and carotid body neural responsiveness. Am J Resp Crit Care Med 1994; 149:1248-53.
12. Wasserman K, Whipp BJ, Casaburi R. Respiratory control during exercise. In: Cherniack NS, Widdicombe J, eds. Handbook of Physiology, The Respiratory System, Vol II. Control of Breathing, Part I. Bethesda: American Physiological Society, 1986:595-620.
13. Dempsey JA, Forster HV, Ainsworth DM. Regulation of hyperpnea, hyperventilation, and respiratory muscle recruitment during exercise. In: Dempsey JA, Pack AI, eds. Regulation of Breathing. 2nd ed. New York: Marcel Dekker, Inc, 1995:1065-1134.
14. Forster HV, Dunning MB, Lowry TF et al. Effect of asthma and ventilatory loading on arterial PCO_2 of humans during submaximal exercise. J Appl Physiol 1993; 75:1385-94.
15. Nakazono Y, Miyamoto Y. Effect of hypoxia and hyperoxia on cardiorespiratory responses during exercise. Jpn J Physiol 1987; 37:447-57.
16. Henson LC, Ward DS, Whipp BJ. Effect of dopamine on ventilatory response to incremental exercise in man. Respir Physiol 1992; 89:209-224.
17. Paterson DJ, Nye PC. The effect of beta adrenergic blockade on the carotid body response to hyperkalemia in the cat. Respir Physiol 1988; 74:229-37.
18. Petersen, ES. Effects of beta-adrenergic blockade on the ventilatory responses to hypoxic and hyperoxic exercise in man. J Physiol London 1987; 393:43-55.
19. Hudgel DW, Kressin NA, Nielsen AM et al. Role of beta adrenergic receptors in carotid body function of the goat. Respir Physiol 1986; 64:203-11.
20. Dempsey JA, Forster HV. Mediation of ventilatory adaptations. Physiol Rev 1982;62:262-346.
21. Engwall MJ, Bisgard GE. Ventilatory responses to chemoreceptor stimulation after hypoxic acclimatization in awake goats. J Appl Physiol 1990; 69:1236-43.
22. Vizek M, Pickett CK, Weil JV. Increased carotid body hypoxic sensitivity during acclimatization to hypobaric hypoxia. J Appl Physiol 1987; 63:2403-10.
23. Ryan ML, Hedrick MS, Pizarro J et al. Carotid body noradrenergic sensitivity in ventilatory acclimatization to hypoxia. Respir Physiol 1993; 92:77-90.

24. Weizhen N, Engwall MJ, Daristotle L et al. Ventilatory effects of prolonged systemic (CNS) hypoxia in awake goats. Respir Physiol 1992; 87:37-48.
25. Smith CA, Engwall MJ, Dempsey JA et al. Effects of specific carotid body and brain hypoxia on respiratory muscle contol in the awake goat. J Physiol London 1993; 460:623-40.
26. Bisgard GE, Busch MA, Forster HV. Ventilatory acclimatization to hypozia is not dependent on cerebral hypocapnic alkalosis. J Appl Physiol 1986; 60: 1011-15.
27. Busch MA, Bisgard GE, Forster HV. Ventilatory acclimatization to hypoxia is not dependent on arterial hypoxemia. J Appl Physiol 1985; 58:1874-80.
28. Bisgard GE, Neubauer JA. Peripheral and central effects of hypoxia. In: Dempsey JA, Pack AI, eds. Regulation of Breathing. 2nd ed. New York: Marcel Dekker, Inc 1995:617-68.
29. Donnelly DF, Haddad GG. Prolonged apnea and impaired survival in piglets after sinus and aortic nerve section. J Appl Physiol 1990; 68:1048-52.
30. Haddad GG, Donnelly DF, Bassy-Asaad AR. Developmental control of respiration: neurobiological basis. In: Dempsey JA, Pack AI, eds. Regulation of Breathing. 2nd ed. New York: Marcel Dekker, Inc 1995:743-796.
31. Lack EE, Perez-Atayde AR, Young JB. Carotid body hyperplasia in cystic fibrosis and cyanotic heart disease. A combined morphometric, ultrastructural, and biochemical study. Am J Path 1985; 119:301-14.
32. Phillipson EA, Kozar LF. Effect of aging on metabolic respiratory control in sleeping dogs. Am Rev Resp Dis 1993; 147: 1521-5.
33. Whipp BJ, Ward SA. Physiologic changes following bilateral carotid-body resection in patients with chronic obstructive pulmonary disease. Chest 1992; 101:656-61.
34. DeBacker W, Vermeire P, Bogaert E et al. Almitrine has no effect on gas exchange after bilateral carotid body resection in severe chronic airflow obstruction. Bull Eur Physiopathol Respir 1985; 21:427-32.
35. Bouverot P, Fitzgerald RS. Role of arterial chemoreceptors in controlling lung volume in the dog. Respir Physiol 1969; 7:203-15.
36. Barer GR, Herget J, Sloan PJM et al. The effect of acute and chronic hypoxia on thoracic gas volume in anesthetized rats. J Physiol London 1978; 277:177-92.
37. Garfinkel F, Fitzgerald RS. The effect of hyperoxia, hypoxia and hypercapnia on FRC and occlusion pressure in human subjects. Respir Physiol 1978; 27:193-206.
38. Nadel JA, Widdicombe JG. Effect of changes in blood gas tensions and carotid sinus pressure on tracheal volume and total lung resistance to airflow. J Physiol London 1962;163:13-33.
39. Tsuchiya Y, Hosokawa T, Kasuya Y. Influence of carotid chemoreceptors on the vagal reflex-induced tracheal constriction. Japan J Pharmacol 1989; 50:403-10.
40. Denjean A, Canet E, Praud JP et al. Hypoxia-induced bronchial responsiveness in awake sheep: role of carotid chemoreceptors. Respir Physiol 1991; 83:201-10.
41. Davis B, Chinn R, Gold J et al. Hypoxemia reflexly increases secretion from tracheal submucosal glands in dogs. J Appl Physiol 1982; 52:1416-19.
42. Alsberge M, Magno M, Lipschutz M. Carotid body control of bronchial circulation in sheep. J Appl Physiol 1988; 65:1152-1156.
43. Van Lunteren E, Haxhiu MA, Cherniack NS. Stimulation of respiratory changes in alae nasi length by chemoreceptor activation. Respir Physiol 1986; 63:361-73.
44. Lung MA, Wang JC. Effects of hypercapnia and hypoxia on nasal vasculature and airflow resistance in the anaesthetized dog. J Physiol London 1986; 373:261-75.
45. England SJ, Harding R, Stradling JR et al. Laryngeal muscle activities during progressive hypercapnia and hypoxia in awake and sleeping dogs. Respir Physiol 1986; 66:327-39.
46. Mifflin SW. Arterial chemoreceptor input to respiratory hypoglossal motoneurons. J Appl Physiol 1990; 69:700-9.
47. Yasuma F, Kimoff RJ, Kozar LF. Abdominal muscle activation by respiratory stimuli in conscious dogs. J Appl Physiol 1993; 74:16-23.

48. Fitzgerald RS. Relationships between tidal volume and phrenic nerve activity during hypercapnia and hypoxia. Acta Neurobiol Exp 1973; 33:419-25.
49. Saupe KW, Smith CA, Henderson KS et al. Respiratory muscle recruitment during selective central and peripheral chemoreceptor stimulation in awake dogs. J Physiol London 1992; 448:613-31.
50. Oku Y, Bruce EN, Richmonds CR et al. The carotid body in the motorneuron response to protriptyline. Respir Physiol 1993; 93:41-9.
51. Gauda EB, Carroll TP, Schwartz AR et al. Mechano- and chemoreceptor modulation of respiratory muscles in response to upper airway negative pressure. J Appl Physiol 1994; 76:2656-62.
52. Martin RJ, van Lunteren E, Haxhiu MA et al. Upper airway muscle and diaphragm responses to hypoxia in the piglet. J Appl Physiol 1990; 68:672-7.
53. Parisi RA, Santiago TV, Edelman NH. Genioglossal and diaphragmatic EMG responses to hypoxia during sleep. Am Rev Respir Dis 1988; 138:610-6.
54. Daly MdeB. Interactions between respiration and circulation. In: Cherniack NS, Widdicombe J, eds. Handbook of Physiology, The Respiratory System, Vol II. Control of Breathing, Part 2. Bethesda: American Physiological Society, 1986: 529-94.
55. Daly MdeB. Chemoreceptor reflexes and cardiovascular control. Acta Physiol Pol 1985; 36:4-20.
56. Marshall JM. Peripheral chemoreceptors and cardiovascular regulation. Physiol Rev 1994; 74:543-94.
57. Downing SE, Remensnyder JP, Mitchell JH. Cardiovascular responses to hypoxic stimulation f the carotid bodies. Circ Res 1962; 10:676-85.
58. Jacobs L, Sampson SR, Comroe JH. Carotid sinus versus carotid body origin of nicotine and cyanide bradycardia in the dog. Am J Physiol 1971; 220:472-76.
59. Rutherford JD, Vatner SF. Integrated carotid chemoreceptor and pulmonary inflation reflex control of peripheral vasoactivity in conscious dogs. Circ Res 1978; 43:200-8.
60. Daly MdeB, Kirkman E, Wood LM. Cardiovascular responses to stimulation of cardiac receptors in the cat and their modification by changes in respiration. J Physiol London 1988; 407:349-62.
61. Franchini KG, Krieger EM. Cardiovascular responses of conscious rats to carotid body chemoreceptor stimulation by intravenous KCN. J Auton Nerv Syst 1993; 42:63-9.
62. Hackett JG, Abboud FM, Mark AL et al. Coronary vascular responses to stimulation of chemoreceptors and baroreceptors. Circ Res 1972; 31:8-17.
63. Kahler RL, Goldblatt A, Barunwald E. The effect of acute hypoxia on the systemic venous and arterial systems and on myocardial contractile force. J Clin Invest 1962; 41:1553-63.
64. Pace JB. Influence of carotid chemoreceptor stimulation on ventricular dynamics. Am J Physiol 1970; 218:1687-96.
65. Rodrigues L, Silva-Carvalho L, Fresta M et al. Primary effect of carotid body stimulation on left ventricular inotropism in swine. Revista Port Cardiol 1992; 11:431-7.
66. Opitz H, Scheufler K. Chemoreflex modification of the myocardial contractility of rabbits. Zeit Exp Chir Transplant Kunst Org 1990; 23:130-6.
67. Kollai M, Koizumi K, Brooks CMcC. Nature of differential sympathetic discharges in chemoreceptor reflexes. Proc Natl Acad Sci USA 1978; 75:5239-43.
68. Dehghani GA, Fitzgerald RS, Mitzner W. The role of the peripheral arterial chemoreceptors in the cardiovascular responses of the cat to acute systemic hypoxia. In: Ribeiro JA, Pallot DJ, eds. Chemoreceptors in Respiratory Control. London: Croom Helm, 1987:209-215.
69. Somers VK, Mark AL, Abboud FM. Potentiation of sympathetic nerve responses to hypoxia in borderline hypertensive subjects. Hypertension 1988; 11:608-12.
70. Tafil-Klawe M, Trzebski A, Klawe J et al. Augmented chemoreceptor reflex tonic drive in early human hypertension and in normotensive subjects with family background of hypertension. Acta Physiol Pol 1985; 36:51-8.
71. Matsumoto H, Osanai S, Nakano H et al. Ventilatory responses in patients with essential hypertension. Jpn J Physiol 1991; 41:831-42.

72. Bonsignore MR, Marrone O, Insalaco G et al. The cardiovascular effects of obstructive sleep apnoeas:analysis of pathogenic mechanisms. Eur Resp J 1994; 7:786-805.
73. Daly IdeB, Daly MdeB. The effects of stimulation of the carotid body chemoreceptors on pulmonary vascular resistance in the dog. J Physiol London 1957; 137:436-446.
74. Daly IdeB, Daly MdeB. The effects of stimulation of carotid body chemoreceptors on the pulmonary vascular bed in the dog, the vasosensory controlled perfused living animal preparation. J Physiol London 1959; 148:201-219.
75. Daly IdeB, Hebb C. Pulmonary and bronchial vascular systems. London: Arnold, 1966.
76. Lejeune P, Vachiery JL, Leeman M et al. Absence of parasympathetic control of pulmonary vascular pressure-flow plots in hyperoxic and hypoxic dogs. Respir Physiol 1989; 78:123-33.
77. Naeje R, Lejeune P, Leeman M et al. Pulmonary vascular responses to surgical chemodenervation and chemical sympathectomy in dogs. J Appl Physiol 1989; 66:42-50.
78. Wilson LB, Levitzky MG. Chemoreflex blunting of hypoxic pulmonary vasoconstriction is vagally mediated. J Appl Physiol 1989; 66:782-91.
79. Chapleau MW, Wilson LB, Gregory TJ et al. Chemoreceptor stimulation interferes with regional hypoxic pulmonary vasoconstriction. Respir Physiol 1988; 71:185-200.
80. Fitzgerald RS, Dehghani GA, Sham JSK et al. Peripheral chemoreceptor modulaltion of the pulmonary vasculature in the cat. J Appl Physiol 1992; 73:20-9.
81. Webber SE, Widdicombe JG. Reflex control of the tracheal vasculature of sheep. J Appl Physiol 1993; 75:2173-9.
82. James IM, MacDonell LA. The role of baroreceptors and chemoreceptors in the regulation of the cerebral circulation. Clin Sci 1975; 49:465-71.
83. James IM, Millar RA, Purves MJ. Observations on the extrinsic neural control of cerebral blood flow in the baboon. Circ Res 1969; 25:77-93.
84. Ponte J, Purves MJ. The role of carotid body chemoreceptors and carotid sinus baroreceptors in the control of cerebral blood vessels. J Physiol Lond 1974; 237:315-40.
85. Bates D, Sundt TM. The relevance of peripheral baroreceptors and chemoreceptors to regulation of cerebral blood flow in the cat. Circ Res 1976; 38:488-93.
86. Hoff JT, Mackenzie ET, Harper IM. Responses of the cerebral circulation to hypercapnia and hypoxia after 7th cranial nerve transection in baboons. Circ Res 1977; 40:258-62.
87. Heistad DD, Marcus ML, Ehrardt JC et al. Effects of stimulation of carotid chemoreceptors on total and regional cerebral blood flow. Circ Res 1976; 38:20-5.
88. Marshall JM, Metcalfe JD. Influences on the cardiovascular response to graded levels of systemic hypoxia of the accompanying hypocapnia in the rat. J Physiol Lond 1989; 410:381-94.
89. Traystman RJ, Fitzgerald RS. Cerebrovascular response to hypoxia in baroreceptor and chemoreceptor denervated dogs. Am J Physiol 1981; 241:H724-H731.
90. Traystman RJ, Fitzgerald RS, Loscutoff SC. Cerebral circulatory responses to arterial hypoxia in normal and chemo-denervated dogs. Circ Res 1978; 42:649-57.
91. Priano LL, Baig H, Rutherford JD et al. Adrenergic and cholinergic control of coronary and cerebral vascular resistance by the carotid chemoreflex in conscious dogs. Circulation 58, Suppl II:8 (abstract), 1978.
92. Vatner SF, Priano LL, Rutherford JD et al. Sympathetic regulation of the cerebral circulation by the chemoreceptor reflex. Am J Physiol 1980; 238:H594-H598.
93. Anwar M, Kissen I, Weiss HR. Effect of chemodenervation on the cerebral vascular and microvascular response to hypoxia. Circ Res 1990; 67:1365-73.
94. Krasney JA, Miki K, McAndrews K et al. Peripheral circulatory responses to 96 hours of hypoxia in conscious sinoaortic-denervated sheep. Am J Physiol 1986; 250:R868-R874.
95. Hanley DF, Wilson DA, Traystman RJ. Effect of hypoxia and hypercapnia on

neurohypophysial blood flow. Am J Physiol 1986; 250:H7-H15.

96. Fitzgerald RS, Dehghani GA. Chemoreceptor control of organ vascular resistance during acute systemic hypoxia. In: Acker H, Trzebski A, O'Regan RG, eds. Chemoreceptors and Chemoreceptor Reflexes. New York: Plenum, 1990:217-22.
97. Stekiel TA, Tominaga M, Bosnjak ZJ et al. The inhibitory effect of halothane on mesenteric venoconstriction and related reflex responses during acute graded hypoxia in rabbits. Anesthesiol 1992; 77: 709-20.
98. Fitzgerald RS, Lahiri S. Reflex responses to chemoreceptor stimulation. In: Cherniack NS, Widdicombe J, eds. Handbook of Physiology, The Respiratory System, Vol II. Control of Breathing, Part 1. Bethesda: American Physiological Society, 1986:529-94.
99. Heistad DD, Abboud FM, Mark AL et al. Interaction of baroreceptor and chemoreceptor reflexes: modulation of the chemoreceptor reflex by changes in baroreceptor activity. J Clin Invest 1974; 53:1226-36.
100. Karim F, Al-Obaidi M. Modification of carotid chemoreceptor-induced changes in renal haemodynamics and function by the carotid baroreflex in dogs. J Physiol London 1993; 466:599-610.
101. Al-Obaidi M, Karim F. Primary effects of carotid chemoreceptor stimulation on gracilis muscle and renal blood flow and renal function in dogs. J Physiol London 1992; 455:73-88.
102. Hainsworth R, Karim F, McGregor KH et al. Hindlimb vascular capacitance response in anaesthetized dogs. J Physiol London 1983; 337:417-28.
103. Marshall JM. Analysis of cardiovascular responses evoked following changes in peripheral chemoreceptor activity in the rat. J Physiol London 1987; 394:393-414.
104. Koehler RC, Traystman RJ, Jones MD Jr. Regional blood flow and O_2 transport during hypoxic and CO hypoxia in neonatal and adult sheep. Am J Physiol 1985; 248:H118-24.
105. Daly MdeB, Kirkman E. Differential modulation by pulmonary stretch afferents of some reflex cardioinhibitiory responses in the cat. J Physiol London 1989; 417:323-41.
106. Sladek M, Grogaard JB, Parker RA et al. Prolonged hypoxemia enhances and acute hypoxemia attenuates laryngeal reflex apnea in young lambs. Ped Res 1993; 34:813-20
107. Daly MdeB, Kirkman E, Wood LM. Cardiovascular responses to stimulation of cardiac receptors in the cat and their modification by changes in respiration. J Physiol London 1988; 407:349-62.
108. Kolobow T, Gattinoni L, Tomlinson TA et al. Control of breathing using an extracorporeal membrane lung. Anesthesiol 1977; 46:138-41.
109. Phillipson EA, Duffin J, Cooper JD. Critical dependence of respiratory rhythmicity on metabolic CO_2 load. J Appl Physiol 1981; 50:45-54.
110. Dorward PK, Burke SL, Janig W et al. Reflex responses to baroreceptor, chemoreceptor and nociceptor inputs in single renal sympathetic neurones in the rabbit and the effects of anesthesia on them. J Auton Nerv Syst 1987; 18:39-54.
111. Share L, Levy MN. Effect of carotid chemoreceptor stimulation on plasma antidiuretic hormone titer. Am J Physiol 1966; 210:157-61.
112. Yamashita H. Effect of baro- and chemoreceptor activation on supraoptic nuclei neurons in the hypothalamus. Brain Res 1977; 126:551-56.
113. Yamashita H. Influence of carotid and aortic baroreceptors on neurosecretory neurons in supraoptic nuclei. Brain Res 1979; 170:259-77.
114. Harris MC. Effect of chemoreceptor and baroreceptor stimulation on the discharge of hypothalamic supraoptic neurones in rats. J Endocrinol 1979; 82: 115-25.
115. Raff H, Shinsako J, Keil LC et al. Vasopressin, ACTH and corticosteroids during hypercapnia and graded hypoxia in dogs. Am J Physiol 1983; 244:E453-E458.
116. Raff H, Tzankoff SP, Fitzgerald RS. ACTH and cortisol responses to hypoxia in dogs. J Appl Physiol 1981; 51:1257-60.
117. Raff H, Fagin KD. Measurement of hormones and blood gases during hypoxia in conscious cannulated rats. J Appl Physiol 1984; 56:1426-30.

118. Lau C. Role of respiratory chemoreceptors in adrenocortical activation. Am J Physiol 1971; 221:602-6.
119. Raff H, Tzankoff SP, Fitzgerald RS. Chemoreceptor involvement in cortisol responses to hypoxia in ventilated dogs. J Appl Physiol 1982; 52:1135-8.
120. Anichkov SV, Malyghina EI, Poskalenko AN et al. Reflexes from carotid bodies upon the adrenals. Arch Int Pharmacodyn Ther 1960; 129:156-65.
121. Critchley JAJH, Ellis P, Ungar A. The reflex release of adrenaline and noradrenaline from the adrenal glands of cats and dogs. J Physiol London 1980; 298:71-78.
122. Critchley, JAJH, Ungar A, Welburn PJ. The release of adrenaline and noradrenaline by the adrenal glands of cats and dogs in reflexes arising from the carotid chemoreceptors and baroreceptors (Abstract). J Physiol London 1973; 244: 111P-112P.
123. Beisold D, Kurosawa M, Sato A et al. Hypoxia and hypercapnia increase the sympatho-adrenal medullary functions in anaesthetized, artificially ventilated rats. Jpn J Physiol 1989; 39:511-22.
124. Bardsley PA, Johnson BF, Stewart AG et al. Natriuresis secondary to carotid chemoreceptor stimulation with almitrine bismesylate in the rat: the effect on kidney function and the response to renal denervation and deficiency of antidiuretic hormone. Biomed Biochim Acta 1991; 50:175-82.
125. Honig A. Peripheral arterial chemoreceptors and reflex control of sodium and water homeostasis. Am J Physiol 1989; 257:R1282-R1302.
126. Hoyt RW, Honig A. Body fluid and energy metabolism at high altitude. In: Fregly MJ, Blatteis CM, eds. Handbook on Adaptation to the Environment. The Terrestrial Altitude Environment. New York: Oxford Univ Press p7, ch. 55. In press.
127. Karim F, Poucher SM, Summerill RA. The effects of stimulating carotid chemoreceptors on renal haemodynamics and function in dogs. J Physiol London 1987; 451:451-63.
128. Swenson ER, Duncan TB, Goldberg SV et al. Diuretic effect of acute hypoxia in humans: relationship to hypoxic ventilatory responsiveness and renal hormones. J Appl Physiol 1995; 78:377-83.
129. Wiersbitzky M, Landgraf R, Gruska S et al. Hormonal and renal responses to arterial chemoreceptor stimulation by almitrine in healthy and normotensive men. Biomed Biochim Acta 1990; 49: 1155-63.
130. Huckstorf C, Habermann G. Cardiovascular and renal responses to systemic hypoxia in conscious chronically instrumented SHR and WKY rats (Abstract). Pfluegers Arch 1994; 426:R133.
131. Ledderhos C, Brauer H, Gens A et al. Renal function in borderline hypertensives in response to arterial chemoreceptor stimulation. Proc Cardiovascular Disease Prevention II 1994:40.
132. Wiersbitzky M, Schuster R, Balke F et al. The reactions of renal excretory function in normotensive and essentially hypertensive men in response to oral administration of almitrine bismesylate. In: Acker H, Trzebski A, O'Regan RG, eds. Chemoreceptors and Chemoreceptor Reflexes. New York: Plenum, 1990: 417-23.
133. Kikuchi Y, Okabe S, Tamura G et al. Chemosensitivity and perception of dyspnea in patients with a history of nearfatal asthma. New Eng J Med 1994; 330:1329-34.

CHAPTER 11

Function of the Carotid Body Intra-utero and in the Postnatal Period

David F. Donnelly

INTRODUCTION

Carotid body chemoreceptors are active in utero and in the newborn period, and play a particularly important role in maintaining a respiratory rhythm in the newborn period. This corresponds to a time during which the response characteristics are radically changing in parallel to the changes in environment and oxygen requirements. Although breathing movements, in utero, serve an important function in lung parenchymal development, they serve no role in maintaining oxygen delivery, and respiration may stop for extended periods of time without liability. However, following birth, the respiratory system is charged with continuous function at PO_2 levels considerably higher than that experienced in utero, i.e., near 100 Torr vs. 29 Torr PaO_2. How this takes place and the importance of the chemoreceptor function in this period are the focus of this chapter.

FUNCTION OF THE CAROTID BODY INTRA-UTERO

Organ Function

Although increases in CO_2 enhance fetal breathing movements, presumably though stimulation of peripheral and central chemoreceptors, hypoxia causes an opposite response, a reduction in fetal breathing movements.[1] This suggests that peripheral chemoreceptor activity is low in the fetus or that it is unresponsive or diminished by hypoxia. Unfortunately, experiments to directly address this conjecture have given inconsistent results. In some laboratory settings, 'normal' chemoreceptor activity in fetal lambs could be readily recorded; this activity was inhibited by hyperoxia and increased by umbilical cord occlusion or maternal hypoxia.[2-4] A decrease in PaO_2 below 20 Torr resulted in a 4-fold increase in discharge frequency.[3] In contrast, other investigators report difficulty in obtaining chemoreceptor spiking activity on the sinus nerve of the fetus,[2] suggesting that the organ is immature and

The Carotid Body Chemoreceptors,
edited by Constancio González.

nonfunctional, in utero. Still others found that spiking activity was present on the sinus nerve but was insensitive to hypoxia (at least in the absence of enhanced sympathetic tone).[2]

This inability to record chemoreceptor activity in several settings raises the possibility that some physiologic factors suppress fetal chemoreceptor discharge. One possible factor is a lack of sympathetic activity, in utero. This is supported by a greatly enhanced ease in recording fetal chemoreceptors following cord compression—a form of artificial birth which stimulates sympathetic activity.[2]

Physiologic Role

During normal oxygenation, the frequency of fetal breathing movements is not affected by chemoreceptor denervation.[4,5] However, the opposite is not true, and CO_2/acidity enhances fetal breathing movement, an affect dependent on both peripheral and central chemoreceptors.[6]

In contrast to CO_2, the affect of hypoxia on fetal breathing movements is complicated. Hypoxia, although stimulating peripheral chemoreceptors,[3] causes a cessation of fetal breathing movement.[1] This inhibition can be overcome by pontine lesion,[7] after which, hypoxia leads to stimulation of fetal breathing, a response dependent on peripheral chemoreceptors.[8] In addition to the respiratory response, chemoreceptor stimulation causes bradycardia and peripheral vasoconstriction.[9]

FUNCTION OF THE CAROTID BODY IN THE POSTNATAL PERIOD

Organ Function

Although peripheral chemoreceptors are not essential for initiation of breathing at birth,[4] they are important in regulating breathing in the neonatal period during which the receptors undergo major maturational changes. At least three processes are initiated at birth: 1) the sensitivity to hypoxia is increased; 2) the response is better sustained; and 3) hypoxia and acidity begin to interact in a multiplicative manner. These changes appear to be triggered by the sharp rise in PaO_2 around the time of birth (from around 30 Torr to 100 Torr) which silences (initially) chemoreceptor discharge.[3] Over the course of hours to weeks, chemoreceptor sensitivity to hypoxia increases to adult levels in which decreases in PaO_2 below 60 Torr lead to a rapid and large increase in discharge activity.[3,5,10]

There is general agreement that maturation of the receptors occurs after birth, but there is considerable disagreement on the time frame of this maturation. Results from some experiments indicated that mature baseline activity and sensitivity to hypoxia is present within a day or two after birth.[11] However, this rapid maturation is in contrast to other data which suggests a slower time frame. Chemoreceptors of cats less than 10 days (d) old were found to be less sensitive to hypoxia (left shifted) compared to older cats.[12,13] Similarly, aortic chemoreceptors of 3d old lambs are left shifted compared to lambs 10-19 d old,[14] and, in piglets, the response of newborns (1-5 d old) is left-shifted compared to older piglets (12-20 d) (Fig. 11.1). This recent data in piglets is especially interesting because action potential recordings were undertaken using microelectrode impalement of the petrosal ganglia. Thus, the efferent sinus nerve fibers remained intact, allowing for the closest approximation to the normal physiologic state. Taken together, this suggests that maturation of a normal response to decreases in PaO_2 occurs, at least, over a 1-2 week time frame.

Not only is the response curve of newborn chemoreceptors left-shifted compared to the mature animal, but the dynamic range (or maximum discharge from a single receptor) is less in the newborn compared to the adult. Recordings from single chemoreceptor fibers in 6 d old piglets demonstrated a dynamic range as PaO_2 was reduced from 300 to 25 Torr of 0.5 to 6 Hz and this increased to 0.5 to 8 Hz in 8 d old piglets.[15] Similarly, in kittens, the discharge rate of single chemoreceptor afferent fibers at P_iO_2 of 55 Torr ($PaO_2 \approx$ 31-44 Torr) increased

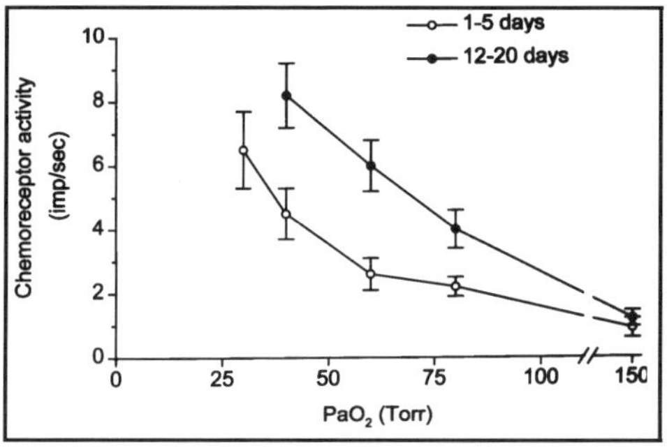

Fig. 11.1. Single-cell carotid chemoreceptor afferent response to isocapnic hypoxia in young (1-5d, N=10) and older (12-20d, N=10) piglets. Chemoreceptor activity was significantly greater in the older group at all PaO_2 levels below 100 Torr (From Mulligan[15]).

from 5.8 ± 0.6 Hz in kittens younger than 10 days to 8.8 ± 1.3 Hz in kittens older than 10 days.[13] In normal adult cats, this decrease in oxygen causes a peak nerve response of approximately 15 Hz,[16] suggesting a further developmental enhancement. However, it is uncertain whether a PaO_2 of 20-25 Torr maximally stimulates spiking activity, especially in the newborn, but further in vivo testing of the O_2 response curve is impractical due to cardiovascular and metabolic complications of severe hypoxia. This question may be better explored in vitro in which nutrient delivery is directly controlled. Under this condition and using an anoxic stimulus, the maximal discharge rate obtained from rat chemoreceptors demonstrated a similar age-dependent enhancement in dynamic range, increasing from about 5 Hz at 1 d of age to about 20 Hz by 15 d of age.[17]

In addition to the enhanced sensitivity to hypoxia, mature chemoreceptors are better able to sustain a response to prolonged stimuli. Recent recordings from piglets, in vivo, showed a "drop out" in about 50% of the active chemoreceptor fibers during sustained stimulation with 8% FiO_2, but this was not observed in recordings from piglets 30 d of age.[15] Similarly, in cats, about 50% of single-fiber chemoreceptors in 2 d old cats demonstrated a biphasic response to hypoxia (P_IO_2=55 torr).[13] Nerve activity peaked about 20 sec following the start of hypoxia, was sustained for approximately 15 sec and subsequently declined for 15 sec until reaching a steady state level. A biphasic response to hypoxia was also reported for two-thirds of cats less than 7d of age.[12]

Like hypoxia, the sensitivity to hypercapnia also appears to increase in the newborn period. In young kittens (<10 d age), an increase in $PaCO_2$ from 38 to 80 Torr caused nerve activity to increase from 0.1 to about 1.5 Hz. In contrast, in older kittens (>10 d age) the same increase in $PaCO_2$ caused activity to increase to 3.5 Hz.[13] The same developmental increase was recently observed using multi-fiber recordings of sinus nerve activity in cats.[12]

Not only does the sensitivity to hypoxia and hypercapnia increase developmentally, but the way these stimuli interact also changes with development. In the adult, hypercapnia is well established to enhance the sensitivity to hypoxia, the so-called multiplicative interaction.[18] This interaction appears to be absent in the newborn period, and does not become significant in the kitten until 4 weeks of age.[12] These studies were recently extended to the rat carotid body, in vitro, in which an enhancement of hypoxia sensitivity by hypercapnia was not significant in carotid bodies harvested from 5-7 d old rats, but was present in adult carotid bodies.[19] Thus, at least part of the maturation of O_2/CO_2 multiplicative interaction occurs independently of the nutritive compartment.

An important correlate of the developmental increase in chemoreceptor activity and responsiveness is the developmental change in the ventilatory response to hypoxia. A few hyperoxic breaths is often used to silence the peripheral chemoreceptors and thus assess their contribution to respiratory drive by measuring the acute decrease in ventilation. Using this assay, peripheral chemoreceptors contribute 5-8% of respiratory drive in the newborn rat, compared to 20% in the 2 week old rat.[20-22] Similarly, in humans, the decrease in ventilation during high oxygen breathing is absent on the day of birth, but significant in the 2-6 d old period.[23] Using the opposite stimulus, hypoxia, it was demonstrated that the ventilatory response to hypoxia is less on the day of birth compared to about one week of life.[24] Taken together, these results suggest that newborn chemoreceptor activity is low and that the contribution to ventilation is less than in the adult of most species. However, rats may be somewhat precocious. Acute hypoxia in rats leads to an immediate hyperventilation which is independent of age over the range of 1-14 d postpartum, suggesting that the early detection system for hypoxia is mature in the rat by 1 day after birth.

Besides a maturation of the magnitude of the respiratory response to hypoxia, the respiratory system matures in its ability to sustain the increased respiratory drive. In the newborn, respiratory drive increases acutely in response to hypoxia but then decreases back to or below baseline with continued hypoxia (biphasic response to hypoxia).[20,25-27] Some of the fall-off of respiratory drive is central in origin,[28] but, as mentioned above, recent observations demonstrate that some adaptation may occur at the receptor level. Approximately half of the recorded chemoreceptor fibers of newborn cats and piglets demonstrate a decrease in activity during progressive or prolonged hypoxia.[13,15] However, it is important to note that these are controversial observations and some investigators see little change in peripheral chemoreceptor activity during hypoxia despite decreases in respiratory drive.[25,29]

The trigger for the above maturation process in chemoreceptor activity appears to be the sharp rise in oxygen at birth. In fact, a premature resetting may be started by exposing the fetus to higher levels of oxygen.[5] Conversely, the maturation process may be delayed by birthing into a low oxygen environment, and rats exposed postnatally to an FiO_2 of 10-12% have an immature respiratory response to hypoxia.[30-32] Unfortunately, it is unclear if the immaturity is due to an impairment at the level of the chemoreceptor. Multi-fiber nerve recordings from rats raised in a hypoxia environment appeared to have a normal O_2 response curve,[30] suggesting that the immature response is of central origin. On the other hand, catecholamine turnover rates in the carotid body remain in an immature pattern in rats raised in a hypoxia environment,[32] suggesting an immaturity in the organ itself. Thus, the reason for the immature hypoxia response in chronically hypoxic rats is not fully resolved.

Mechanism of Postnatal Chemoreceptor Resetting

For analysis purposes, the chemoreceptor unit may be broken into two compartments: a nutritive compartment which regulates tissue oxygen and nutrient delivery, and a transduction compartment (glomus cell/nerve ending complex) directly involved in spike initiation. Maturational changes occur in both compartments and both may contribute to the enhancement of the chemoreceptor response.

Nutritive Compartment

Carotid body tissue PO_2 shows a decrease over the first week after birth and this decrease in PO_2 may be an important factor in explaining the apparent increase in hypoxia sensitivity.[33] It is likely that changes in tissue oxygen reflect changes in blood vessel control since no anatomic change in carotid body vasculature occurs during this time period.[34,35] Since the carotid body receives a major innervation from the superior cervical ganglia (ganglio-glomerular nerve) and a parasympathetic innervation from the sinus nerve[36] (see chapter 1 by A. Verna), the change in tissue O_2 may be directly related to neural blood vessel control. Stimulation of sympathetic and parasympathetic efferents cause ongoing afferent activity to increase[11] and decrease,[37] respectively, and these changes are correlated to blood flow changes within the organ.[33]

Blood borne substances, such as K^+, and neurochemicals may potentially play a major role as modulators of chemosensitivity. A slight increase in K^+, as occurs during exercise, causes a 20-30% increase in discharge sensitivity to hypoxia,[38] but its effects on the newborn are unexplored. Similarly, endorphins are well established to decrease in the newborn period. Since application of exogenous endorphin causes an inhibition of chemoreceptor hypoxia sensitivity, the postnatal increase in sensitivity may be partially due to the decrease in circulating endorphins.[39] Even less well understood is the effect of blood versus artificial plasma on hypoxia sensitivity. This was originally noted by Joels and Neil in 1968 who were studying chemoreceptors, in vitro.[40] They found that chemo-sensitivity decreases over time in saline until the organ is virtually unresponsive to hypoxia. However, addition of as little as 5% blood to the saline restored these 'tired' chemoreceptors and prevented the decline. In the opposite sense, fetal chemoreceptor activity may be sparse, in situ, but readily recorded from the same carotid body, in vitro.[4] Both observations imply that blood borne factors play a major modulatory role in determining the level of chemosensitivity, but identification of the critical substance or their change in the newborn period are presently lacking.

Transduction Compartment

Even in the absence of external modulatory factors (acute hormonal or neural effects), chemosensitivity of the newborn chemoreceptor is less than the adult. As noted above, the dynamic increase in nerve activity of rat carotid bodies, in vitro, following transition from normoxia to severe hypoxia is about four-fold greater in carotid bodies harvested from 20 d old rats compared to 1-2 day old rats.[17] This corresponds well to the maturation pattern of respiratory response to hypoxia in the intact animal[20] and suggests that major maturational changes occur within the carotid body itself, independent of the acute effects of hormones or nerves.

Several histologic, biophysical and neurochemical changes in the glomus cell/nerve ending complex occur in the postnatal period, but interpretation of their significance depends on assumptions of the internal workings of the organ. Although the nature of the chemical transmission between glomus cells and apposed afferent nerve endings is unresolved, the number of synapses increase greatly in the newborn period. In the rat, this increase is of the order of 4-5x between birth and 20 days of age,[41] which is about the same order of increase as the peak nerve response to hypoxia.[17] The synthesis of some purported neurotransmitters are also developmentally linked to chemo-sensitivity. For instance, substance P immunocytochemical staining is sparse in fetal carotid body but rapidly appears after birth.[42] Substance P has been implicated as being a major mediator of the hypoxia response.[43] It is speculated that catecholamines, which are synthesized by glomus cells cause enhanced nerve activity[44] (see chapter 3). If increases in catecholamine secretion mediate the increase in nerve activity, then it would be expected that secretion rates for catecholamine would be lower in the newborn period. This appears to be the case, in that recent measurements of free catecholamine and nerve activity of rat carotid body, in vitro, show a parallel enhancement of the nerve response to hypoxia and the magnitude of catecholamine secretion during anoxia[45](Fig. 11.2).

In addition to the proposed excitatory role for catecholamines, some carotid body catecholamine receptors are, most certainly, inhibitory (see chapters 3 and 7). Exogenous dopamine generally inhibits, not excites, afferent activity, and dopamine blockers generally fail to block hypoxia transduction.[46] Thus, the low sensitivity in the newborn period may be due to high rates of tonic dopamine secretion.[22,32] Indeed, this conjecture is supported by recent data on dopamine turnover rates in the newborn period which show a large increase in the first 6 hours after birth and a gradual decrease over the next 12 hours.[22] As noted above, postnatal hypoxia delays maturation of normal hypoxia sensitivity, and also prolongs the period of enhanced dopamine turnover rate, i.e., chronically hypoxic rats appear to main-

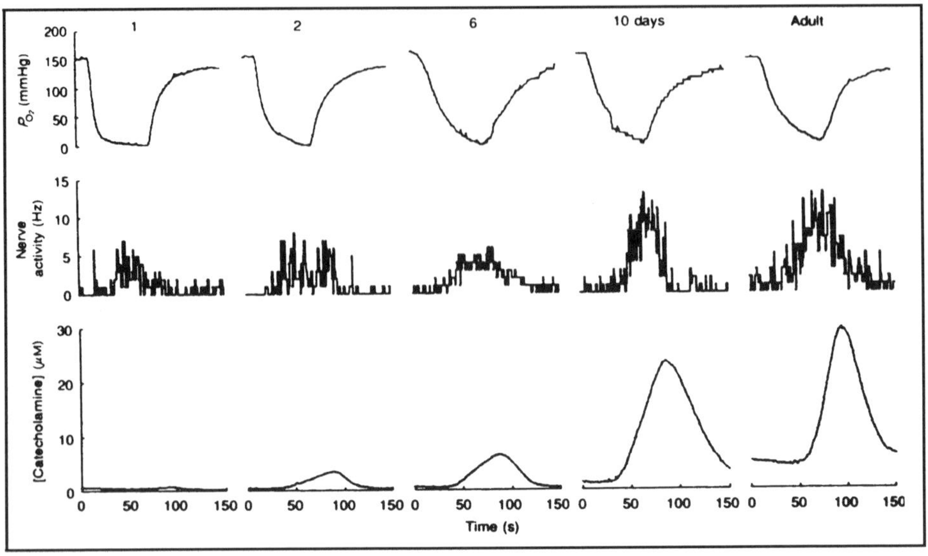

Fig. 11.2. Perfusate PO_2 (top trace), single-fiber nerve activity (middle trace) and free tissue catecholamine (lower trace) measured in rat carotid bodies of different ages, in vitro. Baseline and peak nerve activity during brief anoxia increased with development and this was associated with a greater catecholamine secretory response during hypoxia. (Data from Donnelly[45]).

tain an immature pattern of dopamine secretion.[32]

The maturational increase in chemosensitivity may also be attributed to a maturational change in the biophysical properties of glomus cells. Recent exciting results have shown that the magnitude of the hypoxia-induced increase in intracellular calcium is 3-5x greater in glomus cells from adult compared to newborn rabbits.[47] Presumably, these calcium changes are linked to changes in control of membrane potential. Although no data directly addressing this postulate are presently available , comparison of results between different laboratories may give clues to the result of such a study. In adult rabbit glomus cells, hypoxic transduction appears to be mediated through inhibition of a transient (A-type) K^+ current.[48] However, in neonatal rat glomus cells, hypoxia inhibits a different current, a BK-type calcium-dependent K^+ current.[49] Although comparison among species is problematic, it would be surprising that nature solves the same problem (hypoxia transduction) by modulating entirely different currents, and a maturation from a BK-type to an A-type O_2-sensitive current may be developmentally regulated. Perhaps further confusing the issue is the recent observation that rat glomus cells harvested from rats exposed to postnatal hypoxia develop a unique O_2-sensitive K^+ current, a current which is inhibited by hypoxia but is no longer sensitive to BK-type blocking agents[50] (see chapter 4).

Finally, the maturational increase in hypoxia sensitivity may actually be mediated by chemosensitivity changes in another physiologic stimulus, that is, an enhanced sensitivity to changes in acidity. In rat carotid body, in vitro, hypoxia and CO_2 interact, resulting, for instance, in a nerve response to CO_2 which is enhanced in sensitivity when combined with hypoxia.[51] This enhancement is not present in the newborn[51] and development of the enhancement is delayed by hypoxia after birth.[19] Thus, the greater response of the adult to hypoxia may actually be mediated by an enhanced response to the background (an unchanging) PCO_2.

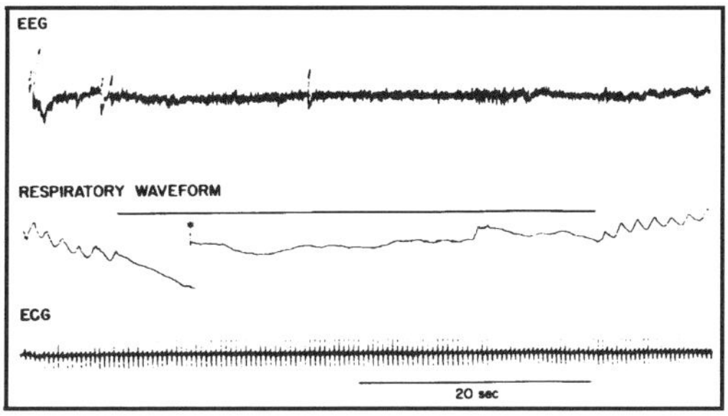

Fig. 11.3. Consequences of denervation in the newborn period on breathing in an unanesthetized, resting piglet. Tracings: EEG (top), respiration (middle, inspiration upward, whole body plethysmography) and ECG (bottom) obtained approximately 24 hrs after surgical denervation in 10d old piglet. Solid bar, spontaneous apnea lasting 42 s. (Data from Donnelly and Haddad[55]).

Physiologic Role

The most obvious role for peripheral chemoreceptors is their role in regulating breathing. As noted, their contribution to eupnic breathing increases from about 5 to 30% in the postnatal period.[21] Under conditions of hypoxia or chronic CO_2 retention, this percentage becomes even greater. Besides an acute regulation of breathing, peripheral chemoreceptors play an important role in maintaining the stability of the respiratory pattern and protecting the newborn against periods of apnea. These essential roles are best discerned by observing the consequences of denervation. Denervation is without major effect on the normal mature subject, outside of a loss of the respiratory response to hypoxia. However, greater consequences are noted in the newborn.

Effect of Denervation on Respiratory Stability

Several anecdotal observations initially suggested that chemodenervated animals have an increased risk of unexpected death. In one report, it was noted that after being returned to the farm, 30% of denervated lambs died weeks or months following the surgery.[52] More systematic observations in other species demonstrated sleep-related respiratory impairments. Rats denervated at 2 weeks of age produced atypical respiratory patterns characterized by pauses and gasps confined to REM sleep.[53] Denervation at 3-5 d of age caused frequent apneas and, more importantly, a mortality rate of 62%.[54] Similarly, denervation in piglets at 5-7 d of age results in spontaneous respiratory pauses and desaturation (Fig. 11.3). Ultimately, nearly 50% of the piglets died by 2 weeks after surgery.[55]

This window of vulnerability which is opened by denervation in the newborn period gives support to the speculation that Sudden Infant Death syndrome (SIDS) may be due to peripheral chemoreceptor malfunction[56,57] (see chapter 12 by Pásaro and Ribas). Although no direct information is presently available to support or refute this speculation, it is intriguing that histologic and neurochemical abnormalities are often present in the carotid body tissue of SIDS victims.[56,57]

CONCLUSIONS AND FUTURE DIRECTIONS

Carotid body chemoreceptors represent the major sensor for early detection of hypoxia and evoke a number of reflexes which serve to defend against further hypoxia. Two important characteristics of the maturational process are a decreasing dependence with age on peripheral chemoreceptor input in sustaining a continuous respiratory rhythm and an increase with age in the magnitude of the nerve response to hypoxia.

Although it is relatively well established that an increase in chemosensitivity occurs in the postnatal period and that this is triggered by the increase in PaO_2 at birth, the mechanism remains unknown. Most likely, these answers will be forthcoming with a better understanding of the nature of transmitters elaborated by the glomus cells and better understanding of the biophysical changes of glomus cells. Dopamine, in particular, is well established to be secreted in close association with the increase in nerve activity, but whether this leads to nerve excitation or only inhibition is uncertain.

Several laboratories are focused on changes in glomus cell membrane currents harvested from cats, rats and rabbits. Although a direct examination of developmental changes has not been undertaken in any one species, these types of studies are on the horizon and should give an important insight to the basis of chemosensitivity. Once understood, an enhancement of the maturation process through pharmacologic manipulation promises a therapeutic improvement for the treatment of developmental respiratory difficulties, such as apnea of prematurity, hypoventilation syndromes and pulmonary hypertension.

References

1. Boddy K, Dawes GS, Fisher R et al. Foetal respiratory movements, electrocortical and cardiovascular responses to hypoxaemia and hypercapnia in sheep. J Physiol (London) 1974; 243:599-616.
2. Biscoe TJ, Purves MJ, Sampson SR. Types of nervous activity which may be recorded from the carotid sinus nerve in the sheep fetus. J Physiol (London) 1969; 202:1-23.
3. Blanco CE, Dawes GS, Hanson MA et al. The response to hypoxia of arterial chemoreceptors in fetal sheep and newborn lambs. J Physiol (London) 1984; 351:25-37.
4. Jansen AH, Purves MJ, Tan ED. The role of sympathetic nerves in the activation of the carotid chemoreceptors at birth in the sheep. J Dev Physiol 1980; 2:305-321.
5. Blanco CE, Hanson MA, McCooke HB. Studies of chemoreceptor resetting after hyperoxic ventilation of the fetus in utero. In: JA Riberio, DJ Pallot, eds. Chemoreceptors in Respiratory Control: Croom Helm, 1988:221-227.
6. Hohimer AR, Bissonnette JM, Richardson BS et al. Central chemical regulation of breathing movements in fetal lambs. Respir Physiol 1983; 52:88-111.
7. Gluckman PD, Johnston BM. Lesions in the upper lateral pons abolish the hypoxic depression of breathing in unanaesthetized fetal lambs in utero. J Physiol (London) 1987; 382:373-383.
8. Koos BJ, Chao A, Doany W. Adenosine stimulates breathing in fetal sheep with brain stem section. J Appl Physiol 1992; 72:94-99.
9. Giussani DA, Spencer JAD, Moore PJ et al. Afferent and efferent components of the cardiovascular reflex responses to acute hypoxia in term fetal sheep. J Physiol (London) 1993; 461:431-449.
10. Hanson MA, Kumar P, McCooke HB. Post-natal resetting of carotid chemoreceptor sensitivity in the lamb. J Physiol (London) 1987; 382:57P.
11. Biscoe TJ, Purves MJ. Carotid body chemoreceptor activity in the new-born lamb. J Physiol (London) New York: 1967; 190: 443-454.
12. Carroll JL, Bamford OW, Fitzgerald RS. Postnatal maturation of carotid chemoreceptor responses to O_2 and CO_2 in the cat. J Appl Physiol 1993; 75:2383-2391.
13. Marchal F, Bairam A, Haouzi P et al. Carotid chemoreceptor response to natural stimuli in the newborn kitten. Respir Physiol 1992; 87:183-193.
14. Kumar P, Hanson MA. Re-setting of the hypoxic sensitivity of aortic chemoreceptors in the new-born lamb. J Dev Physiol 1989; 11:199-206.
15. Mulligan EM. Discharge properties of carotid bodies: developmental aspects. In: Haddad GG, Farber JP, eds. Developmental Neurobiology of Breathing. Marcel Dekker, 1991:321-340.
16. Fitzgerald RS, Dehghani GA. Neural responses of the cat carotid and aortic bodies to hypercapnia and hypoxia. J Appl Physiol 1982; 52:596-601.
17. Kholwadwala D, Donnelly DF. Maturation of carotid chemoreceptor sensitivity to hypoxia: in vitro studies in the newborn rat. J Physiol (London) 1992; 453:461-473.
18. Lahiri S, DeLaney RG. Relationship between carotid chemoreceptor activity and ventilation in the cat. Respir Physiol 1975; 24:267-286.
19. Pepper DR, Landauer RC, Kumar P. Postnatal development of CO_2-O_2 interaction in the rat carotid body in vitro. J Physiol (London) 1995; 485:531-541.
20. Eden GJ, Hanson MA. Maturation of the respiratory response to acute hypoxia in the newborn rat. J Physiol (London) 1987; 392:1-9.
21. Hanson MA. Peripheral chemoreceptor function before and after birth. In:

Johnson BM, Gluckman PD, eds. Respiratory Control and Lung Development in the Fetus and Newborn. New York: Perinatology Press., 1986:311-330.
22. Hertzberg T, Hellstrom S, Lagercrantz H et al. Development of the arterial chemoreflex and turnover of carotid body catecholamines in the newborn rat. J Physiol (London) 1990; 425:211-225.
23. Calder NA, Williams BA, Kumar P et al. The respiratory response of healthy term infants to breath-by-breath alterations in inspired oxygen at two postnatal ages. Ped Res 1994; 35:321-324.
24. Belenky DA, Standaert TA, Wooddrum DE. Maturation of hypoxic ventilatory response of the newborn lamb. J Appl Physiol 1979; 47:927-930.
25. Blanco CE, Hanson MA, Johnson P et al. Breathing pattern of kittens during hypoxia. J App Physiol 1984; 56:12-17.
26. Bureau MA, Begin R. Postnatal maturation of the respiratory response to O2 in awake newborn lambs. J Appl Physiol 1982; 52:428-433.
27. Bureau MA, Cote A, Blanchard PW et al. Exponential and diphasic ventilatory response to hypoxia in conscious lambs. J Appl Physiol 1986; 61:836-842.
28. Goiny M, Lagercrantz H, Srinivasan M et al. Hypoxia-mediated in vivo release of dopamine in nucleus tractus solitarii of rabbits. J Appl Physiol 1991; 70: 2395-2400.
29. Schwieler GH. Respiratory regulation during postnatal development in cats and rabbits and some of its morphological substrate. Acta Physiol Scand 1968; 72:1-123.
30. Eden GJ, Hanson MA. Effects of chronic hypoxia from birth on the ventilatory response to acute hypoxia in the newborn rat. J Physiol (London) 1987; 392: 11-19.
31. Hanson MA, Kumar P, Williams BA. The effect of chronic hypoxia upon the development of respiratory chemoreflexes in the newborn kitten. J Physiol (London) 1989; 411:563-574.
32. Hertzberg T, Hellstrom S, Holgert H et al. Ventilatory response to hyperoxia in newborn rats born in hypoxia--possible relationship to carotid body dopamine. J Physiol (London) 1992; 456:645-654.
33. Acker H, Lubbers DW, Purves MJ et al. Measurement of the partial pressure of oxygen in the carotid body of foetal sheep and newborn lambs. J Dev Physiol 1980; 2:323-338.
34. Clarke JA, deBrugh Daly M, Ead HW. Comparison of the size of the vascular compartment of the carotid body of the fetal, neonatal and adult cat. Acta Anat 1990; 138:166-174.
35. Moore PJ, Clarke JA, Hanson MA et al. Quantitative studies of the vasculature of the carotid body in fetal and newborn sheep. J Dev Physiol 1991; 15:211-214.
36. McDonald DM. Peripheral chemoreceptors: structure-function relationships of the carotid body. In: Hornbein TF, ed. Regulation of Breathing. Mercel Decker, 1991:105-320.
37. Neil E, O'Regan RG. The effects of electrical stimulation of the distal end of the cut sinus and aortic nerves on peripheral arterial chemoreceptor activity in the cat. J Physiol (London) 1971; 215:15-32.
38. Band DM, Linton RAF. Plasma potassium and the carotid body chemoreceptor in the cat. J Physiol (London) 1984; 345:33.
39. Pokorski M, Lahiri S. Effects of naloxone on carotid body chemoreception and ventilation in the cat. J Appl Physiol 1981; 51:1533-1538.
40. Joels N, Neil E. The idea of a sensory transmitter. In: Torrance R, ed. Arterial Chemoreceptors Oxford: Oxford Univ Press 1968:153-178.
41. Kondo H. An electron microscopic study on the development of synapses in the rat carotid body. Neurosci Lett 1976; 3:197-200.
42. Scheibner T, Read DJ, Sullivan CE. Distribution of substance P-immunoreactive structures in the developing cat carotid body. Brain Res 1988; 453:72-78.
43. Prabhakar NR, Runold M, Yamamoto Y et al. Effect of substance P antagonist on the hypoxia-induced carotid chemoreceptor activity. Acta Physiol Scand 1984; 121:301-303.
44. González C, Almaraz L, Obeso A et al. Oxygen and acid chemoreception in the carotid body chemoreceptors. TINS 1992; 15:146-153.

45. Donnelly DF, Doyle TP. Developmental changes in hypoxia-induced catecholamine release from rat carotid body, in vitro. J Physiol (London) 1994; 475: 267-275.
46. Donnelly DF, Smith EJ, Dutton RE. Neural response of carotid chemoreceptors following dopamine blockade. J Appl Physiol 1981; 50:172-177.
47. Sterni LM, Bamford OS, Tomares SM et al. Developmental changes in intracellular Ca^{2+} response of carotid chemoreceptor cells to hypoxia. Am J Physiol 1995; 268:L801-L808.
48. Lopez-Barneo J, Lopez-Lopez JR, Urena J et al. Chemotransduction in the carotid body: K current modulated by pO_2 in type I chemoreceptor cells. Science 1988; 241:580-582.
49. Peers C. Hypoxic suppression of K^+ currents in type I carotid body cells: selective effect on the Ca^{2+}-activated K^+ current. Neurosci Lett 1990; 119:253-256.
50. Wyatt CN, Wright C, Bee D et al. O_2-sensitive K^+ currents in carotid body chemoreceptor cells from normoxic and chronically hypoxic rats and their roles in hypoxic transduction. Proc Natl Acad Sci 1995; 92:295-299.
51. Landauer RC, Pepper DR, Kumar P. Effect of chronic hypoxaemia from birth upon chemosensitivity in the adult rat carotid body in vitro. J Physiol (London) 1995; 485:543-550.
52. Bureau MA, Lamarche J, Foulon P et al. Postnatal maturation of respiration in intact and carotid body-denervated lambs. J Appl Physiol 1985; 59:869-874.
53. Hofer MA. Sleep-wake state organization in infant rats with episodic respiratory disturbance following sinoaortic denervation. Sleep 1985; 8:40-48.
54. Hofer MA. Lethal respiratory disturbance in neonatal rats after arterial chemoreceptor denervation. Life Sci 1984; 34: 489-496.
55. Donnelly DF, Haddad GG. Prolonged apnea and impaired survival in piglets after sinus and aortic nerve section. J Appl Physiol 1990; 68:1048-1052.
56. Naeye RL, Fisher R, Ryser M et al. Carotid body in sudden infant death syndrome. Science 1976; 191:567-569.
57. Perrin DG, Cutz E, Becker LE et al. Sudden infant death syndrome: increased carotid body dopamine and noradrenaline content. Lancet 1984; Sept 8: 535-537.

CHAPTER 12

Physiopathology of the Carotid Body and its Role in the Development of Sudden Infant Death Syndrome

Rosario Pásaro and Juan Ribas

INTRODUCTION: AN OVERVIEW OF CAROTID BODY PATHOLOGY

The established facts on the abnormal or pathological function of the carotid body (CB) are fragmentary compared to our knowledge of the normal significance of this chemoreceptor organ. In adulthood, the only primary established pathology of the CB is that related to CB tumors. Carotid body tumors are infrequent. They exhibit some familial tendency and a greater prevalence in highlanders; they are rarely malignant, and only occasionally do they exhibit systemic manifestations in the form of catecholamine-secreting tumors. In most occasions the capital clinical sign of the CB tumors is a mobile local mass of a variable size in the neck, and in some other occasions hoarseness, dysphagia, or carotid sinus syndrome are the complaints that bring patients to the hospital.[1] Most surgeons would agree that the most relevant aspects of these rare tumors are related to their location, and thereby to the functional alterations produced by their surgical management, which include severe hemorrhage, loss of baroreceptor function, paralysis of the vocal cords, or resections of the vagus or the hypoglossal nerves.[2,3] Since the frequency of sequels resulting from the surgical treatment of the CB tumors is proportional to the size of the tumors, it follows that prompt diagnosis and surgical treatment in very specialized centers are critical.[2] Alterations in the CB function, in the form of chemoreceptor hyper-reactivity, have been suggested to be involved in the genesis or early manifestations of essential hypertensive disease.[4] Alterations in the CB structure, secondary to several systemic diseases, have been described in necropsies,[1] but the physiopathological significance of those alterations remains to be elucidated.

The main thrust of this chapter will be to summarize the abnormalities, both at the structural and functional level, which result in an anomalous drive to the central respiratory

The Carotid Body Chemoreceptors,
edited by Constancio González.

controller. Particular attention will be given to alterations in the CB chemoreceptors sensitivity, their afferent inputs, the central outputs to the respiratory muscles, and their possible role in the genesis of the Sudden Infant Death syndrome (SIDS). Since SIDS involves a failure of respiration and affects infants in their early postnatal months, we will make frequent references to the maturational changes occurring in the CB. Similarly, we shall describe the central projections of the carotid sinus nerve and their maturational changes, and also the central neuronal networks involved in the control of respiration during early postnatal ages (see also chapters 9 and 11 by Katz et al and Donnelly, respectively). Morphological alterations in victims of SIDS, probably reflecting maturational deficits, have been described at all levels of the control of respiration. Possible influences of environmental factors in the abnormal maturation of the CB and the central respiratory controllers, and their possible relation to the genesis of SIDS, will also be discussed.

THE SUDDEN INFANT DEATH SYNDROME

Clinical and Epidemiological Features

Over the past 25 years there has been a steady fall in infant mortality in developed countries. It has reached a constant rate of about 2 per 1,000 live births.[5] SIDS represents the major cause of death in infants after the first week of age. The definition of SIDS most widely used today is the one first proposed by Beckwith.[6] According to this author, SIDS is '*the sudden death of an infant or young child which is unexpected by history, and in which a thorough postmortem examination fails to demonstrate an adequate cause of death*'. This definition implies that most diagnoses of SIDS are made postmortem, and by exclusion. However, in the clinical history of infants dying of SIDS it is common to find episodes of cyanosis and apneas while the babies were quietly sleeping, and there are vivid descriptions of "near misses" in which babies have been resuscitated from episodes of prolonged apneas. These near-miss infants are at great risk of dying of SIDS and special vigilance should be imposed in closely monitoring these infants.

The cause of death in SIDS may be the result of multiple determining factors with an interaction between physiological and environmental elements. SIDS is rare in babies of less than 1 month and over 6 months of age, with a peak incidence at 2-4 months of age. This epidemiological fact might suggest that there is a particularly vulnerable stage in the development of respiratory control between these ages.[7] Infants with low weight at birth, or born prematurely, are at increased risk of SIDS, as are infants of multiple births and newborns of higher birth order.[8] The incidence of SIDS varies with the season, with more deaths occurring during the winter months, suggesting some infectious component in triggering SIDS. Maternal risk factors include: young maternal age, poor prenatal care, bleeding during pregnancy and smoking. Furthermore, there is evidence that household exposure to tobacco smoke has an independent additive effect.[9,10] Parental drug misuse (aside from smoking) has an additional small but significant effect.[11] These and other environmental factors, as for example infections, may work in combination with a vulnerable stage of physiological development, to precipitate death.[12]

SIDS is closely associated with sleep. The relationship between SIDS and sleeping position has been examined in several epidemiological studies. Most of those studies, but not all, found that the prone position during sleep was more common in babies dying of SIDS than in control babies. The mechanism on the apparently significant association between the prone position for sleep and the risk for SIDS is unknown, but an impaired ventilatory control and arousal responsiveness has been suggested.[13]

Respiratory failure has long been recognized to be involved in SIDS. There are several hypotheses implicating a deficient function of the peripheral chemoreceptors in the etiology of SIDS.[14,15] Also an unstable respiratory activity during sleep, prolonged sleep apneas, and oropharyngeal/laryngeal dysfunction induced by liquid stimulation of the upper airways have been postulated to be involved in the genesis of SIDS.[16-18] It has been found that infants with the aborted syndrome ("near-miss" infants), in comparison with normal infants, hypoventilated during quiet sleep, and their ventilatory response to carbon dioxide breathing during quiet sleep was impaired.[19] However, the underlying mechanisms are unknown. Clearly, however, there is some malfunction in the respiratory control if breathing ceases during sleep, and if arousal and hyperventilation do not occur despite the development of asphyxia.

Abnormal development or delayed maturation of the neural components involved in the control of respiration may induce changes in excitability or connectivity. These abnormalities would finally impair the normal drive for breathing. Certainly, during transition from fetal to infant life, rapid functional changes have to occur to allow adaptation to distinct environmental conditions[20] (see chapter 11 by Donnelly). Early in the postnatal periods, the CBs have to readjust, or reset, their sensitivity to O_2. This resetting is imposed by the great increase in the arterial PO_2 that occurs immediately upon birth (Fig. 12.1). In addition to O_2 sensitivity, CB sensitivity to CO_2, pH, plasma K^+ and hormone levels also change in the postnatal period (see chapter 11 by Donnelly). In the adult, superimposed with the chemical drive to breathe, inputs from the somatosensory system, including mechanoreceptors and thermoreceptors, and inputs from higher centers in the central nervous system also participate in the final setting of the output of the brainstem controllers of respiration.[21] In the postnatal period some of these costimuli might not be developed, or might be greatly reduced by the completely different living conditions in the postnatal period.

The Carotid Bodies in the Sudden Infant Death Syndrome

Peripheral arterial chemoreceptors pathology, mainly pathology of the CB, has been suggested to be involved in the etiology and/or clinical expression of SIDS.[17] This suggestion is supported by the findings that carotid body denervation caused unexpected death in lambs at 4-5 weeks of age.[22] Similarly, sinoaortic denervations in rats of 3-21 days of age resulted in very prolonged episodes of apnea during sleep and an increased rate of mortality in operated vs. nonoperated animals.[23,24] Comparable observations have been made in piglets.[25] In this later animal species it has recently been reported that CB denervation at about 2 weeks, but not at 1 or 3 weeks of age, caused life-threatening apneic events during sleep associated with severe hypoxemia, implying that a critical period exists in the maturation process during which the malfunction of the CB can be fatal.[26] The overall clinical picture observed in the denervated piglets in this study[26] greatly recalls symptomatology described in infant victims of SIDS: prolonged apneas during quiet sleep, profound reductions in blood oxygen content, tachycardia, rise in blood pressure, and eventually, a flattening of the electroencephalogram.

Denervation studies, however, do not clarify the primary cause of apneic events that eventually develop to fatal apnea in SIDS. To propose a cause-effect relationship, one must postulate an abnormal function of the CB, probably due to an abnormal development or failure to mature of this chemoreceptor organ. Early histological studies have provided valuable information on the size and cellular composition of CB in the fetus, and on the changes occurring in the early postnatal period, i.e., on the changes occurring as a result of the change in PO_2 associated to birth.[1] According to these authors, the fetal, immature or progenitor chemoreceptor cells in the CB would disappear after birth, leading to the appearance of the functionally mature light and dark variants of chemoreceptor cells. Biopsies of the CB belonging to some SIDS victims have shown a greater percentage of immature cells, in comparison to age-matched controls, leading to the suggestion that the CBs are functionally immature. Another common finding in CBs of SIDS victims is an abnormal proliferation of sustentacular cells or fibroblasts with the consequent percentile decrease of chemoreceptor cells; in other words, even if the total mass of the CB is normal it would be a reduction of the noble parenchymal chemoreceptor cells. Additionally, some authors have found that the size of the CBs in SIDS victims is small in comparison to controls, but others have found no differences.[1] These variable findings might be genuine, and probably are related to the frequently unknown previous clinical history of the victim. Thus, a victim having a prolonged clinical history of episodes of apnea, and therefore of hypoxemia, or a clinical history of previous respiratory diseases might have developed CB hypertrophy as a response to the hypoxic episodes. On the contrary, an infant dying after only a reduced number of hypoxemic episodes may have a normal CB size or even a reduced size if the organ was originally underdeveloped. The observations made in adults whose CB has been invaded by metastasis of carcinoma of the tongue are some extent, consistent with the histopathological changes found in the CB of victims of SIDS, as well as with their clinical history. These patients have a clinical history severe episodes of apnea as a very relevant symptom, and may suffer fatal cardio-respiratory syncope.[27,28]

Physiopathology of the CB Maturation Process

The ventilatory response to hyperoxia, in the form of a few breaths of pure O_2, also known as chemical or functional denervation of the CB, is frequently used to silence the CB arterial chemoreceptors, and thereby to assess their contribution to the overall respiratory drive. This test has also been used as a marker for development of peripheral chemoreceptor function, it being found that in normal infants of 1 day (d) of age CBs do not contribute to the respiratory drive but that at 1 week of age there is a clear but small contribution (see chapter 11). Using this suppression test it has been found that premature infants with chronic lung disease showed a delayed development of their chemosensitivity. This implies that these infants are unprotected against hypoxia and have an increased risk for SIDS.[29] As mentioned above, CB chemoreceptors sensitivity to hypoxia resets during the postnatal period, and it seems well established that the resetting process is triggered by the increase in arterial blood PO_2 which occurs after birth. This is true for both mature and premature neonates. On the basis of observations made in highland residents that exhibit a blunted response to hypoxic tests,[30] it was reasoned that if neonates suffer frequent episodes of hypoxia, there the normal resetting of the CB function might not develop or might be delayed, leading to an impaired defense against hypoxic episodes at ages when the role of the CBs to maintain an adequate drive for breathing during sleep may be critical[26] (see above). Clinical observations seem to support this suggestion, as it has been reported that normal infants born at high altitudes, as well as infants suffering from chronic hypoxemic illness have diminished responses to hypoxic tests.[31] Experimental evidence also supports contention. Thus, several animal species kept in hypoxic environments after birth do not develop an adequate response to hypoxic tests, i.e., hypoxia after birth prevents the normal resetting of the CB function.[20] These arguments would explain satisfactorily the increased incidence of SIDS among infants who have suffered hypoxemia due to respiratory or cardiocirculatory pathology in the postnatal period, but what is the cause of the hypoxemia in infants threatened by SIDS with an *unexpected clinical history*? We are forced to invoke a deficient control of the respiratory function at birth. Whether that deficiency or lack of maturation affects the CB chemoreceptor tissue, the wiring of the central projections of the carotid sinus nerve, the organization of the neuronal respiratory groups of the medulla, or the connections of other CNS nuclei with the respiratory controllers of the medulla is a question on debate. Although an alteration at any of those levels is capable of generating infants with apparently unresetted CB function, the possibility exists that deficiencies in SIDS victims occur at more than one level.

Brady and McCann[32] studied the ventilatory response to hypoxia (17% oxygen) and hypercapnia (4% carbon dioxide) in subsequent siblings of SIDS victims. They found that after 5 weeks of age, siblings of SIDS had a normal response to hypercapnia but responded to mild hypoxia with periodic breathing. When the infants were sleeping, arousal occurred during 25% of the hypoxic challenges in the control group, but was not seen in the siblings of SIDS victims. The significance of periodic breathing and absence of arousal is not clear, but it is thought that this instability of ventilation may lead to profound apnea and SIDS in the presence of other predisposing factors such as an upper respiratory tract infection or overheating. It is well known that in the normal CB of adult animals, exists a positive interaction between hypoxic and hypercapnic stimuli (see chapter 6). In neonates this positive interaction at the level of the CB is minimal. This aspect of the CB physiology has recently been studied by Kumar and coworkers.[33,34] They had found that in rats of 5-7 days of age some degree of interaction is already evident, and, what is more important in the present context, that the maintenance of the pups in a hypoxic environment (about 12% O_2) for up to 5 weeks greatly attenuated the positive CO_2-O_2 interaction at the level of the CB. These findings would imply that infants suffering from chronic hypoxemia would present a reduced CB respiratory drive during the episodes of apnea of quiet sleep.

As described in detail by Donnelly, (see chapter 11) the ventilatory response to hypoxic stimulus in neonatal animals is biphasic, an initial and transient increase in ventilation followed by an undershoot in ventilation below the prehypoxic levels (see Fig. 12.1). In neonatal lambs (1-4 weeks of age), nicotine administration produced, in comparison to adult animals, a paradoxical effect that consisted in a decrease of the initial hyperventilation produced by hypoxia. Additionally, nicotine produced an increase in the ventilatory depression induced by a hyperoxic suppression test.[35] The authors concluded that these paradoxical effects of nicotine in neonatal animals CB- and centrally-mediated. Whether peripheral or central in origin, these paradoxical effects of nicotine could explain the higher risk of SIDS for infants living in an environment rich in nicotine or being born from smoking mothers (see Fig. 12.1).

So far, clinical, epidemiological and experimental evidence indicates that whenever the CB function in the neonatal period is impaired, the risk for SIDS increases. However, the question remains—is there any subtle CB alteration in real unexpected SIDS? It is well known that the CB blood flow is higher than in any other body organ when blood flow is referred to weight units. It also appears that this very high blood flow (and thereby small arteriovenous O_2 difference) enables the CB to obtain enough oxygen to work at maximal capacity during intense hypoxia (see chapter 2). In this context, it may be suggested that the high CB blood flow plays a significant role in the resetting of the CB function in the postnatal period, as it facilitates the CB to be exposed high PO_2, the apparent resetting signal. Therefore, it is conceivable that an abnormal angiogenic development in the CB, leading to a reduced blood flow through the organ, would impair its physiological maturation. Recent data obtained by Zhong and Nurse[36] may render some support to that suggestion. These authors found that after culturing fetal chemoreceptor cells in the presence of basic fibroblast growth factor (bFGF) for two days, they exhibited a significant increase in the density of both, the transients inward Na^+ and the outward K^+ currents, i.e., bFGF increased the excitability of chemoreceptor cells as reflected by the fact that they readily fire action potentials following depolarization. Since bFGF is a potent angiogenic factor, the authors suggested that different degrees of expression of this growth factor during fetal life in the CB of

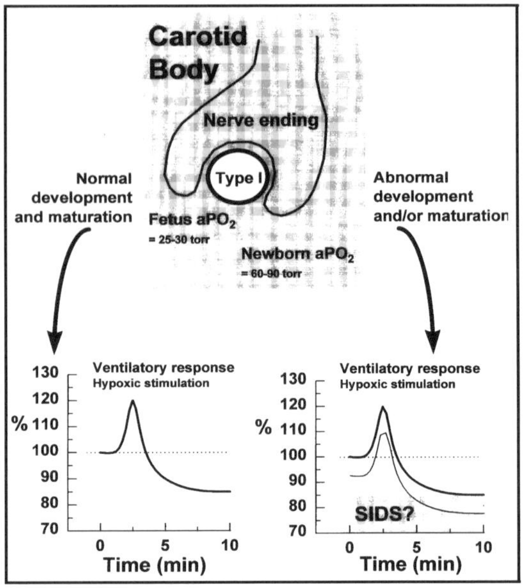

Fig. 12.1. Schematic drawing showing changes leading to depression of the ventilatory response to hypoxia, in the newborn. Different ranges of arterial PO_2 in fetus and newborn (*upper panel*) trigger normal changes in oxygen sensitivity in the carotid body chemoreceptors during the early postnatal weeks (months in humans), which lead to the normal hypoxic ventilatory response to hypoxic stimulation in this early postnatal period (*left, bottom panel*), and which ultimately culminate in the genesis of the normal hypoxic ventilatory response observed in adult animals. An abnormal development of the carotid body, or an abnormal process of maturation, would generate a depressed sensitivity to hypoxia in the early postnatal period (thin trace in *right, bottom panel*) which eventually might lead to SIDS.

different species, could contribute to the genesis of the known species differences in CB chemoreceptor excitability. In the same framework we are prone to suggest that a deficient expression of bFGF (or some other angiogenic factor) could be responsible for the inadequate (or slow) functional maturation of the CB that normally culminates in the resetting of its sensitivity to hypoxia.

Although the real significance of K^+ current inhibition in the transduction of the hypoxic stimulus remains to be fully clarified, it is a constant that chemoreceptor cells from every animal species tested, and at any age, exhibit O_2-sensitive K^+ currents. In addition, pulmonary artery smooth muscle cells, which react to similar levels of hypoxia than chemoreceptor cells, also exhibit O_2-sensitive K^+ currents (see chapter 5). Therefore, the presence of O_2-sensitive K^+ currents in a cell type has been taken as an index of O_2-sensing capacity. When rat pups are reared in hypoxic environments, their chemoreceptor cells showed a significant decrease in potassium current density, when compared to cells obtained from age-matched animals grown in normoxic atmospheres. The reduced K^+ current density was mainly due to a lack of charybdotoxin-sensitive Ca^{2+}-dependent K^+ channels, which in rats are the main O_2-sensitive K^+ channels.[37] Certainly this absence would reduce CB excitability if we accept the above-mentioned index (but see Donnelly[38]).

Neurotransmitters and Neuromodulators and the Carotid Body Function in the Postnatal Period

A large number of neuroactive substances that may act as transmitters or modulators in the chemoreception process have been found in the carotid body[4,39] (see also chapter 3). The significance of those neurotransmitters in the normal function of the adult CB is controversial, in spite of the large effort devoted to their study. As a consequence, the significance of the neurotransmitters in neonatal CBs, where the studies are scarce, and even further in the physiopathology of the neonatal CB, is largely speculative. Quite frequently, the studies suggesting the involvement of a given neurotransmitter in the CB function are pharmacological, and the conclusions reached involve suggestions on the neurotransmitter dynamics that are not known, or if they are known, might be in contradiction to the suggestions.

The only CB neurotransmitter that has attracted the attention of a large of number of researchers in perinatal CB is dopamine (DA). On the basis of pharmacological responses, DA is generally considered to be an inhibitory neurotransmitter at the CB chemoreceptors (see chapter 7), but some authors, based on the dynamics of DA in relation to the natural stimulation and the location of the receptors for DA in the CB, propose that this DA can act as an excitatory neurotransmitter (see chapter 4). Pharmacological studies in newborn kittens reveal that DA produces mainly excitatory effects, especially during hypoxic stimulation.[40] In neonatal rats Donnelly and Doyle[41] have shown that there is a maturational increase in the release of DA and carotid sinus response to hypoxia as the age of the animals increases from 7 to 30 days. Bairam et al[42] have made a similar observation in neonatal rabbits. In this latter species the CBs challenged with hypoxia (perfusion with 8% O_2-equilibrated solutions) do not release DA in amounts different from normoxia until 25 days of age. Paralleling these observations on neurotransmitter dynamics, Sterni et al[43] have shown that increase in intracellular Ca^{2+} elicited by hypoxic/anoxic stimuli was considerably (3-5 x) lower in chemoreceptor cells from newborn rabbits in comparison to adult animals; the same was true if the stimulus was NaCN. These studies clearly indicate that the release of DA induced by hypoxia runs in parallel to the resetting of the CB function. Therefore, to propose that an increased dopaminergic activity is responsible for the low hypoxic sensitivity in the neonatal period seems unsupported by experimental observations. Increased concentration of biogenic amines in carotid bodies from SIDS victims, with very high levels of DA, have been found in CBs of SIDS victims.[14] However, the interpretation of this static finding is ambiguous. Increased DA levels may reflect an increased turnover of DA with an increased rate of synthesis and an increased, but smaller, rate of release; this is the normal response of the DA stores in the CB of adult animals when they are chronically exposed to hypoxia.[39] Alternatively, high DA stores in the CB of SIDS victims may be the result of a normal rate of synthesis associated to a reduced rate of release.

As already mentioned, epidemiological studies have shown a clear relationship between maternal smoking and SIDS.[10] Nicotine in adult animals is a well known chemostimulant agent capable of increasing ventilation, and it is known to release catecholamines from chemoreceptor cells in amounts that parallel the action potential frequency elicited in the carotid sinus nerve.[44,45] However, in neonatal lambs nicotine has paradoxical effects on breathing (see above). It might be suggested that the paradoxical effect of nicotine on ventilation is the result of a parallel paradoxical decrease in the release of catecholamines. However, a recent report by Holgert et al[46] would suggest the opposite. These authors found that nicotine exposure to rat pups results in an impaired hypoxic respiratory drive, when compared to age-matched pups (3 days of age), which is associated with a decrease of DA in the CB and with an increased expression of tyrosine hydroxylase mRNA. Although increased mRNA levels for TH do not necessarily mean an increased TH activity or an increased rate of DA synthesis, the authors concluded that nicotine had produced, in parallel, an increase in the turnover rate of DA in the CB and a decrease in hypoxic drive.

Central Respiratory Control and the Sudden Infant Death Syndrome

An Overview of the Central Respiratory Control

Respiration (ventilation) is a complex motor act that requires precise coordination of numerous muscle groups and thereby of numerous neuronal circuits. The integrating centers and pathways for the control of ventilation, cardiac activity and blood pressure are located in the brainstem, especially in the reticular formation of the ventrolateral medulla.[21-49] The neural respiratory network in mammals is represented bilaterally, as columns extending rostrocaudally throughout the ventrolateral medulla. The principal respiratory oscillator is localized

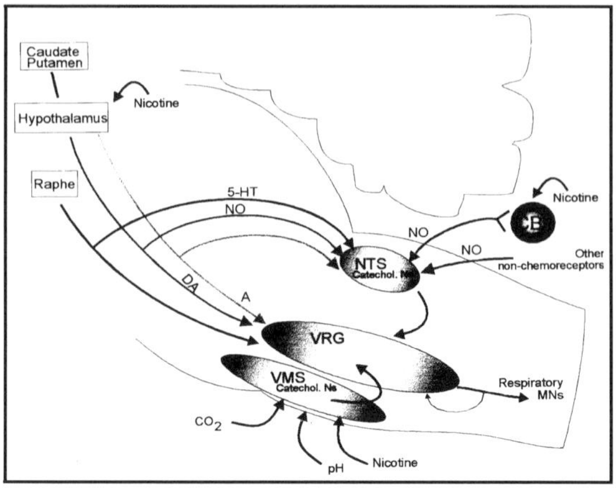

Fig. 12.2. Schematic diagram of the brainstem showing the regions involved in control of breathing and their afferent and efferent inputs. The diagram includes neurotransmitter systems that have been found altered in SIDS victims, and the sites of action of nicotine which in an important epidemiological factor in triggering SIDS. CB, carotid body. MNs, motorneurons; Ns, neurons NTS, nucleus of the tractus solitarius; VMS, ventral medullary surface; VRG, ventral respiratory group; DA, dopamine; NO, nitric oxide.

in a region termed the ventral respiratory group[21,47,50] (Fig. 12.2).

Also involved in respiratory control is the dorsomedial medulla containing the nucleus of the tractus solitarius (NTS; Fig. 12.2), which is the primary relay nucleus for carotid chemoreceptors and baroreceptors. Therefore the NTS is essential for the reflex adjustment of the respiratory and cardiovascular systems. The hypoglossal nucleus innervating the pharyngeal and tongue muscles also plays a critical role in respiratory control. The afferent fibers from the CB enter the lateral aspect of the medulla towards the ipsilateral NTS terminating most densely in the medial and commissural subnuclei (see chapter 9 by Katz et al). The distribution of afferent terminals is consistent with the role of this relatively restricted region of NTS in mediating the hypoxic ventilatory response.[51-53] However, it should be noted that there is evidence suggesting that the synaptic and cellular mechanisms underlying respiratory rhythmogenesis in the adult mammal are different from those of the neonate.[54,55]

The precise location of the central chemosensitive area is debated, but there is a substantial evidence supporting that the arcuate nucleus of the ventral medullary surface (VMS) participates in the ventilatory response to carbon dioxide and hydrogen ions; this nucleus also plays a prominent role in cardiorespiratory coupling, and in the genesis of pressor responses[56] (Fig. 12.2). Neurons in the VMS are intimately associated with the ventrolateral neurons of the brainstem that integrate ventilatory, pressor, and depressor responses. Direct application of cholinergic agonists to the VMS stimulates ventilation, whereas application of antagonists results in decreased ventilation.[57] Consistent with these findings, the effects of breathing high CO_2 on the expression of *c-fos* have demonstrated the existence of CO_2-responsive neurons in the ventral medulla, including the VMS, and that the targets of these neurons include brainstem and spinal neurons.[58-60] In this context, it should also be noted that *c-fos* immunohistochemistry has similarly been used to locate brainstem neurons activated by hypoxia or electrical stimulation of the carotid sinus nerve. In the cat, both types of stimuli induced an increase in the expression of *c-fos* in the intermediate VMS; on the contrary, systemic hyperoxia reduced the activity in the same area. Consistent with these findings, denervation of the CB markedly delayed the onset of this hypoxic response.[61] The afferent projections of CB where overlapping with the pattern of expression of the immediate early gene of *c-fos*, following hypoxia or carotid sinus nerve stimulation, which imply that at least some of the *c-fos* labeled neurons within the NTS and the VMS are likely to be the second-order neurons in the chemosensory pathways[62] (see also chapter 9).

Neurons of the NTS with inputs from arterial chemoreceptors, can be inhibited by electrical or glutamate stimulation of the locus coeruleus and nucleus raphe magnus, suggesting that these catecholaminergic and serotoninergic nuclei play a role in controlling chemosensory input at the NTS[63] (Fig. 12.2). There is evidence in the literature of a mutual facilitatory interaction between the arterial chemoreceptor reflex and the alerting stage of the defense reaction, particularly in relation to the patterning of cardiopulmonary activity. Neurons within the NTS display excitatory responses to stimulation of the hypothalamic defense area as well as arterial chemoreceptor stimulation.[64]

Development of Central Respiratory Network and Pathological Findings in the Sudden Infant Death Syndrome

Within the medulla oblongata, neuronal maturation occurs slightly earlier in the ventral reticular formation than in the dorsal vagal nucleus.[65,66] Reports of morphological abnormalities in the brainstem of victims of SIDS include focal astrogliosis, a persistence of dendritic spines in proximal segments of dendrites and hypomyelinization.[7,17,67] These anatomical regions are susceptible to pathology in infants who have been exposed to severe hypoxic-ischemic episodes during gestation or in the early postnatal period.[7,68] On the other hand, with normal gestational growth, the dendrites become long, the spines increased in number and their distribution assumed a mature pattern in the medullary reticular formation, vagal and tractus solitarius nuclei with the number of spines increasing on the distal dendrite segments. Some of the SIDS victims have abnormal respiratory control before the terminal event, suggesting an abnormal maturation of the respiratory network.

During the first 2 weeks of life in rats and mice there are profound changes in both, the rhythmic pattern of hypoglossal motoneurons and the sensitivity of the respiratory rhythm to strychnine blockade of glycine receptors.[69] Developmental changes in strychnine-sensitive receptors are vital to maturation of the respiratory network, and it has been suggested that a disturbance in their development may be lethal. As an index of the neuronal changes during maturation, motoneurons of the genioglossus in rats from 1-6 days of age and later in development (13-15 and 19-30 days),[70,71] as well as phrenic motoneurons in kittens (2 to 14 weeks)[72] exhibit membrane properties, branching pattern and spine distribution which are different from those of adult animals. In addition, some SIDS infants have minor signs of autonomic dysfunction and behavioral disorders before death. These minor signs may also be related to abnormal dendritic and neurotransmitter development of the brainstem.[73] Since the autonomic control of respiration is essential to maintain the normal respiratory pattern during sleep, a developmental failure of this control mechanism may also be associated with SIDS.[74]

Recently, there had been identified ependymal alterations in preterm and neonates who died suddenly and unexpectedly without any other cause or explanation found at autopsy. The histological changes consisted of denudation, vacuolization, macro- and microglial nodules and gliosis.[75] The physiopathological significance of these alterations is presently unknown. Conversely, no quantitative evidence of astrocytosis was found in the hypoglossal nuclei of SIDS infants.[76]

Neurotransmitters and Neuromodulators in the Central Respiratory Network. Findings in the Sudden Infant Death Syndrome

The identity of all the neurotransmitters involved in the mediation of the afferent signals to the central respiratory neurons is far from elucidated. Fast switching neurotransmitters like acetylcholine, amino acids (glutamic acid, aspartic acid) and monoamines are probably of major importance.[77] A few studies have sought to determine if SIDS victims exhibit any abnormalities that may indicate a deficiency in neurotransmitter function. A predominance of inhibitory neurotransmitters in the brainstem has been found in SIDS victims.[78]

The catecholaminergic neurons of the ventrolateral and dorsal medulla are part of the complex circuitry involved in autonomic regulation and chemoreceptive function[79] (Fig. 12.2). No synaptic contacts were found between carotid sinus nerve afferents and catecholaminergic dendrites or perkarya in the commissural nucleus of the NTS, implying that it is unlikely that second-order neurons of either the chemo- or baroreceptor reflex are catecholaminergic.[80] However, there is solid evidence to support a role for catecholaminergic neurons in the integration of the chemoreceptor reflex. For example, electrical stimulation of carotid sinus nerve and physiological stimulation of the carotid bodies by hypoxia induced c-fos-like immunoreactivity in cathecolaminergic neurons containing TH or phenylethanolamine-N-methyl transferase (PNMT) in the ventrolateral medulla and to a lesser extent in the dorsal vagal complex.[62] Furthermore, in the commissural nucleus of the NTS there is evidence for axo-axonic synapses between tyrosine-hydroxylase positive carotid sinus nerve afferent terminals (which are chemoreceptor fibers; see chapter 9) and central terminals positive to TH.[80] Then, a disturbance of developmental patterns of cathecolaminergic neurons in the medulla may be involved in the genesis of an altered cardiopulmonary control and, therefore, in the genesis of SIDS. Several recent studies have been conducted on the immunocytochemical distribution of TH and PNMT in the medullas of SIDS victims.[81,82] In SIDS victims there was an absence of PNMT positive neurons in the NTS, but TH positivity displayed a similar distribution between SIDS victims and control medullas. They suggested that SIDS victims may have a specific alteration of adrenergic neurons in the NTS, which might be primarily responsible for cardiopulmonary dysfunction. Furthermore, the catecholaminergic neurons of SIDS victims showed a delayed dendritic maturation in the ventrolateral medulla, which might suggest a genetic mechanism in the pathogenesis of SIDS.[7] Abnormalities within the monoamine-containing neurons were also observed in other CNS neurons of SIDS victims. Based on the rich innervation of the human basal ganglia by monoaminergic afferents from cell bodies in the substantia nigra, Kalaria et al[83] studied the synaptic chemistry of cathecolamine and associated neurons of the putamen. They found smaller concentrations of DA and TH protein and an altered ratio of serotonin to DA catabolites in SIDS infants, suggesting specific changes in dopaminergic neurons originating in the midbrain or alterations in monoaminergic metabolism in the terminal arborization of the brainstem nuclei, or both (Fig. 12.2).

Sparks and Hunsaker[84] reported serotonergic and cholinergic abnormalities in the hypothalamus of SIDS infants. Cholinergic muscarinic activity in the human arcuate nucleus in the VMS is postulated to be involved in cardioventilatory control[57] (Fig. 12.2). A significant decrease in [^{3}H] quinuclidinilbenzilate (a muscarinic antagonist) binding in the arcuate nucleus of the VMS, in comparison to infants dying acutely of known causes, occurred in SIDS infants. In infants with chronic oxygenation abnormalities, binding is low in other nuclei, as well as in the arcuate nucleus. The binding deficit observed in the arcuate nucleus of SIDS infants could be correlated to the cardiorespiratory failures occurring during sleep in these infants.[85]

In recent years, the role of neuromodulators during the fetal and neonatal periods has been reported to be more important than during adult life.[86] The finding that endorphins and somatostatin strongly inhibit breathing in animal models suggested the possibility that these neuropeptides could be involved in SIDS. It has been proposed the existence of an endorphinergic tonic inhibition in the fetus and the neonate, which diminishes after the neonatal period, and higher concentrations of endorphins have been found in asphyxiated newborn infants.[86] Monti et al[87] have correlated the effects of adenosine analogues with the incidence of sleep apneas, and have concluded that a decrease in adenosine receptors in central structures might increase the apneic index during sleep. Finally, Substance P, which appears to be a central cotransmitter of the chemosensory afferents of the CB, has been found to enhance the effect of serotonin, in depolarizing respiratory neurons,[86] but there is not information relating SP and SIDS.

Independently of the role of NO in the functioning of the CB in the hypoxic responses (see chapter 8), central nitrergic mechanisms also appear to contribute importantly to the respiratory responses elicited by hypoxia. Hypoxia leads to activation of a NO-cGMP pathway in the CNS, which contribute to the induction and maintenance of hypoxia-induced increases in respiratory output.[88] These effects of NO appear to involve the inhibition of inhibitory synapses which are directly activated by CNS hypoxia, and do not appear to be related to the peripheral chemoreceptor inputs.[88] Nitrergic inputs of central and peripheral origin have been demonstrated in the dorsal vagal complex (NTS-X). The medial parvicellular subdivision of the paraventricular hypothalamic nucleus and peripheral afferents, including those of the CB, were found to be the origin of these inputs. It is possible that NO of peripheral and central origin modulate the viscerosensory signal processing in the NTS-X and autonomic reflex function[89] (Fig 12.2). However, a possible relationship between NO and SIDS has not been explored.

As mentioned in the clinical and epidemiological description of SIDS, drug abuse in mothers is associated with an increased incidence of SIDS. We have been making references to nicotine in dealing with the possible role of the CB in the pathogenesis of SIDS (see references 9 and 10), and here we shall mention some additional, potentially pathogenic effects of nicotine acting at the CNS. Human fetuses are exposed to significant amounts of nicotine, the primary psychoactive ingredient in cigarette smoke, by both active smoking of their mothers and exposure to passive smoke.[90] Clegg et al[91] showed that administration of nicotine induced the expression of *c-fos* within the maternal habenula and hypothalamic paraventricular nucleus, whereas in the fetal brain, *c-fos* was induced in both these structures and in the suprachiasmatic nucleus. It was suggested that nicotine during the postnatal period can induce alterations in the composition or number of the nicotinic receptors, or in the subsequent intracellular transduction cascade leading to *c-fos* expression. Finally, other drugs (e.g., cocaine, amphetamine, lysergic acid) which so profoundly affect the systems of neurotransmitters in the CNS, can alter, without a doubt, not only the psychomotor behavior of the mother, but also the CNS of the fetus, and affect the process of maturation of the neuronal circuits containing the neurotransmitter systems affected. In this way, these drugs can create imbalances in the circuitry controlling cardiopulmonary functions. In this regard, it should be mentioned that cocaine can induce the expression of *c-fos* in the fetal CNS, through stimulation of dopamine D1 receptors.[92]

CONCLUSIONS

The main core of SIDS physiopathology rests on impaired developmental processes in the CB chemoreceptors as well as in central nervous system, including their neurotransmitter systems. Some environmental factors have a well established role in the genesis of those alterations. At the functional level SIDS implies a defective (slowness or incompleteness) resetting of the CB sensitivity to hypoxia and hypercapnia and/or a defective processing of signals in the cardiorespiratory centers of the brainstem. A normal infant's nervous system gets prompt information on a progressive hypercapnia and hypoxia event, and a new respiration or arousal is triggered; in infants with CB or VMS defects these protective reflexes are not initiated at normal levels of hypoxia and hypercapnia, and prolonged apneas develop until blood gas alterations reach a higher level capable of initiating the new respiration or arousal. These prolonged apneas may lead to fatal apneas and sudden death. However, whether these alterations are unique or primary in triggering SIDS is not known.

It should be mentioned that other alterations have been described in some SIDS victims. For example, an increase in the medial muscle mass of small arteries, increased eosinophilia and elevated immunoglobulins in mucus secretion have been described in the lungs of SIDS victims.[93] Some victims of SIDS present higher iron concentration than normal newborns in their livers. However, the increase in the liver iron concentration likely occurs after birth. It is not presently known if the increase in the blood iron and ferritin concentration is a cause or an effect (or it is not related) of abnormal management of oxygen, including the sensitivity to low oxygen.[93] These findings give rise to the possibility that, independent of the quality of CNS orders, final effectors for the respiratory output might be too inefficient to respond. Other authors have emphasized the importance of coordination in motor orders to diaphragm and pharyngolaryngeal muscles that help to maintain the upper airways open;[94,95] a deficit in the premotor outputs at the medullary controller can lead to respiratory obstructions and contribute to episodes of hypoxemia that would slow the resetting of the CB function.

As a final conclusion, we should state that today we know many facts related to SIDS, and yet we are forced to recall that the definition of SIDS given at the outset of this chapter as infant death without a cause is, unfortunately, still valid.

Acknowledgments

This work was supported by grant PB94/1443 from the Spanish DGICYT.

References

1. Heath D, Smith P. The Carotid Body in Fetus, Neonate and Infants. London: Springer-Verlag 1992:1-41.
2. Biga LA, Netterville, JL. Care of the patient with carotid body tumors. ORL Head Neck Nurs 1994; 12:11-6.
3. Netterville JL, Reilly KM, Robertson, D et al. Carotid body tumors: a review of thirty patients with forty six tumors. Laryngoscope 1995; 105:115-26.
4. Fidone SJ, González C. Initiation and control of chemoreceptor activity in the carotid body. In: Fishman AP, Cherniack NS, Widdicombe JG eds. Handbook of Physiology: The Respiratory System. Control of Breathing Part 1. Bethesda: American Physiological Society 1986:247-312.
5. Finlay FO, Rudd PT. Current concepts of the aetiology of SIDS. British J Hosp Med 1993; 49:727-732.
6. Beckwith JB. Discussion of terminology and definition of Sudden Infant Death Syndrome. In: Bergman AB, Beckwith JB, Ray CG, eds. Proc Second Int Confe Causes Sudden Death Infants. Seattle: University of Washington Press 1970: 14-22.
7. Takashima S, Mito T, Yamanouchi H. Developmental brain-stem pathology in sudden infant death syndrome. Acta Paediatr Jap 1994; 36:317-20.
8. Guntheroth WG, Spiers PS, Naeye RL. Redefinition of the sudden infant death syndrome: the disadvantages. Pediatr Pathol 1994; 14:127-32.
9. Naeye R, Ladis B, Drage J. Sudden infant death syndrome: a prospective study. Am J Dis Child 1976; 130:1207-10.
10. Taylor JA, Sanderson M. A reexamination of the risk factors for the sudden infant death syndrome. J Pediatr 1995; 126:887-91.
11. Blair PS, Flemming PJ, Bensley D et al. Smoking and the sudden infant death syndrome: results from 1993-5 case-control study for confidential inquiry into stillbirths and deaths in infancy. Brit Med J 1996; 313:195-8.
12. Golding J, Limerick S, Macfarlane A. Summary of epidemiological findings. In: Golding J, Limerick S, Macfarlane A. eds. Sudden Infant Death: Patterns, Puzzles and Problems. Shepton Mallet, England: Open Book 1985:38-40.
13. Hunt CE, Shannon DC. Sudden infant death syndrome and sleeping position. Pediatr 1992; 90:115-8.
14. Perrin DG, Cutz E, Becker LE et al. Sudden infant death syndrome: increased carotid-body dopamine and noradrenaline content. Lancet 1984; 2:535-7.
15. Hertzberg T, Srinivasan M, Lagercrantz H. Disturbed chemical neurotransmis-

sion and sudden infant death syndrome —the peripheral arterial chemoreceptor as an example. Acta Paediatr Suppl 1993; 389:63-6.
16. Cherniak NS. Sleep apnea and its causes. J Clin Invest 1984; 73:1501-6.
17. Naeye RL. Hypoxemia and sudden infant death syndrome. Science 1974; 186: 837-838.
18. Steinschneider A, Weinstein SL, Diamond E. The sudden infant death syndrome and apnea obstruction during neonatal sleep and feeding. Pediatrics 1982; 70:858-63.
19. Shannon DC, Kelly DH, O'Connell K. Abnormal regulation of ventilation in infant at risk for sudden infant death syndrome. N Engl J Med 1977; 297: 747-50.
20. Hanson M, Kumar P. Chemoreceptor function in the fetus and neonate. In: O'Regan RG, Nolan P, McQueen DS et al. eds. Arterial Chemoreceptors. Cell to System. New York: Plenum Press 1994: 99-108.
21. Bianchi AL, Denavit-Saubié M, Champagnat J. Central control of breathing in mammals: neuronal circuitry, membrane properties, and neurotransmitters. Physiol Rev 1995; 75:1-10.
22. Blanco CE, Dawes GS, Hanson MA et al. The response to hypoxia of arterial chemoreceptors in fetal sheep and newborn lambs. J Physiol 1984; 351:25-37.
23. Hofer MA. Lethal respiratory disturbances in neonatal rats after arterial chemoreceptor denervation. Life Sci 1984; 34:389-96
24. Hofer MA. Sleep-wake organization in infant rats with episodic respiratory disturbance following sinoaortic denervation. Sleep 1985; 59:40-48
25. Donnelly DF, Haddad GG. Prolonged apnea and impaired survival in piglets after sinus and aortic nerve section. L Appl Physiol 1990: 68:1048-52
26. Cote A, Porras H, Meehan B. Age-dependent vulnerability to carotid chemodenervation in piglets. J Appl Physiol 1996; 80:323-31.
27. Metersky ML, Castriotta RJ, Elnaggar A. Obstructive sleep apnea due to a carotid body paraganglioma. Sleep 1995; 18:53-4.
28. Molinary L, Altieri PI, Trinidad J et al. Syncope produced by metastatic carcinoma of the tongue to the carotid body. Proc Health Sci J 1996; 15:49-50.
29. Katz-Salamon M, Eriksson M, Jonsson B. Development of peripheral chemoreceptor function in infants with chronic lung disease and initially lacking hyperoxic response. Archiv Dis Childh Fetal Neonatal Edi 1996; 75:F4-9.
30. Weil JV. Ventilatory control at high altitude. In: Cherniack NS and Widdicombe JG, eds. Handbook of Physiology: The Respiratory System. Control of Breathing Part 1. Bethesda: American Physiological Society 1986:703-728.
31. Sorensen SC, Severinghaus JW. Respiratory insensitivity to acute hypoxia persisting after correction of tetralogy of Fallot. J Appl Physiol 1968; 25:221-3
32. Brady JP, McCann EM. Control of ventilation in subsequent siblings of victims of sudden infant death syndrome. J Pediatr 1985; 106:21-17.
33. Landauer RC, Pepper DR, Kumar P. Effect of chronic hypoxaemia from birth upon chemosensitivity in the adult rat carotid body in vitro. J Physiol (London) 1995; 485: 543-50.
34. Pepper DR, Landauer RC, Kumar P. Postnatal development of CO_2-O_2 interaction in the rat carotid body in vitro. J Physiol (London) 1995; 485:531-41.
35. Milerad J, Larsson H, Lin J et al. Nicotine attenuates the ventilatory response to hypoxia in the developing lamb. Pediatr Res 1995; 37:652-60.
36. Zhong H, Nurse C. Basic fibroblast growth factor regulates ionic currents and excitability of fetal rat carotid body chemoreceptors. Neurosci Lett 1995; 202:41-4.
37. Wyatt CN, Wright C, Bee D et al. O_2-sensitive K^+ currents in carotid body chemoreceptor cells from normoxic and chronically hypoxic rats and their roles in hypoxic chemotransduction. Proc Natl Acad Sci USA 1995; 92:295-9.
38. Donelly DF. Modulation of glomus cell membrane currents of intact rat carotid body. J Physiol (London) 1995; 489: 677-88.
39. González C, Almaraz L, Obeso A, Rigual R. Carotid body chemoreceptors: From

natural stimuli to sensory discharges. Physiol Rev 1994; 74:829-898
40. Marchal F, Bairam A, Haouzi P et al. Dual responses of carotid body chemosensory afferents to dopamine in the newborn kitten. Respir Physiol 1992; 90:173-83
41. Donnelly DF, Doyle TP, Developmental changes in hypoxia-induced catecholamine release from rat carotid body. J Physiol (London) 1994; 475:267-275
42. Bairam A, Basson H, Marchal F et al. Effects of hypoxia on carotid body dopamine content and release in developing rabbits. J Appl Physiol 1996; 80:20-4
43. Sterni, LM, Bamford OS, Pomares SM et al. Developmental changes in intracellular Ca^{2+} response of carotid chemoreceptor cells to hypoxia. Am J Physiol 1995; 268:L801-8
44. Dinger B, González C, Yoshizaki K et al. Localization and function of cat carotid body nicotine receptors. Brain Res 1985; 339:295-304.
45. González C, Almaraz L, Obeso A et al. Oxygen and acid chemoreception in the carotid body chemoreceptors. TINS 1992; 15:146-53.
46. Holgert H, Hökfelt T, Hertzberg T et al. Functional and developmental studies of the peripheral arterial chemoreceptors in rat: effects of nicotine and possible relation to sudden infant death syndrome. Proc Natl Acad Sci USA 1995; 92:7575-9.
47. Bianchi AL, Pasaro R. Organization of central respiratory neurons. In: Miller AD, Bianchi AL, Bishop B eds. Neural Control of the Respiratory Muscles. Boca Raton: CRC Press 1996:77-89.
48. Lipski J, Kanjhan R, Kruszewska B et al. Cardiovascular and respiratory neurons in the rostral ventrolateral medulla of the rat. In: Trouth CO, Millis RM, Kiwul-Shöne HF, Schläfke ME eds. Ventral Brainstem Mechanisms and Control of Respiration and Blood Pressure. Lung Biology in Health and Disease vol 82. New York: Marcel Dekker, 1995:437-52.
49. Millhorn DE, Eldridge FL. Role of ventrolateral medulla in regulation of respiratory and cardiovascular system. J Appl Physiol 1986; 61:1249-63.
50. Bianchi AL. Localisation et étude des neurones respiratoires bulbaires. Mise en jeu antidromique par stimulation spinale ou vagale. J Physiol (Paris) 1971; 63:5-40.
51. Donogue S, Felder RB, Gylbey MP et al. Postsynaptic activity evoked in the nucleus tractus solitarius by carotid sinus and aortic nerve afferents in the cat. J Physiol 1985; 360:261-73.
52. Finley JC, Katz DM. The central organization of carotid body afferent projections to the brainstem of the rat. Brain Res 1992; 572:108-16.
53. Jean A. Le noyeau du faisceau solitaire: aspects neuroanatomiques, neurochimiques et fonctionnels. Arch Int Physiol Biochim Biophys 1991; 99:A3-A52.
54. Feldman JL, Smith JC. Cellular mechanisms underlying modulation of breathing pattern in mammals. Ann NY Acad Sci 1989; 563:114-30.
55. Onimaru H, Arata A, Homma I. Inhibitory synaptic inputs to the respiratory rhythm generator in the medulla isolated from newborn rats. Pflügers Arch 1990; 417:425-32.
56. Trouth CO, Odek-Ogunde M, Holloway SA. Morphological observations on superficial medullary CO_2-chemosensitive areas. Brain Res 1982; 246:35-45.
57. Nattie EE, Li A, Coates EL. Central Chemoreceptor location and the ventrolateral medulla. In: Trouth CO, Millis RM, Kiwul-Shöne HF, Schläfke ME eds. Ventral Brainstem Mechanisms and Control of Respiration and Blood Pressure. Lung Biology in Health and Disease vol 82. New York: Marcel Dekker, 1995: 131-150.
58. Haxhiu MA, Erokwu B, Martin RJ. Medullary chemosensory neurons can be identified by expression of c-fos protein during early postnatal life. Pediatr Res 1992; 31:1842.
59. Cherniack NS, Ernsberger P, Mitra J et al. The role of the ventral medulla in hypoxic respiratory depression and sympathetic excitation. In: Trouth CO, Mills RM, Kiwull-Schöne HF, et al, eds. Ventral Brainstem Mechanisms and Control of Respiration and Blood Pressure. Lung Biology in Health and Disease vol 82 New York: Marcel Dekker 1995:103-29.

60. Nattie E. Central chemoreception. In: Dempsey JA, Pack AI, eds. Regulation of Breathing. Lung Biology in Health and Disease vol 79 New York: Marcel Dekker 1995:473-510.
61. Aljadeff G, Gozal D, Carroll JL et al. Ventral medullary surface responses to hypoxic and hyperoxic transient ventilatory challenges in the cat. Life Sci 1995; 5:319-24.
62. Erickson JT, Millhorn DE. Hypoxia and electrical stimulation of the carotid sinus nerve induce fos-like immunoreactivity within cathecholaminergic and serotoninergic neurons in the rat brainstem. J Comp Neurol 1994; 348:161-82.
63. Perez H, Ruiz S. Medullary responses to chemoreceptor activation are inhibited by locus coeruleus and nucleus raphe magnus. Neuroreport 1995; 6:1373-6.
64. Silva-Carvalho L, Dawid-Milner MS, Goldsmith GE et al. Hypothalamic modulation of the arterial chemoreceptor reflex in the anaesthetized cat: role of the nucleus tractus solitarii. J Physiol (London) 1995; 487:751-60.
65. Cherniak V, Warshaw JB, Kiley JP. Developmental neurobiology of respiratory control. Ann Rev Respir Dis 1989; 139: 1295-301.
66. Takashima S, Becker LE. Prenatal and postnatal maturation of medullary respiratory centers. Dev Brain Res 1986; 26:173-7.
67. Becker LE, Zhang W. Vagal nerve complex in normal development and sudden infant death syndrome. Can J Neurol Sci 1996; 23:24-33.
68. Haddad CG, Mellis RB. Hypoxia and respiratory control in early life. Ann Rev Respir Physiol 1988; 46:629-43.
69. Paton JFR, Ramirez JM, Richter DW. Mechanisms of respiratory rhythm generation change profoundly during early life in mice and rats. Neurosci Lett 1994; 170:167-70.
70. Nuñez-Abades PA, Spielmann JM, Barrionuevo G et al. In vitro electrophysiology of developing genioglossal motoneurons in the rat. J Neurophysiol 1993; 70:1401-11.
71. Nuñez-Abades PA, He F, Barrionuevo G et al. Morphology of developing rat genioglossal motoneurons studied in vitro: changes in length, branching pattern, and spatial distribution of dendrites. J Comp Neurol 1994; 339:401-20.
72. Cameron WE, Jodkowski JS, He F et al. Electrophysiological properties of developing phrenic motoneurons in the cat. J Neurophysiol 1991; 3:671-9.
73. Yamanouchi H, Takashima S, Becker LE. Increased substance P-positive nerve fibers in the brainstem of victims of sudden infant death syndrome. Neuropediatr 1993; 24:200-203.
74. Armstrong D, Sachis P, Bryan C et al. Pathological features of persistent infantile sleep apnea with reference to the pathology of sudden infant death syndrome. Ann Neurol 1982; 12:169-74.
75. Lucena J, Cruz-Sanchez FF. Ependymal changes in sudden infant death syndrome. J Neuropathol Exp Neurol 1996; 55:348-56.
76. Pamphlett R, Treloar L. Astrocytes in the hypoglossal nuclei of sudden infant death syndrome (SIDS) infants: a quantitative study. Neuropathol. Appl Neurobiol 1996; 22:136-43.
77. Eldridge FL, Millhorn DE. Central regulation of respiration by endogenous neurotransmitters and neuromodulators. Ann Rev Physiol 1981; 43:121-35.
78. Lagercrantz H, Milerad J, Walker DW. Control of ventilation in the neonate. In: Crystal RG, West JB, Barnes PJ, eds. The Lung: Scientific Foundations. New York: Raven Press 1991:1711-22.
79. Arango V, Ruggiero DA, Callaway JL et al. Catecholaminergic neurons in the ventrolateral medulla and nucleus of the solitary tract in the human. J Comp Neurol 1988; 273:224-40.
80. Massari VJ, Shirahata M, Johnson TA et al. Carotid sinus nerve terminals which are tyrosine hydroxylase immunoreactive are found in the commissural nucleus of the tractus solitarius. J Neurocytol 1996; 25:197-208.
81. Chigr R, Najimi M, Jordan D et al. Absence of adrenergic neurons in medulla oblongata in sudden infant death syndrome. CR Acad Sci Paris 1989; 309: 543-9.
82. Kopp N, Chigr F, Denory L et al. Absence of adrenergic neurons in nucleus tractus solitarius in sudden infant death syndrome. Neuropediatr 1993; 24:25-9.

83. Kalaria RN, Fiedler C, Hunsaker JC III et al. Synaptic neurochemistry of human striatum during development: changes in sudden infant death syndrome. J Neurochem 1993; 60:2098-105.
84. Sparks DL, Hunsaker JC III. Sudden infant death syndrome: altered aminergic-cholinergic synaptic markers in hypothalamus. J Child Neurol 1991; 6:335-9.
85. Kinney HC, Filiano JJ, Sleeper LA et al. Decreased muscarinic receptor binding in the arcuate nucleus in sudden infant death syndrome. Science 1995; 269: 1446-50.
86. Lagercrantz H. Neuromodulators and respiratory control during development. TINS 1987; 10:368-72.
87. Monti D, Carley DW, Radulovacki M. Adenosine analogues modulate the incidence of sleep apneas in rat. Pharmacol Biochem Behav 1995; 51:125-31.
88. Haxhiu MA, Chang CH, Dreshaj IA et al. Nitric oxide and ventilatory response to hypoxia. Respir Physiol 1995; 101: 257-66.
89. Ruggiero DA, Mtui EP, Otake K et al. Central and primary visceral afferents to nucleus tractus solitarii may generate nitric oxide as a membrane permeant neuronal messenger. J Comp Neurol 1996; 364:51-67.
90. Eliopoulos C, Klein J, Phan MD et al. Hair concentrations of nicotine and cotinine in women and their newborn infants. J Am Med Assoc 1994; 27:621-3.
91. Clegg DA, O'Hara BH, Heller HC et al. Nicotine administration differentially affects gene expression in the maternal and fetal circadian clock. Dev Brain Res 1995; 84:46-54.
92. Weaver R, Rivkees SA, Reppert SM. D1 dopamine receptors activate c-fos expression in the fetal suprachiasmatic nuclei. Proc Natl Acad Sci 1992; 89:9201-4.
93. Raha-Chowdbhury R, Moore CA, Bradley D et al. Blood ferritin concentrations in newborn infants and the sudden infant death syndrome. J Clin Pathol 1996; 49:168-70.
94. Gauda EB, Miller MJ, Carlo WA et al. Genioglossus response to airway occlusion in apneic versus nonapneic infants. Pediatr Res 1987; 22:683-7.
95. Remmers JE, Degroot WJ, Sauerland EK et al. Pathogenesis of upper airway occlusion during sleep. J Appl Physiol 1978; 44:931-42.

INDEX

D

E

F

G